SCIENCE OF STRETCHING

Michael J. Alter, MS

Human Kinetics Books
Champaign, Illinois

Library of Congress Cataloging-in-Publication Data

Alter, Michael J., 1952–
    Science of stretching.

    Bibliography: p.
    Includes index.
    1. Stretch (Physiology) I. Title. [DNLM: 1. Joints—
physiology. 2. Movement. 3. Muscles—anatomy & histolo-
gy. 4. Muscles—physiology. 5. Physical Education and
Training. QT 255 A466s]
QP310.S77A45   1988   612'.76   87-2952
ISBN 0-87322-090-0

Developmental Editor: Sue Wilmoth, PhD
Production Director: Ernie Noa
Projects Manager: Lezli Harris
Copy Editor: Lise Rodgers
Assistant Editor: Julie Anderson
Proofreader: Judith Edelstein
Typesetter: Brad Colson
Text Design: Keith Blomberg
Text Layout: Gordon Cohen
Cover Photo: Courtesy of Paul and Diane Taylor,
    photographer Greg Merhar, American Running & Fitness
    Association and model Karen Lips
Printed By: Braun-Brumfield

ISBN: 0-87322-090-0

Printed in the United States of America

10 9 8 7 6 5 4 3 2

Human Kinetics Books
A Division of Human Kinetics Publishers, Inc.
Box 5076, Champaign, IL 61825-5076
1-800-DIAL-HKP
1-800-334-3665 (in Illinois)

To my parents, Frieda and Moses Alter

Acknowledgments

The author wishes to express his deep gratitude to the many people who made this work possible. My thanks go to the American Academy of Orthopaedic Surgeons; the American Alliance for Health, Physical Education, Recreation, and Dance; the American Orthopaedic Association; the American Physiological Society; the Associated Press; Jerome V. Ciullo, M.D.; the F. A. Davis Company; the H. P. Publishing Company; Mrs. F.P. Kendall; Lea and Febiger, Publishers; Little, Brown and Company; the Pergamon Press; the staff of *The Physician and Sportsmedicine*; the W.B. Saunders Company; Systems DC; Charles C Thomas, Publishers; John Wiley and Sons, Inc.; and the Williams and Wilkins Company, all of whom generously gave permission to quote passages and reproduce drawings, photographs, and other illustrative material. All of the above added greatly to the content, clarity, and usefulness of the text.

The author appreciates the excellent work of the artist, Michael Richardson. Michael drew over 250 clear and concise stretching illustrations. The drawings reflected patient craftsmanship and added immeasurably to the final product.

I am also indebted to Baxter Venable for his generous counsel, to Shirley Beer and Art Lipman for their advice on word processing, and to the numerous reviewers for their kind encouragement, insightful suggestions, and sometimes deservedly blunt criticisms.

I am also grateful to Human Kinetics Publishers, Inc., who made this project possible. Human Kinetics' genuine interest in the project and its desire to produce an educationally useful text contributed enormously to its success.

Lastly, I wish to acknowledge the patience, skill, and loyal support and assistance of my editor, Dr. Sue Wilmoth, and all other members of the Human Kinetics staff for their helpfulness throughout the production of this book.

Michael J. Alter

Contents

Preface

Many factors influence flexibility and its development during childhood, adolescence, adulthood, and later life. To develop optimal flexibility one must understand what these factors are and how they interact. The importance of understanding flexibility became apparent to me during the course of my career in gymnastics as a competitor, coach, and nationally certified judge. Why can some individuals perform splits while others cannot? Why are females generally more flexible than males? Can one get hurt by stretching, and if so, to what degree? What is the elusive secret to developing optimal flexibility?

In search of answers to questions like these, I first turned to books on Hatha Yoga. At the time this approach seemed practical and relevant, and the materials were quite accessible. My satisfaction was not fulfilled, however, because much of the information in these books was not based on scientific research and offered a general "how to" approach to stretching. As I searched further, I found that many stretching programs were based on information passed down from teacher to student and then retaught in rote fashion. Questions were rarely asked, and if the exercises seemed to work they were accepted and taught without further exploration.

Interest in flexibility and stretching has increased greatly during the last few years. The general explosion in physical fitness has produced advances in many sport science areas that have stimulated research in flexibility and stretching. Despite the tremendous amount of material, however, most of it was either too difficult to locate, too fragmented, or too technical to be of any real value to most readers. There appeared to be no single source that covered the theory and practice of stretching for the interested individual, coach, and physical educator. The purpose of this text is to provide you with a general survey of current knowledge on flexibility in terms of its limitations and optimal development.

To present each particular aspect of flexibility, the text has been divided into three parts. Part I analyzes the factors related to flexibility and stretching. Part II is devoted to functional anatomy, methods of stretching, and causes of injury. Regions of the body are analyzed in terms of their structure, function, and limitations to range of motion. To facilitate the reader's understanding of the concepts presented, the text is liberally illustrated. References and recommendations for further reading are provided for those who wish to investigate the material presented in greater depth. In addition, chapters 1–15 conclude with questions designed to help you apply the information in each chapter to your own stretching program. Part III presents a systematic method of developing flexibility using over 200 exercises and warm-up drills. Illustrations on how free weights can be used to enhance flexibility are also included.

I have long been fascinated by the importance of stretching to muscular flexibility and physical fitness. I hope that my research and this book will motivate you to pursue your own stretching and flexibility program.

Michael J. Alter

PART I

Factors Related to Flexibility and Stretching

An Overview of Flexibility

The outcome of any flexibility program can be made more predictable and less haphazard if certain biological and biomechanical principles are understood and applied. In evaluating one's flexibility and formulating a flexibility training program, one must consider not only the benefits of increased flexibility but also the potential for injury and impairment of function and performance if progress is allowed to occur under suboptimal conditions. All individuals, including coaches, instructors, trainers, physical therapists, artists, athletes, and participants, should take advantage of every opportunity to manipulate the various factors that affect the development of optimal flexibility.

The Nature of Flexibility

Flexibility has been variously defined as mobilization, freedom to move, or, technically, the range of motion (ROM) available in a joint or group of joints (Holland, 1968). ROM may be measured in either linear units (e.g., inches or centimeters) or angular units (degrees). There is unanimous agreement that flexibility is *specific* (Bryant, 1984; Corbin & Noble, 1980; Harris, 1969a; Sigerseth, 1971). The amount or degree of range of motion is *specific* for each joint. Thus ROM in the hip does not ensure ROM in the shoulder. Similarly, ROM in one hip may not be highly related to ROM in the other hip.

There are two basic types of flexibility. *Static flexibility* relates to ROM about a joint with no emphasis on speed. For example, static flexibility is utilized when one performs a split. In contrast, *dynamic flexibility* corresponds to the ability to use a range of joint movement in the performance of a physical activity at either a normal or a rapid speed (Corbin & Noble, 1980). A split leap in

gymnastics or dance exemplifies this type of flexibility. Here, too, flexibility is specific. Thus static and dynamic flexibility are not necessarily related.

The Flexibility Training Program

To obtain maximum benefits from a flexibility training program, you must know and understand what can and what cannot be achieved by using it properly. Before we examine the value of such a program, we need to differentiate a flexibility training program from a flexibility warm-up/cool-down program. A *flexibility training program* is defined as a planned, deliberate, and regular program of exercises that can permanently and progressively increase the usable range of motion of a joint or set of joints over a period of time (Aten & Knight, 1978; Corbin & Noble, 1980). Conversely, a *flexibility warm-up/cool-down program* is defined as a planned, deliberate, and regular program of exercises that are done immediately before and after an activity to improve performance or reduce the risk of injury in that activity.[1] Consequently, a flexibility warm-up/cool-down program alone will not improve flexibility during the following weeks of activity (Aten & Knight, 1978; Corbin & Noble, 1980).

The Benefits of a Flexibility Training Program

When one begins a flexibility training program, the potential benefits are virtually unlimited. The qual-

---

[1]The term *cool-down* is synonymous for *warm-down*.

ity and quantity of these benefits are ultimately determined by two factors. The first of these factors is the individual's *ends*. The ends are an individual's goals or objectives. These may be based on a wide range of contexts, such as biological, psychological, sociological, and philosophical. The second factor, the *means*, determines how and whether the ends are achieved. The means are the methods and techniques used to attain one's goals. Obviously, if one's ends are purely emotional or psychological as opposed to biological or physiological, then certain stretching techniques would be employed and others would not. What then can one expect from a flexibility training program? In light of the recent proliferation of material on the subject, we will now examine the purported benefits of flexibility training.

Union of the Body, Mind, and Spirit

From a purely esoteric point of view, a flexibility training program can serve to unify one's body, mind, and spirit. Of the many disciplines that claim to seek the perfection and harmony of the body, mind, and spirit, yoga is probably the most widely known. The word yoga is derived from the Sanskrit root *yuj*, meaning "to bind, attach, and yoke; to direct and concentrate one's attention; to use and apply." It also means *union* or *communion* (Iyengar, 1979, p. 19).

The many books on yoga emphasize the following basic principles that are mystical and transcendental yet highly logical and rational:

* The body is a temple that houses the Divine Spark.
* The body is an instrument of attainment.
* The yogi masters the body by the practice of *asanas* (postures).
* The yogi performs *asanas* to develop complete equilibrium of the body, mind, and spirit.
* The body, mind, and spirit are inseparable.

Iyengar (1979) explained yoga as follows:

To the yogi, his body is the prime instrument of attainment. If his vehicle breaks down, the traveller cannot go far. If the body is broken by ill-health, the aspirant can achieve little. Physical health is important for mental development, as normally the mind functions through the nervous system. When the body is sick or the nervous system is affected, the mind becomes restless or dull and inert and concentration or meditation becomes impossible. (pp. 24-25)

Relaxation of Stress and Tension

Stress can be generally described as "the wear and tear of life." Stress occurs in varying degrees and different forms—mental, emotional, and physical. All forms of stress affect the individual in ways that are sometimes good and sometimes harmful to health. Normal levels of stress are healthy and desirable. Love and work, for example, involve stress. Intense and persistent stress, however, such as continuous anger, fear, frustration, inhibition, or tension, can become bottled up inside ourselves and threaten health. This buildup of stress without release of tension is what leads to problems.

As stated earlier, "the body, mind, and spirit are inseparable." One of the advances of modern medicine is the increasing recognition or rediscovery of the major influence of emotions upon physical health. In fact, the knowledge that illness must be considered and treated in relation to *the whole person* forms the basis for psychosomatic medicine (psyche-mind; soma-body). Today many scientists believe that prolonged emotional tensions play a major role in triggering ailments such as high blood pressure, peptic ulcer, headache, and joint and muscular pains (Larson & Michelman, 1973).

When you are upset, angry, or frustrated, you can try to reduce these negative feelings through exercise. The literature contains abundant evidence that therapeutic exercise alleviates stress (de Vries, 1975; de Vries, Wiswell, Bulbulion, & Moritani, 1981; Levarlet-Joye, 1979; Morgan & Horstman, 1976; Sime, 1977). Just as exercise has been found to be immeasurably therapeutic for many people, empirical evidence indicates that individualized flexibility training programs may be similarly beneficial.

Muscular Relaxation

One of the most important benefits of a flexibility program is the promotion of relaxation. From a purely physiological perspective, *relaxation* is the cessation of muscular tension. Undesirably high levels of muscular tension in the human organism result in several negative side effects. Excessive muscular tension tends to decrease sensory awareness of the world and raise blood pressure (Larson & Michelman, 1973). It also wastes energy; a contracting muscle obviously requires more energy than a relaxed muscle. Furthermore, habitually tense muscles tend to cut off their own circulation. Reduced blood supply results in a lack of oxygen and essential nutrients and causes toxic waste products to accumulate in the cells. This predisposes one to fatigue, aches, and even pain. Common sense and everyday experience show that a relaxed muscle is less susceptible to these and many other ailments.

Our chief concern, however, is flexibility. When a muscle stays partially contracted, an abnormal state of prolonged contraction called *contracture* develops. Contracture and chronic muscle tension not only shorten the muscle but also make the muscle less supple, strong, and able to absorb the shock and stress of various types of movement. Consequently, undue muscular tension can produce excessive muscular tightness. Here, too, common sense indicates that the most appropriate remedy for such a disorder would be to facilitate muscular relaxation and immediately follow with some type of stretching. In support of this position, de Vries and Adams (1972) found exercise to be more effective than medication in decreasing muscular tension.

Self-Discipline

Most of us live undisciplined lives; that is, we are creatures of habit and tend to live *conditioned* lives. Self-discipline is a necessity of life because sustained effort is required to attain any goal. When the goal is success (e.g., performing a split), effort must be backed up with unflagging persistence that does not recognize failure. The goal must be pursued until it is achieved.

Because the body is controlled by the mind, if the body is to be disciplined or mastered, then the mind must be disciplined or mastered. Herein lies the fundamental importance of the *asanas* in yoga. The yogi masters the body by the practice and self-discipline or *asanas* and thus makes the body a fit vehicle for the spirit. This also holds true for the athlete, artistic performer, and lay person. If one aspect of life can be disciplined, then there is no limit to anything in one's life that can be mastered. A flexibility training program offers an ideal opportunity to seek mastery over oneself. Stretching can give one something to struggle for and against, just as a marathon race presents a runner with elements to struggle for and against.

Another benefit of stretching is that it offers a unique opportunity for spiritual growth. A stretching program provides quiet intervals for thought, meditation, or self-evaluation. During such moments you can also listen to and monitor your own body—something most of us today seldom do. Thus a stretching program provides the opportunity to get in touch with yourself or with the cosmos. And the beauty of stretching is that it can be done anywhere at any time.

Finally, one of the most helpful benefits of a stretching program (or any exercise program) is that it can enable you to understand your own development and abilities. Stretching can teach you lessons about your own human limits and provide opportunities to test yourself physiologically. Not everyone can perform a split or touch his toes with the legs kept straight. Each of us has different abilities and talents. Yet this is something that many people have failed to recognize.

In the world of artistic performance and sports, individuals' successes and failures are visible for all to see and the measures of success are objectively accurate. One can do little to hide a poor arabesque or a failed split jump. There is no use in trying to cover up or explain away a failed performance. The world delivers its verdict loudly and clearly. Thus we learn to realize our own limitations while continuing to grow and develop our skills and abilities.

Body Fitness, Posture, and Symmetry

The desire to be healthy and attractive is almost universal. The best way to improve bodily measurements and proportions is through a combination of appropriate diet and exercise. To develop body symmetry and good posture, one should engage in gross motor activities rather than specialize in an activity that develops only one area of the body. By incorporating an individualized flexibility program into an overall fitness program, you can improve not only your appearance but also your physical fitness and health. Physical fitness is multidimensional and includes flexibility, cardiorespiratory endurance, strength, and muscular endurance.

The relationship of flexibility to good posture is mainly theoretical and clinical. Corbin and Noble (1980), however, suggest that an imbalance in muscular development and a lack of flexibility in certain muscle groups can contribute to poor posture. Rounded shoulders, for example, are thought to be associated with poor flexibility in the pectoral muscles of the frontal chest area and lack of muscular endurance in the scapular girdle adductors (i.e., rhomboids and middle trapezius).

Physical fitness and health can be greatly enhanced by daily physical activity. When physical activity is not a regular part of one's life, many ailments and debilitating conditions are more likely to occur. Among these are *asthenia* (loss of strength), *ataxia* (inability to coordinate bodily movements), and *hypokinesis* (diminished ability to move), to mention only a few (Larson & Michelman, 1973). Conversely, if one makes physical activity a regular part of one's life, many of these conditions can be avoided. Depending on the method and technique of stretching that are employed, individuals can enhance their agility, coordination, flexibility, and muscular strength.

Flexibility and Low Back Pain

Low back pain is one of the most prevalent complaints afflicting people in modern society. Thousands of people seek relief from low back pain by various treatments every year. In fact, most people will probably be affected by low back pain at some point in their lives. Numerous articles and books on the problem appear annually.

Although the etiology of low back pain disorders remains controversial, strong evidence supports the need for adequate mobility of the trunk. Farfan (1978), for example, reported that flexibility of the lumbar spine provides a mechanical advantage for function and efficiency. Jackson and Brown (1983), however, point out that clinical assessment of sufficient mobility remains undefined. Consequently, until adequate flexibility can be scientifically defined and the clinical means are developed to measure the achievement of goals, the use of mobility/flexibility exercises will remain on an empirical basis.

Relief of Muscular Soreness

Everyday experience and research appears to indicate that slow stretching exercises can reduce and sometimes eliminate muscular soreness. Two types of pain are associated with muscular exercise: (a) pain during and immediately after exercise, which may persist for several hours and (b) delayed, localized soreness, which usually does not appear for 24 to 48 hours following exercise. Currently, there is still disagreement regarding the physiological cause or causes of muscular soreness and how stretching reduces or eliminates it.

Regardless of the theoretical reasons for it, slow stretching has proven effective in reducing muscular soreness both during and immediately after exercise. For example, it is well known that a cramp is immediately relieved by stretching the involved muscle and holding the stretch. Furthermore, electromyographic (EMG) recordings by de Vries (1966) have shown that static stretching relieves muscle soreness and significantly decreases electrical activity in the muscle to bring

symptomatic relief. Similarly, static stretching appears to be effective in relieving delayed localized soreness.

Static stretching is also recommended in cases of dysmenorrhea (painful menstruation). The findings of Billig and Lowendahl (1949) and Golub and Christaldi (1957) indicate that painful menstruation can be prevented or at least reduced in severity through regular stretching of the pelvic region.

Enhancement of Physical and Athletic Skills

Today flexibility is generally recognized as a crucial factor in skilled movement. Practical and everyday experience indicates that flexibility enhances and optimizes the learning, practice, and performance of skilled movement. Therefore, some skills may be enhanced more effectively by purposefully increasing or decreasing the range of motion around certain joints until what appears to be optimal flexibility is reached (Sigerseth, 1971).

Experts on physical exercise universally recognize that any exercise period should be preceded by a series of calisthenics and loosening exercises to warm up the muscle masses. The benefits of warm-up exercises are believed to be derived from the increased body and muscle temperature. This topic will be discussed later in greater detail.

From an aesthetic point of view, flexibility is definitely a requirement for skilled movement. This is especially true in disciplines such as dance, gymnastics, and karate to mention only a few. Flexibility allows the individual to create an appearance of ease, smoothness of movement, graceful coordination, self-control, and total freedom. It also helps the individual to perform more skillfully and with greater self-assurance, elegance, and amplitude. Without a supple body, highly skilled performance is impossible. The difference between good skill and excellent skill is simply a matter of degree. Flexibility can provide the critical difference between average and outstanding performance.

Another factor in skilled movement is the importance of flexibility as a biomechanical parameter. *Biomechanics* is the study of the application of mechanical laws to living structures. It examines the forces that act on a body and the effects of these forces. For example, in tennis an increased range of motion allows one to apply forces over greater distances and longer periods of time. This can increase velocities, energies, and momenta involved in physical performance (Ciullo & Zarins, 1983). Conversely, Craig (1973) points out that

Baseball pitchers and quarterbacks may lose force (i.e., speed) from their throws because of the limited flexibility of the rotator cuff (shoulder) muscles. This results in limited range of motion in the windup. The loss of range of motion causes a subsequent loss in the amount of momentum that an athlete can generate. (p. 148)

Furthermore, an increased range of motion can permit a greater stretch on the involved muscles. As a result, those muscles can produce even greater forces. This is because a prestretched muscle can exert more force than a nonstretched muscle. Prestretched muscles function with greater efficiency because elastic energy is stored in the muscle tissue during stretching and is recovered during the subsequent shortening (Asmussen & Bonde-Petersen, 1974; Boscoe, Tarkka, & Komi, 1982; Cavagna, Dusman, & Margaria, 1968; Cavagna, Saibene, & Margaria, 1965; Ciullo & Zarins, 1983; Grieve, 1970; Komi & Boscoe, 1978). Ciullo and Zarins compare this phenomenon to cocking an air rifle. They point out, however, that Hill (1961) found that when relaxation of the muscle takes place between the stretching and shortening, the preloaded condition is not taken advantage of and the stored elastic energy is dissipated as heat. Thus time is an all-important component.

Injury Prevention

The use of stretching exercises to increase flexibility is commonly based on the idea that it may decrease the incidence, intensity, or duration of musculotendinous and joint injury (Arnheim, 1971; Aten & Knight, 1978; Bryant, 1984; Corbin & Noble, 1980; Davis, Logan, & McKinney, 1961). More than minimal joint extensibility appears to be advantageous in some sports to prevent severe muscle strain and/or joint sprain. In other words, there seems to be an "ideal or optimal" range of flexibility that will prevent injury when muscles and joints are accidentally overstretched. However, this should *not* be interpreted to mean that *maximum* joint flexibility will prevent injury. In further elaborating this point, the question must be asked whether there is any benefit in stretching a muscle to an extreme ROM. In addressing this question, Hubley-Kozey and Stanish (1984) point out that some athletes such as gymnasts must be able to reach an extreme ROM without damaging the surrounding tissues. Not *all* athletes, however, need this extreme ROM. Runners, for example, require a much smaller ROM. Nevertheless, their range of motion should

be adequate to allow them to run without excessive soft-tissue resistance.

Insufficient data are currently available to assess the average ROMs required for different athletic activities. Furthermore, only normal ROMs have been determined for healthy, nonathletic patients. Thus physicians and therapists must rely on their

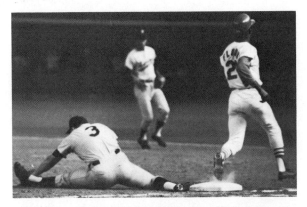

Figure 1.1a. Harmon Killebrew, first baseman for the Minnesota Twins in the 1966 All-Star game, makes a long stretch to take a short throw.

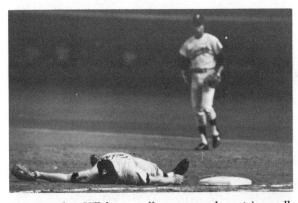

Figure 1.1b. Killebrew suffers a severe hamstring pull.

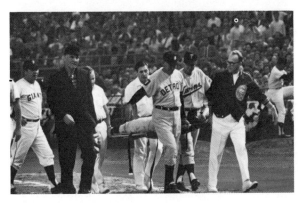

Figure 1.1c. Killebrew was out of action for an extended period of time. Photos courtesy of AP/World Wide Photos.

empirical experience and knowledge of a particular sport when suggesting how far an athlete should stretch. Thus, in determining whether there is any benefit in stretching a muscle to an extreme ROM, Hubley-Kozey and Stanish (1984) concluded that "most athletes do not need, and therefore should not attempt to reach, maximum or extreme ranges of motion" (p. 26). Furthermore, available data do not document if a lack of flexibility predisposes one to injury or the minimal amount of flexibility that is necessary to prevent such injuries.

In summarizing the research, Corbin and Noble (1980) state that a wealth of clinical data support the need for flexibility training to prevent muscle and connective tissue injuries. Furthermore, conventional wisdom suggests that shortness of muscle and connective tissue limits joint mobility and may predispose that muscle or connective tissue to injury. Thus, although "a wealth of empirical data on the subject is lacking, common sense suggests that adherence to lengthening (stretching) and strengthening programs for athletes, vocational or avocational, would be wise" (p. 59) (see Figure 1.1).

Enjoyment

Developing and following a flexibility training program provides many physical and mental advantages. And added to these benefits is the enjoyment and personal gratification that one receives from doing so.

Potential Disadvantages of Flexibility Training

Although it may be assumed that flexibility and/or joint looseness can reduce the incidence of injury, many researchers contend that flexibility training might actually increase the risk of injury! Surburg (1983) points out that flexibility may be thought of as a continuum. At one end is no flexibility or movement, as in individuals diagnosed with ankylosis (stiffness or fixation of a joint by disease, injury, or surgery). At the opposite end of the continuum is extreme flexibility or instability, that is, subluxation or dislocation. Obviously, between these two extremes lies an optimal level of flexibility that allows efficient execution of movement and diminishes the risk of certain types of injuries.

Several authorities (Bird, 1979; Lichtor, 1972; Nicholas, 1970) believe that increased joint laxity or looseness increases the likelihood of ligament injury, joint separation, and dislocation. This position has been variously rationalized. Lichtor (1972) found that individuals with loose joints do not have normal bodily control and coordination. Therefore, such persons are not usually seen in professional sports, having been eliminated early by injury or poor performance. Similarly, another study (Barrack, Skinner, Brunet, & Cook, 1983) concluded that joint hypermobility may be a factor in decreased position sense that may indicate below normal protective reflexes, and thus increase the risk of acute or chronic injury. Another argument (Gomolak, 1975) is that tight-jointed individuals are better protected from severe injury because their characteristically bulky builds limit the ROM of their joints. Finally, along a similar line of thought, some studies have suggested that in looser individuals the amount and quality of stabilizing fibrous tissue that resists the impact is such that the joints lose their parallelism when they are hit, especially when the body or legs are fixed (Nicholas, 1970; Sutro, 1947).

A vital question that must be addressed is whether joint looseness and/or flexibility training is potentially detrimental for some individuals. Some authorities believe that too much flexibility or ROM can be as dangerous as inadequate flexibility (Barrack, Skinner, Brunet, & Cook, 1983; Bird, 1979; Corbin & Noble, 1980; Gomolak, 1975; Nicholas, 1970).

The basis of this hypothesis is that excessive flexibility may destabilize joints (Balaftsalis, 1982/1983; Corbin & Noble, 1980; Nicholas, 1970). For example, Klein (1961) contended that the deep squatting of weight lifters tends to weaken the ligaments and hence make the knee more vulnerable to injury. Similarly, Nicholas (1970) reported that "independent of many other factors responsible for injury in football, an increased likelihood of ligamentous rupture of the knee occurred in loose-jointed football players" (p. 2239). Here too, however, other researchers (Grana & Moretz, 1978; Kalenak & Morehouse, 1975; Moretz, Walters, & Smith, 1982) found no correlation between ligamentous laxity and the incidence or type of injury. Because so many other factors are involved, a correlation between flexibility and injury is almost impossible to establish.

Another point of controversy is the relationship of joint laxity to osteoarthritis (i.e., that joint hyperlaxity predisposes one to premature osteoarthritis). Beighton, Grahame, and Bird (1983) present two possible explanations. First, "the particular collagen structure [that] contributes to hyperlaxity may be identical to that which leads to osteoarthritis." Second, that biomechanical factors assist in the "pathogenesis of the degenerative change" (p. 39). Beighton, Grahame, and Bird believe that the truth may lie in a combination of these two theories because there is evidence to support both hypotheses.

Recently, some studies have also suggested that individuals participating in regular physical exercise may avoid osteoarthritis (Beighton, Grahame, & Bird, 1983; Bird, 1979; Bird, Hudson, & Wright, 1980). This view is based on the premise that regular physical exercise may protect lax joints from osteoarthritis by stabilizing joints through increased muscular tone. Beighton, Grahame, and Bird (1983), however, point out that "surveys of professional sportsmen show that osteoarthritis tends to develop in those who have had surgery or injuries to a joint, causing incongruity of the articulating surfaces or stretching of the ligaments" (p. 40).

Thus, three possible courses of action appear to be prudent based on empirical evidence. First, in joints where excessive flexibility is evident, the ROM should be reduced (Sigerseth, 1971). Second, preventive and compensatory exercises should be incorporated into the training program to enhance the strength and stability of the joints (Arnheim, 1971; Corbin & Noble, 1980; Javurek, 1982; Kalenak & Morehouse, 1975; Moretz, Walters, & Smith, 1982; Sigerseth, 1971). Third, a flexibility training program (i.e., stretching) is *not* indicated when the joint or joints in question are hypermobile (Corbin & Noble, 1980; Sigerseth, 1971).

Summarizing the research, the following statements can be made:

- Sufficient data are not presently available to conclusively determine whether exercises that stretch ligaments are detrimental to ligaments (Booth & Gould, 1975; Corbin & Noble, 1980; Craig, 1973).
- Restricting athletic participation on the basis of ligamentous laxity testing is not warranted (Grana & Moretz, 1975).
- Individuals with loose ligaments need to increase strength through a strength training program. The muscle-tendon unit is the "first line of defense" in protecting ligaments. Strengthening not only increases the muscle power that a person may use in performing an activity but also probably protects the joint ligaments (Javurek, 1982; Kalenak & Morehouse, 1975; Moretz, Walters, & Smith, 1982).

- Individuals with less ROM need to increase their flexibility through a flexibility training program.

Summary

Simply stated, *flexibility* is the range of motion available in a joint or group of joints. Flexibility is usually classified into two components. *Static flexibility* relates to the ability to move through a range of motion with no emphasis on speed or time. *Dynamic flexibility* corresponds to the ability to move through a range of motion with emphasis on speed or time. Both types of flexibility are *specific*; that is, the amount or degree of range of motion is specific for each joint. Thus flexibility in one hip does not ensure flexibility in the other, and a flexible hip does not ensure a flexible back. To develop flexibility, one should participate in a *flexibility training program*. This is defined as a planned, deliberate, and regular program of exercises that can permanently and progressively increase the usable range of motion of a joint or set of joints over a period of time.

Flexibility training programs can result in benefits that can be *qualitative* and/or *quantitative*. Among the benefits associated are:

- Union of the body, mind, and spirit.
- Relaxation of stress and tension.
- Muscular relaxation.
- Spiritual growth and learning about oneself.
- Improvement in bodily fitness, posture, and symmetry.
- Reduction of low back pain.
- Relief from muscular soreness.
- Enhanced performance of certain skills.
- Reduced risk of injury.
- Personal enjoyment and gratification.

Some literature suggests that joint looseness and/or flexibility training are potentially detrimental for some individuals. This opinion is based on the idea that excessive flexibility may destabilize joints and increase the risk of injury. Because so many factors are involved, however, a direct correlation between increased flexibility and increased risk of injury cannot be established. Other researchers have suggested a relationship between joint laxity and predisposition to osteoarthritis. Empirical evidence indicates that stretching should be avoided in a hypermobile situation and that a strength training program should be initiated. For those who are physically able, common sense suggests participating in *both* flexibility training and strength training programs.

Review Questions

1. Define the term *flexibility*.

2. Compare and contrast a *flexibility training program* and a *flexibility warm-up/cool-down program*.

3. Explain how a lecture on flexibility and stretching for housewives would differ from a lecture to a group of high school varsity athletes, college athletes, and professional athletes.

4. Explain how stretching may enhance skilled movement.

5. You are a coach of distance runners. Explain to your athletes why they do not need to be able to perform a split.

6. Explain the relationship between flexibility and injury prevention.

7. You are the coach of an athlete who has been identified with ligamentous laxity in the knees. Prescribe an appropriate exercise regime. Give specific exercises and procedures to be followed.

8. What guidelines would you follow as a coach when selecting training programs for athletes?

9. You are giving a lecture to your team. In one paragraph, explain the concept of *specificity of training* as it relates to flexibility and stretching.

10. Identify a situation where excessive flexibility would be detrimental for a (a) gymnast, (b) platform diver, (c) archer, and (d) runner.

Answers

1. Flexibility has been variously defined as mobilization, freedom to move, or, technically, the range of motion available in a joint or group of joints.

2. A *flexibility training program* is a planned, deliberate, and regular program of exercises that can permanently and progressively increase the usable range of motion of a joint or set of joints over a period of time. In contrast, a *flexibility warm-up/cool-down program* represents a planned, deliberate, and regular program of exercises that are done immediately before or after an activity to improve performance or reduce the risk of injury in that activity. A flexibility training program will increase the individual's flexibility, but a flexibility warm-up/cool-down program will not.

3. A lecture on flexibility and stretching to housewives would differ from one to a group of high school varsity athletes, college athletes, and professional athletes in terms of both the ends (i.e., goals) and the means (i.e., methods and techniques) utilized.

4. Stretching enhances skilled movement physiologically (e.g., increased body and muscle temperature), psychologically, and biomechanically (e.g., forces can be applied over greater distances and times).

5. Runners do not need to reach an extreme range of motion because it is not specific. One needs adequate flexibility to run without excessive soft-tissue resistance.

6. Currently, there are no conclusive data that document whether a lack of flexibility predisposes one to injury and, if so, the minimal amount of flexibility necessary to prevent such injuries.

7. All athletes should incorporate a series of general warm-up exercises before performing. These should be followed with a set of stretching exercises. Excessive strain on the joints involved should be avoided. For example, one should avoid the hurdler's stretch, excessive flexion or hyperextension of the joint(s) involved, and ballistic types of movements. Strengthening exercises could include 2–3 sets of 10 repetitions of half squats, hamstring curls, and quadriceps extensions.

8. Avoid stretching in a hypermobile situation and incorporate a strength training program and vice versa.

9. Flexibility is specific. If one wanted to run a marathon, one would not run sprints. If one wanted to be a high jumper, one would not practice the shot put. If one wanted to

improve flexibility, one must incorporate a flexibility training program.

10. (a) Gymnast: Hyperextended elbow, support movements on the parallel bars.
    (b) Platform diver: Excessively loose back, unable to lock out the body.
    (c) Archer: Hyperextended elbow, contact with the string when pulled back.
    (d) Runner: Joint instability in the ankles and knees; joints may give way when running on rough and uneven surfaces.

Recommended Readings

Bird, H. A., Brodie, D. A., & Wright, V. (1979). Quantification of joint laxity. *Rheumatology and Rehabilitation, **18**(3), 161-166.

Brodie, D. A., Bird, H. A., & Wright, V. (1982). Joint laxity in selected athletic populations. *Medicine and Science in Sports, **14**(3), 190-193.

Fixx, J. F. (1977). *The complete book of running.* New York: Random House.

Grahame, R. (1971). Joint hypermobility: Clinical aspects. *Proceedings in the Royal Society of Medicine, **64**, 692-694.

Grahame, R., & Jenkins, J. M. (1972). Joint hypermobility: Asset or liability? *Annals of the Rheumatic Diseases, **31**(2), 109-111.

Key, I. A. (1927). Hypermobility of joints. *The Journal of the American Medical Association, **58**, 1701-1712.

Klemp, P., & Learmonth, I. D. (1984). Hypermobility and injuries in a professional ballet company. *British Journal of Sports Medicine, **18**(3), 143-148.

Marshall, J. L., Johnson, N., Wickiewicz, T. L., Tischler, H. M., Koslin, B. L., Zeno, S., & Meyers, A. (1980). Joint looseness: A function of the person and the joint. *Medicine and Science in Sports, **12**(3), 189-194.

Schellock, F. G., & Prentice, W. E. (1985). Warming-up and stretching for improved physical performance and prevention of sports-related injuries. *Sports Medicine, **2**(4), 267-278.

Scott, D., Bird, A., & Wright, V. (1979). Joint laxity leading to osteoarthritis. *Rheumatology and Rehabilitation, **18**(3), 167-169.

Seyle, H. (1956). *The stress of life.* New York: McGraw-Hill.

Shyne, K. (1982). Richard H. Dominguez, M.D: To stretch or not to stretch? *The Physician and Sportsmedicine, **10**(9), 137-140.

CHAPTER 2

Contractile Components of Muscle: Limiting Factors of Flexibility

Muscles vary in shape and size. The central portion of a whole muscle is called the *belly*. The belly is comprised of smaller compartments called *fasciculi*. Each fasciculus consists in turn of approximately 100 to 150 individual muscle fibers that range from 1 to 40 millimeters in length and 10 to 100 microns in diameter.[1] Each muscle fiber constitutes a single muscle cell.

As illustrated in Figure 2.1, each muscle fiber is actually composed of many smaller units called *myofibrils*. Myofibrils range in diameter from 1 to 2 microns. They are grouped in clusters and run the length of the muscle fiber. The myofibrils are the elements that *contract* (shorten), *relax*, and *elongate* (stretch) the muscle. Myofibrils are comprised of even smaller structures called *myofilaments*. Below the myofilaments is the molecular dimension. This dimension includes the *amino acids*, the building blocks of all proteins. The synthesis of amino acids is under the control of deoxyribonucleic acid (DNA). The amino acids are comprised of their subparts, the *molecules* and *atoms*.

Composition of Myofibrils and Their Constituents

When viewed under a microscope, individual muscle fibers are seen to have a banded or striated structure. This banding pattern of the muscle fiber reflects the ultrastructural organization of each myofibril. Thus, to understand how muscles contract, relax, and elongate, we must understand the structure of the myofibril.

The Ultrastructure of the Myofibrils

Myofibrils are characterized by alternating light and dark areas (see Figure 2.1). The light or translucent areas are called *I-bands*. The I-bands measure approximately 1.5 microns in length. The dark areas are called *A-bands*. The A-bands measure approximately 1.0 micron in length. These bands are named according to their translucence in polarized light.

The center of each A-band is occupied by a relatively lighter area the *H-zone*. The H-zone is less dense than the rest of the band. Its size depends upon the muscle length, or the extent of overlap of the myofilaments. In the middle of each I-band is a darker and denser line called the *Z-line* (from the German word *zwischen*, meaning *between*). The segments between two successive Z-lines are the functional units of the myofibrils. They are termed *sarcomeres*. Sarcomeres are approximately 2.3 microns in length and repeat themselves in a specific pattern in each myofibril.

Under extremely high magnification, each myofibril of a sarcomere is seen to consist of a bundle of thick and thin interlocking *myofilaments*. The thinner myofilament is called *actin*, and the thicker one is called *myosin*. In the I-bands, only the thin myofilaments are present. Hence the I-bands appear translucent. Actin has a diameter of about 60 angstroms and a length of about 2 microns. They begin at the Z-line, run continuously through the I-bands, and extend into the A-bands. Thus the

---

[1]One millimeter equals .03937 of an inch; 1 inch equals about 25.4 of a millimeter. 1 micron equals .000039 of an inch.

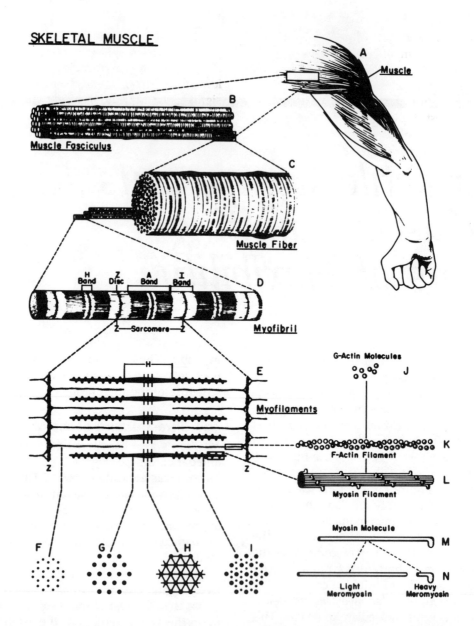

SKELETAL MUSCLE

Figure 2.1. Organization of skeletal muscle from gross to the molecular level. F, G, H, and I are cross sections at the levels indicated. *Note*. From *A Textbook of Histology* (10th ed., p. 206) by W. Bloom and D. Fawcett, 1975, Philadelphia: W.B. Saunders. Copyright 1962 by W.B. Saunders Company. Reprinted by permission.

actin myofilaments are free at the opposite end. Actin myofilaments have been found to consist of bead-like molecules that are connected together in a double helical form. Furthermore, they have been found to consist of the proteins actin, troponin, and tropomyosin.

In contrast, the myosin myofilaments are thicker (about 100 angstroms in diameter) and shorter (about 1.5 microns in length). Furthermore, the myosin myofilaments are free at both ends. Myosin myofilaments are also unique in that they possess numerous short lateral projections that extend

toward the actin myofilaments. These important projections are called *cross-bridges*.

When analyzed in greater detail, the cross-bridges consist of two parts: a *head* and a *tail*. The tail has been termed *light meromyosin*, or *LMM* for short. The LMM attach to each other to form the myosin myofilaments. The heads are known as *heavy meromyosin*, or *HMM*. The HMM are what actually form the cross-bridges. Therefore, the HMM bind with the active sites on the actin myofilaments. The significance of these structures will be explained later in this chapter.

Another interesting aspect of the HMM is that the two sides of the myofilaments oppose each other. Furthermore, a projection-free area can be seen in the center of the HMM. This projection-free region corresponds with the H-zone of the sarcomere. In contrast, the presence of both the actin and myosin myofilaments in the denser portions of the A-bands is what gives them their characteristic darkness.

The Sarcotubular System

The *sarcotubular system* consists of two components (see Figure 2.2). The first is the *sarcoplasmic reticulum*. It envelops each of the contractile elements of

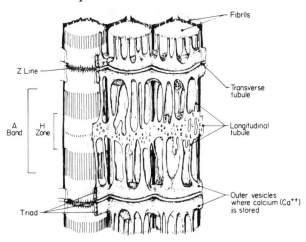

Figure 2.2. The sarcotubular system. *Note.* From *The Physiological Basis of Physical Education and Athletics* (3rd ed., p. 87) by D. Matthews and E. Fox, 1981, Philadelphia: CBS College Publishers. Copyright 1981 by W.B. Saunders Company. Reprinted by permission.

the sarcomeres and is the site of calcium storage. The second component is the *T-system*. The T-system derives its name from the fact that it consists of tubules that run across or transversely into the sarcoplasm. At the Z-line of the sarcomere, two portions of the sarcoplasmic reticulum come in close contact with a transverse tubule of the T-system to form a *triad*. The basic function of the T-system is communication. When the sarcolemma (i.e., the sarcomere's tubular sheath) is excited by an incoming nerve impulse, it undergoes *depolarization*. Simultaneously, the entire T-system also depolarizes, thus communicating an electrical impulse to all sarcomeres in the muscle fiber.

The impulse is then transmitted to a sleeve-like system of sacs and tubules of the sarcoplasmic reticulum. Here is where the calcium ions are actually stored. When the T-system depolarizes,

however, this change is transmitted to the membrane of the sarcoplasmic reticulum and causes it to become more permeable. As a result, calcium ions escape from the sacs of the reticulum. The significance of this process will soon become apparent.

Muscular Contraction, Relaxation, and Elongation

Muscles can be contracted, relaxed, or elongated. These actions can be described both physically and chemically and will be analyzed and discussed in the following section.

The Theory of Contraction

The function of muscle is to develop or generate tension. This process of "tension generation" is called *contraction*. The primary function of muscular contraction is to produce movement. Two other essential functions associated with contraction are (a) to maintain posture and (b) to produce body heat. Once a muscular contraction is initiated, a reversible chain of physical and chemical events is set into motion.

The Ultrastructural (Physical) Basis of Contraction. The mechanism by which muscles contract, relax, or elongate can be explained by the ultrastructure of the sarcomere. The exact mechanism that regulates the contractile elements, however, is not yet completely understood. The currently accepted theory is the interdigitation or sliding of myofilaments theory (see Figure 2.3).

When maximally contracted, a sarcomere may shorten from 20 to 50%. When passively stretched, it may extend to about 120% of its normal length. Careful microscopic measurements of the length of the A-bands and I-bands in intact muscle in the contracted, relaxed, and elongated states have conclusively proven that the A-bands, and thus the thick myofilaments, always remain constant in length. Similarly, the distance between the Z-line and the edge of the H-zone also remains constant at all stages of a normal contraction. This indicates that the thin myofilaments likewise undergo no change in length. Based on these observations, researchers have concluded that changes in muscle length must be due to the sliding of the thick and thin myofilaments along each other.

Thus when a muscle contracts, the actin and myosin myofilaments slide over each other so that each fiber shortens. For this to occur, the Z-line

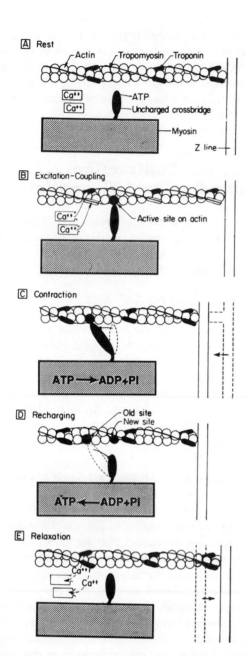

Figure 2.3. Proposed method of the sliding filament theory. (A) At rest, uncharged ATP cross-bridges are extended, actin and myosin are uncoupled, and Ca⁺⁺ is stored in the reticulum. (B) During excitation-coupling, stimulation releases Ca⁻⁻, which then binds to troponin, "turning on" actin active sites; actomyosin is formed. (C) During contraction, ATP is broken down, releasing energy that swivels the cross-bridges; actin slides over the myosin, tension is developed, and the muscle shortens. (D) During recharging, ATP is resynthesized and actin and myosin uncouple and are recycled. (E) When stimulation ceases, Ca⁺⁺ is restored in the reticulum by the calcium pump, and the muscle relaxes. *Note.* From *The Physiological Basis of Physical Education and Athletics* (3rd ed., p. 87) by D. Matthews and E. Fox, 1981, Philadelphia: CBS College Publishers. Copyright 1981 by W.B. Saunders Company. Reprinted by permission.

of the sarcomere must be drawn in towards the A-band. This results in the gradual narrowing and eventual elimination of the I-bands and H-zone.

The Molecular (Chemical) Basis of Contraction.

When nerve impulses arrive at a skeletal muscle fiber, they spread over its sarcolemma and move inward via its T-tubules. This increases the permeability and triggers the release of *calcium ions* (Ca^{+2}) from the sacs of the sarcoplasmic reticulum in the sarcoplasm. In resting muscle fiber, the actin and myosin myofilaments are inhibited from interacting with each other due to the presence of a protein called *troponin*. When calcium ions are released, however, they bind with the troponin and inhibit its action. This occurs because, with two positive charges, the calcium ions are attracted to the negative charges of the actin myofilaments and myosin cross-bridges (like charges repel each other, and opposing charges attract each other). This process creates an *electrostatic bond* between the actin and myosin myofilaments. Specifically, the cross-bridges of myosin attach to the actin myofilaments. The cross-bridges then collapse, whereupon the actin myofilaments are pulled toward the center of the sarcomere. Consequently, the muscle shortens and tension is generated. The immediate source of energy for muscular contraction is the compound adenosine triphosphate (ATP). Thus it is apparent that *muscles are completely and totally subservient to nerve impulses for activation. Without a nerve impulse, no muscular tension can be generated.*

The Theory of Muscular Relaxation

The ability of muscle to relax is essential for optimal movement and health. Hence the process of muscular relaxation has been studied intensively at both the physical and chemical levels. Like contraction, the exact mechanism of relaxation is not yet fully understood. The physical and chemical basis of relaxation will be analyzed in the following section.

The Ultrastructural (Physical) Basis of Relaxation.

Muscular relaxation is completely passive. When muscle fibers no longer receive nerve impulses, they relax. Thus relaxation is basically a cessation of the production of muscular tension. Consequently, as the cross-bridges detach and separate at relaxation, the internal elastic force that accumulated within the myofibrils during contraction is released. Thus the recoil of the elastic components is what restores the myofibrils to their uncontracted lengths (Gowitzke & Milner, 1980).

The Molecular (Chemical) Basis of Relaxation.

The chemical reactions associated with relaxation are not yet fully understood. Most scientists believe that relaxation is brought about by a reversal of the contraction process. In relaxation, *calcium-troponin* combinations separate, and the calcium ions reenter the sacs of the sarcoplasmic reticulum. Because the troponin is no longer bound to the calcium, it inhibits the actin and myosin from interacting. This allows for disassociation of actin and myosin and "resliding" of the myofilaments. In short, contraction is turned on by the release of calcium and turned off by its withdrawal.

The Theory of Muscular Elongation

Muscular fibers are incapable of lengthening, or stretching, themselves. For lengthening to occur, a force must be received from outside the muscle itself. Among these forces are (a) the force of gravity, (b) the force of momentum (motion), (c) the force of antagonistic muscles on the opposite side of the joint, and/or (d) the force provided by another person or by some part of one's own body. The latter can be accomplished by a pushing or pulling force, either manually or through the use of special equipment. In any event, the result is that the two myofilaments slide further apart.

Ultrastructural Limitations of Sarcomere Elongation

The theoretical limitation of a muscle cell's contractile component to stretch can be determined by extremely careful analysis of the microscopic measurements of the length of the (a) sarcomere, (b) myosin myofilaments, (c) actin myofilaments, and (d) the H-zone. For example, consider the following measurements:

	Length (in microns)		Length (in angstroms)
Sarcomere	2.30	or	23,000
Myosin	1.50	or	15,000
Actin	2.00	or	10,000
H-zone	.30	or	3,000

When a sarcomere is maximally stretched to the point of rupture, it can reach a length of approximately 3.60 microns. A rupture of the sarcomere, however, is undesirable. Our main concern is to stretch the sarcomere to a length where at least one cross-bridge can be maintained between the actin and myosin myofilaments. This length has been found to be approximately 3.50 microns. Thus the contractile component of the sarcomere (muscle cell) is capable of increasing 1.20 microns (3.50 − 2.30 = 1.20). This represents an incredible increase from the resting state of over 50%. If the sarcomere's length is given at 2.10 microns and all other factors remain constant, the contractile component of the muscle can then increase by an amazing 67% from its resting length. This enables our muscles to move through a wide range of motion (see Figure 2.4). In the next chapters we will examine how the connective tissue and the nervous system (i.e., muscle spindles) limit range of motion.

Improper Muscle Balance as a Limiting Factor

Healthy muscles maintain a structural homeostasis. A key to this structural balance is an equal pull by antagonistic muscles. Due to the attachments of muscles, an imbalance in the structural homeostasis of a muscle can cause direct lever action on the process and affect range of motion. Muscle imbalance can be due to several factors, including the presence of *hypertonic muscles* (i.e., muscles in a state of contracture and/or spasm) and/or *weak muscles* (see Figure 2.5).

At times a muscle may be hypertonic because of a primary functional weakness of its antagonist. As explained by Walther (1981), a classic example of a muscle contracting when unopposed is the rupture of the biceps brachii tendon. Depending on which tendons are severed, the muscle that is unopposed bunches up in the upper or lower arm. This is obviously an example of a total loss of resisting pull against the muscle. Thus "the amount of hypertonicity in a poorly opposed muscle from ineffective antagonistic function will be in direct relation to the amount of weakness in the antagonist" (p. 13). Orthodox treatments of hypertonic muscles include diathermy and other forms of heat, ultrasound, and massage. Walthers points out, however, an interesting aspect of using physical therapy to treat a muscle that is hypertonic secondary to weakness: "If the treatment is successful, the patient will then have two weak muscles" (p. 30).

Another method to correct a muscle imbalance is the use of manipulation (this will be discussed later in more detail). Occasionally, relief through manipulation may only be temporary. For example, when a muscle imbalance is present, the structure being held in place may deviate from normal. The

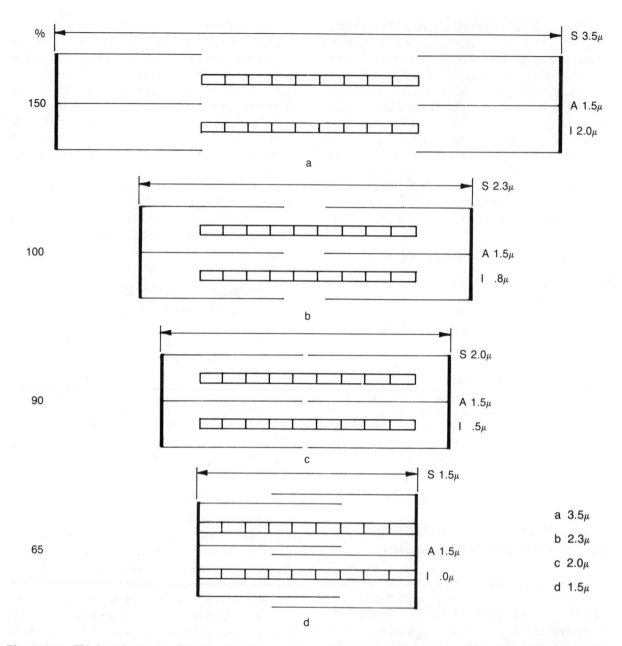

Figure 2.4. The lengthening and shortening of the sarcomere. (a) Stretched to approximately 150% rest length, (b) at rest, 100% rest length, (c) contracted to approximately 90% rest length, and (d) contracted to approximately 65% rest length. Sarcomere lengths (S) and A and I band lengths are given to the right of the diagrams. Lengths of sarcomeres expressed on % of rest length are given to the left.

structure cannot be returned to a permanent balance until the muscle imbalance is corrected. Simply stated, "a structure can be manipulated into balance, but if the muscular imbalance is not corrected, the structure held by the muscles will not remain balanced" (Walther, 1981, p. 30). This concept can be easily demonstrated by holding the ends of two rubber bands in each hand and suspending a button in the center. The rubber bands represent the muscles pulling on the button, which represents the vertebrae. If the pull is equal on both sides, the button will stay in the center. If you release one of the rubber bands, however, the pull will be stronger on one side and the button will slide off the center. This exemplifies the condition that results from weak muscles. The vertebrae is pulled out of place, and no matter how many times it is centered by manipulation, it will not stay balanced until the cause of the muscle imbalance is corrected. Obviously, the key is to correct the primary *cause* of the muscle imbalance (in this instance, a muscle weakness) (Walther, 1981).

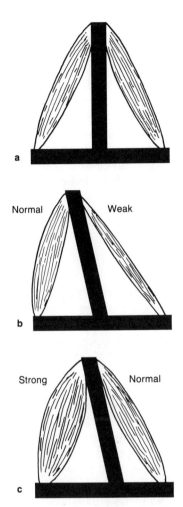

Figure 2.5. Muscle balance. (a) Balance in muscle gives structural balance. (b) Balance is most often lost because one muscle is weak. (c) Sometimes balance is lost because a muscle is too strong. *Note.* From *Applied Kinesiology: Vol. 1. Basic Procedures and Muscle Testing* by D.W. Walther, 1981, Pueblo, CO: Systems DC. Copyright 1981 by Systems DC. Reprinted by permission.

Inadequate Muscle Control as a Limiting Factor

Even if a person is endowed with natural flexibility and suppleness, local muscular control may still be inadequate to execute specific flexibility skills. This is because many flexibility skills are comprised of additional components. For our needs, *muscular control* will be considered to be the presence of adequate balance, coordination or control of one's body part(s), and/or sufficient muscular strength to perform a given skill. For example, to perform a skill as delicate as an arabesque (scale) one must have the necessary balance. One must also have enough strength to be able to raise, support, and maintain the desired position. To perform more intricate skills such as ballet or karate movements, sufficient coordination, rhythm, or timing may also be necessary. More complex motor skills can be performed only with the proper combination of all the required skill and fitness components.

The Effects of Aging on Muscle

The normal aging process brings about an almost imperceptible diminution in normal muscle functions. These include muscular strength, endurance, agility, and flexibility. When compounded by deconditioning of inactivity and complicated by disease and injury, these functions decline rapidly. Physiologically, one of the most conspicuous degenerative changes associated with aging is the progressive *atrophy*, or wasting away, of muscle mass. This is due to the reduction in both size and number of the muscle fibers (Grob, 1983; Gutmann, 1977; Rockstein & Sussman, 1979). The age at which these changes in the muscles begin is highly variable. These changes also vary in degree depending on the muscles involved and their degree of use as one grows older. The number of nerve cells in the musculoskeletal system decreases with age (Gutmann, 1977). Lastly, as muscle fibers atrophy, fatty and fibrous (collagen) tissue replacement occurs. Collectively, these changes appear to be partly responsible for the age-related loss of flexibility.

The Effects of Immobilization

The ability of muscle to adapt in length was demonstrated early by the experiments of Marvey (1887). Approximately 40 years later, Steindler (1932) related this ability in an equation. Recently, the mechanisms of length adaptation have been studied at the cellular and ultrastructural levels. Research by Goldspink (1968, 1976) and Williams and Goldspink (1971) has shown that the increase in fiber length during normal growth is associated with a large increase in the number of sarcomeres along the length of the fibers. Because the length of the actin and myosin filaments is constant, the adaptation of adult muscles to a different functional length presumably must involve the production or removal of a certain number of sarcomeres in series in order to maintain the correct sarcomere length in relation to the whole muscle (Goldspink, 1976; Tabary, Tabary, Tardieu, Tardieu, & Goldspink, 1972).

When adult cat soleus muscle is immobilized in a lengthened position by plaster casts, it adapts to its new length. Tabary et al. (1972) found that this is accomplished by a production of approximately 20% more sarcomeres in series. Williams and Goldspink (1973) found that the new sarcomeres are added on to the ends of the existing myofibrils. In the case of denervation and immobilization in a lengthened state, 25% more sarcomeres in series were produced (Goldspink, Tabary, Tabary, Tardieu, & Tardieu, 1974). Upon removal of the plaster cast, both the normal and denervated muscles rapidly readjusted to their original length (Goldspink et al., 1974; Tabary et al., 1972; Williams & Goldspink, 1976).

On the other hand, when the limb was immobilized with the muscle in its shortened position, the muscle fibers were found to have lost 40% of the sarcomeres in series (Tabary et al., 1972). With denervation and immobilization in its shortened position, a 35% reduction of sarcomeres in series was found (Goldspink et al., 1974). Here, too, these muscles were found to adjust rapidly to the original position with respect to their sarcomere number (Goldspink et al., 1974; Tabary et al., 1972).

Thus the results for the normal and denervated muscles immobilized in both the extended and shortened positions indicated that the adjustment of sarcomere number to the functional length of the muscles does *not* appear to be directly under neuronal control. Rather, it appears to be a myogenic response to the amount of passive tension to which the muscle is subjected (Goldspink, 1976; Goldspink et al., 1974; Williams & Goldspink, 1976).

Associated with the changes in fiber length and the number and length of the sarcomeres, researchers found a reduced extensibility (increase in passive resistance) of the muscles immobilized in the shortened position (Goldspink, 1976; Goldspink & Williams, 1978; Tabary et al., 1972). This was true whether or not the muscle was denerved (Goldspink, 1976). Along this line, Goldspink and Williams (1978) found that connective tissue was lost at a slower rate than muscle fiber tissue. Hence the relative amount of connective tissue increased (Goldspink, 1976; Goldspink & Williams, 1978; Tabary et al., 1972).

The decrease in extensibility appears to be a safety mechanism that prevents the muscle from being suddenly overstretched (Goldspink, 1976; Goldspink & Williams, 1978; Tabary et al., 1972). This mechanism is particularly important in the shortened muscle (i.e., muscles that have lost sarcomeres) because stretching even through the normal range of movement would cause the sarcomeres to be pulled out to the point where the myosin and actin myofilaments do not interdigitate or overlap, thus causing permanent damage to the muscle (Goldspink, 1976; Tabary et al., 1972). In contrast, changes in the elastic properties of the muscle immobilized in the lengthened position do not appear to be necessary because the adaptation is in the reverse direction and the chance of the muscle being overstretched is no greater than in the case of a normal muscle (Tabary et al., 1972).

Summary

Muscle tissue is comprised of progressively smaller units. The largest units (in descending order) are the (a) muscle *bundle*, (b) muscle *fasciculus*, and (c) muscle *fiber*. Each fiber is composed of smaller units called *myofibrils*. The myofibril can be resolved into a series of repeating light and dark patterns called *sarcomeres*. The sarcomere is the functional unit of a myofibril. The myofibrils are composed of still smaller units called *myofilaments*. Analysis of the myofilaments has found that they are primarily composed of two types of proteins. The thicker and shorter myofilaments are made of *myosin* and are free at both ends. The thinner and longer myofilaments are made of *actin* and terminate at the edge of the sarcomere. Extending from the myosin myofilaments are a number of short lateral projections called *cross-bridges*. At the molecular level, the ultimate building blocks of muscles are amino acids.

At present, muscle is hypothesized to work via the *sliding myofilament theory*. According to this theory, a muscle fiber receives a nerve impulse that spreads throughout the entire cell via the *T-system*. The T-system consists of tubules that run transversely into the sarcomere. The reception of a nerve impulse induces the release of calcium ions that are stored in the *sarcoplasmic reticulum* of the muscle. In the presence of adenosine triphosphate (ATP), a high energy source, the calcium ions bind with actin and myosin myofilaments to form an *electrostatic bond*. This bond can be likened to two opposing magnets attracting each other. As a result, the cross-bridges collapse and the actin and myosin myofilaments slide over one another. This causes the muscle fiber to shorten and develop tension. Later, when the muscle fiber ceases to receive nerve impulses, it *relaxes*. The key point to remember and understand is that *muscles are totally subservient to nerve impulses for activation. Without a nerve impulse, no muscular tension can be generated.*

The theoretical limitation of a muscle cell's (sarcomere's) ability to elongate and still maintain at least one cross-bridge between the actin and myosin myofilaments exceeds 50%. Thus the contractile elements of a muscle are capable of increasing over 50% from resting length, thereby allowing muscles to move through a wide range of motion.

Research has demonstrated that muscle tissue is very adaptable. In particular, sarcomere number, fiber length, and sarcomere length have been shown to adjust to the functional length of the whole muscle. For example, when adult muscle is immobilized in its lengthened position, it adapts to its new length by producing more sarcomeres in series. The new sarcomeres are added on to the ends of the existing myofilaments. In contrast, when muscle is immobilized in its shortened position, it loses sarcomeres in series. The physiological significance of this process is apparent when one considers that maximum contractile tension and the maximum rate of shortening of the muscle are obtained at the sarcomere length at which there is maximum interaction/overlap of the myosin cross-bridges with the actin myofilaments. In other words, muscle is able to adjust its sarcomere number to give the maximal functional overlap of the myosin cross-bridges and actin myofilaments. This adjustment does *not* appear to be directly under neuronal control. Instead, it appears to be a myogenic response to the amount of passive tension to which the muscle is subjected.

Review Questions

1. Draw a diagram and label the parts of the structure of a muscle.

2. Draw a diagram of a sarcomere and label its respective parts.

3. Draw a diagram and describe a sarcomere in a state of (a) elongation, (b) relaxation, and (c) contraction.

4. Explain the statement, ''Muscles never push; they always pull.''

5. Briefly explain the current theory about the role of calcium ions in muscle contraction and relaxation.

6. Explain whether or not you agree with the statement, ''There is no such thing as a tight muscle.''

7. Select a specific skill that requires a degree of strength, flexibility, and balance. Describe how best to improve an individual's performance of that skill. Cite specific exercises and procedures to be followed.

8. Explain how aging reduces a person's flexibility.

9. Explain to an athlete who is about to have a cast removed from a healed broken arm the physiological changes that have occurred.

10. Explain the consequences of immobilizing a muscle in a lengthened position.

Answers

1. Identify the following structures: (a) muscle belly, (b) fasciculus, (c) muscle fiber, (d) myofibril, and (e) myofilament. See Figure 2.1.

2. Identify the following structures: (a) actin myofilaments, (b) myosin myofilaments, (c) the Z-line (disc), (d) the H-zone, (e) the A-band, and (f) the I-band. See Figure 2.1.

3. See Figure 2.4.

4. During contraction, actin slides over the myosin, tension is developed, and the Z-lines are contracted or drawn closer together. Pulling is associated with a bringing in toward or after itself. In contrast, pressing is associated with pushing forward.

5. A nerve impulse received in the muscle cell via the T-system initiates the release of Ca^{+2} ions stored in the sarcoplasmic reticulum. The Ca^{+2} ions bind with troponin and this ''turns on'' actin active sites. A contraction then follows. When stimulation ceases, Ca^{+2} ions separate from the troponin and the ions reenter the sarcoplasmic sacs. As a result of this withdrawal, actin can no longer interact with myosin. This permits ''resliding'' of the myofilaments, and thus relaxation occurs.

6. There is no such thing as a ''tight'' muscle. Muscles are completely and totally subservient to nerve impulses for activation. Without a nerve impulse, no muscular tension can be generated.

7. Performing a Y-scale requires a degree of strength, flexibility, and balance. To master

this skill, one should work on stretching the adductors (see Exercises 63-90). The stretches should be in sets of 10-15 repetitions, or the static stretch position should be maintained between 30–60 seconds. In terms of strength, one must concentrate on working the erector spinae, abdominal, hip flexor, and hip abductor muscles. This can be accomplished by performing sit-ups, leg extensions against a resistance and a set of Y-scale lifts with a partner who can provide both support and resistance.

8. Aging results in decreased flexibility due to the replacement of muscle tissue with collagen.

9. Physiologically, the muscles have atrophied (i.e., become smaller), and the number of sarcomeres has decreased.

10. Immobilizing a muscle in the lengthened position will increase the number of sarcomeres in series. After demobilization, the number of sarcomeres will return to normal.

Recommended Readings

Etemadi, A.A., & Hosseini, F. (1968). Frequency and size of muscle fibers in athletic body build. *Anatomical Record*, **162**(3), 269-273.

Flint, F.W., & Hirst, D.G. (1978). Cross-bridge detachment and sarcomere "give" during stretch of active frog's muscle. *Journal of Physiology* (London), **276**, 449-465.

Gossman, M.R., Sahrmann, S.A., & Rose, S.J. (1982). Review of length-associated changes in muscle. *Physical Therapy*, **62**(12), 1799-1808.

Herring, S.W., Grimm, A.F., & Grimm, B.R. (1984). Regulation of sarcomere number in skeletal muscle: A comparison of hypotheses. *Muscle & Nerve*, **7**(2), 161-173.

Hill, D.K. (1968). Tension due to interaction between the sliding filaments in resting striated muscle: The effect of stimulation. *Journal of Physiology* (London), **199**, 637-684.

Hoyle, G. (1970). How muscle is turned on and off. *Scientific American*, **222**(4), 84-93.

Huxley, A.F., & Simmon, R.M. (1971). Proposed mechanism of force generation in striated muscle. *Nature*, **233**(5321), 533-538.

Huxley, H.E. (1965). The mechanism of muscular contraction. *Scientific American*, **213**(6), 18-28.

Jones, R.H. (1984). Physiological basis of rehabilitation therapy. In T.F. Williams (Ed.), *Rehabilitation in the aging* (pp. 97-109). New York: Raven Press.

Murray, J.M., & Weber, A. (1974). The cooperative action of muscle proteins. *Scientific American*, **230**(2), 58-71.

Shephard, R.J. (1982). *Physiology and biochemistry of exercise*. New York: Praeger.

Vallbona, C., & Baker, S.B. (1984). Physical fitness prospects in the elderly. *Archives of Physical and Medical Rehabilitation*, **65**, 194-200.

Williams, P.L., & Warwick, R. (1980). *Gray's anatomy* (36th British ed.). Philadelphia: W. B. Saunders.

CHAPTER 3

Connective Tissue as a Limiting Factor of Flexibility

In this chapter we will review the present state of knowledge about the mechanical properties, mechanical ultrastructure, biochemical constituents, and effects of aging and immobilization on connective tissues. Our goal will be to understand how these variables affect and determine the function of connective tissues. This will provide important information to enable us to better understand the behavior of connective tissue, which to a major extent determines our degree of flexibility.

Connective tissue contains a wide variety of specialized cells. Different types of cells perform the functions of defense, protection, storage, transportation, binding, connection, and general support and repair. In this chapter we will concentrate on the cells that perform the latter half of these functions.

Two types of connective tissue can significantly affect range of motion: *fibrous connective tissue* and *elastic connective tissue*. Fibrous connective tissue forms aponeuroses, fascia, membranes, ligaments, and tendons. Fibrous connective tissue consists predominantly of *collagenous fibers (collagen)*.

Collagen

Collagen is generally regarded as a primary structural component of living tissues. In fact, collagen is probably the most abundant protein in the animal kingdom. In higher vertebrates, for example, collagen constitutes one-third or more of the total body proteins. The two major physical properties of collagen fibers are their great tensile *strength* and relative *inextensibility*.

Collagenous fibers appear virtually colorless or off-white. They are arranged in bundles and, except under tension, run a characteristically wavy course. Collagen fibers are capable of only a slight degree of extensibility. They are, however, very resistant to tensile stress. Therefore, they provide the basis for structures such as ligaments and tendons that are subjected to a pulling force.

The Ultrastructure of Collagen

The structural organization of collagen is analogous to that of muscle (see Table 3.1 and Figure 3.1). However, the classification system is not widely agreed upon due to a lack of consistent terminology used in the field (Kastelic, Galeski, & Baer, 1978). When viewed under a microscope, individual collagen fibers are seen to have a banded or striated structure. The characteristic pattern of cross-striations of collagen reflects its ultrastructural organization. Knowledge of this pattern is fundamental to understanding the mechanism of collagen's two major physical properties: its great tensile strength and relative inextensibility.

The collagen of a tendon is arranged in wavy bundles called the *fascicle* (see Figure 3.1). A fascicle varies from 50 to 300 microns in diameter. The fascicle is in turn composed of bundles of *fibrils*, each of which is approximately 500 to 5,000 angstroms in diameter. The fibrils are in turn composed of bundles of collagen *subfibrils*, each of which is approximately 100 to 200 angstroms in diameter. Each subfibril is comprised of bundles of collagen *microfibrils* or *filaments*, each of which is approximately 35 angstroms in diameter. The sizes of the

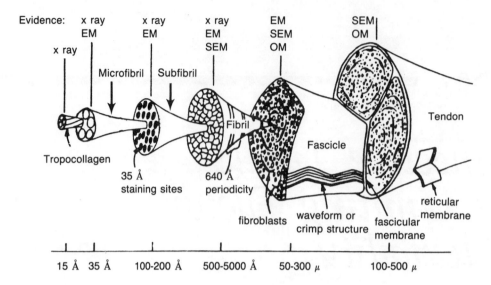

Figure 3.1.   Collagen hierarchy. *Note.* From "The Multicomposite Structure of Tendon" by J. Kastalic, A. Galeski, and E. Baer, 1978, *Connective Tissue Research*, **6**(1), p. 21. Copyright 1978 by Gordon and Breach Science Publishers, Inc. Reprinted by permission.

Table 3.1   A Comparison of Muscle and Collagen Structures

Muscle	Collagen
Muscle belly	Tendon
Muscle bundles (fasiculus)	Fascicle
Muscle fibers	Fibril
Myofibrils	Subfibril
Myofilaments	Microfibril
Sarcomeres (functional unit)	Collagen molecules (functional unit)
Actin	Alpha$_1$ chains (2)
Myosin	Alpha$_2$ chain (1)
Cross-bridges	Cross-links

filaments in a given tissue vary with age and other factors.

The collagen microfibril is composed of regularly spaced, overlapping *collagen molecule* units (see Figure 3.2b). (The term *tropocollagen* is now considered obsolete.) These units are analogous to the sarcomeres of muscle cells. The collagen molecules are in turn made of *coiled helices* of *amino acids*. The collagen molecules are very small; they measure about 2,800 angstroms in length and 15 angstroms in diameter (see Figure 3.2c). They lie in parallel alignment with a staggered overlap of almost one-fourth their length. Actual measurements indicate that a gap or hole of about 410 angstroms occurs

between the end of one collagen molecule and the beginning of the next in the same line. This overlapping is what creates the prominent cross-bands or striations. Collagen fibrils have a cross-band periodicity of from 600 to 700 angstroms depending on the source and degree of hydration.

Upon extreme magnification, the collagen molecule is seen as three polypeptide chains that are coiled in a unique type of rigid helical structure. Of the three intertwining amino acid chains in human collagen, two (the *alpha$_1$ chains*) are identical and one (the *alpha$_2$ chain*) is distinct. The three chains are thought to be held together by hydrogen bonds that form cross-links (see Figure 3.2d).

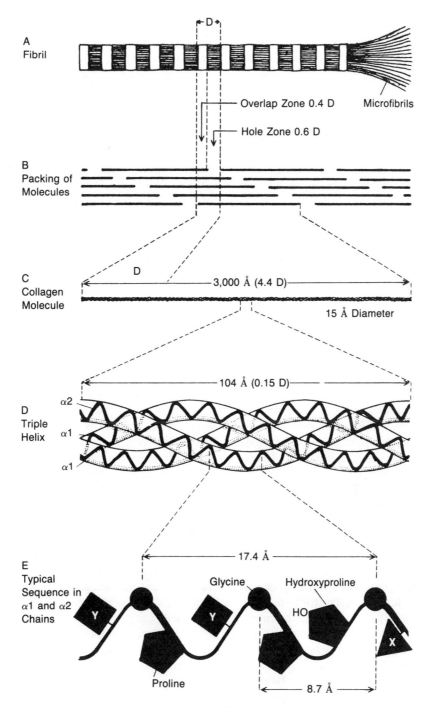

Figure 3.2. Collagen ultrastructure. Many tiny collagen fibrils make up a collagen fiber (a). The cross-striations in the fibril result from the overlapping of collagen molecules (b). The collagen molecule itself (c) is composed of three polypeptide chains that are organized into a rope-like triple helix (d). The amino acid sequence of these polypeptide chains is unique in having glycine as every third amino acid (e). The X position following glycine is frequently proline and the Y position preceding glycine is frequently hydroxyproline. *Note.* From "Collagen Diseases and the Biosynthesis of Collagen" by D.J. Prockop and N.A. Guzman, 1977, *Hospital Practice,* **12**(12), p. 62. Copyright 1977 by HP Publishing Company. Reprinted by permission. (Drawing by B. Tagawa.)

Cross-links

A major factor that adds tensile strength to collagenous structures is the presence of both *intra-molecular cross-links* between the alpha₁ and alpha₂ chains of the collagen molecule and the *inter-molecular cross-links* between collagen subfibrils, filaments, and fibers. In a sense, cross-links act to weld the building blocks (i.e., the molecules) into a strong, rope-like unit. Generally, the shorter the length between one cross-link and the next and/or the larger the number of cross-links in a given distance, the higher the elasticity or resistance to stretch will be (Alexander, 1975).

Researchers currently speculate that the number of cross-links relates to a collagen turnover; that is, collagen is continuously and simultaneously being produced and broken down. If collagen production exceeds collagen breakdown, more cross-links are established and the structure is more resistant to stretching. Conversely, if the collagen breakdown exceeds collagen production, then the opposite holds true. Some research has suggested that exercise or mobilization can decrease the number of cross-links by increasing the collagen turnover rate (Bryant, 1977; Shephard, 1982). Recent findings have also suggested that exercise or mobilization may play a determining factor in preventing cross-linking. This topic will be discussed later in this chapter.

The Biochemical Composition of Collagen

The collagen molecule is a complex helical structure whose mechanical properties are due to both its biochemical composition and the physical arrangement of its individual molecules. Although collagen is comprised of many complex molecules called *amino acids*, three stand out. These are the amino acids *glycine*, which comprises one-third, and *proline* and *hydroxyproline*, each of which comprise one-fourth or more (see Figure 3.2e). The presence of proline and hydroxyproline is what keeps the rope-like packing arrangement of collagen stable and resistant to stretching. Thus the higher the level of these amino acids, the higher the resistance of the molecules will be. This is because the nitrogen of the proline is fixed in a ring structure. Consequently, its presence prevents easy rotation of the regions in which they are located (Grant, Prockop, & Darwin, 1972; Gross, 1961). To help visualize this idea, think of these amino acids as being comparable to the adding of eggs to a meat loaf or the chemical combining of tin to copper to make bronze. In both cases, the result is increased rigidity and stability to the end product.

Groundsubstances

A major factor affecting the mechanical behavior of collagen is the presence of *groundsubstances*. Groundsubstances are widely distributed throughout connective and supporting tissues. At many sites, they are known as *cement substances*. They form the nonfibrous element of the matrix in which cells and other components are embedded. This viscous gel-like element is composed of glycoaminoglycans (GAGs), plasma proteins, a variety of small proteins, and water. The four major GAGs found in connective tissue are hyaluronic acid, chrondroitin-4-sulfate, chrondroitin-6-sulfate, and dermatan sulfate. Generally, GAGs are bound to a protein and collectively referred to as proteoglycan. In connective tissue, proteoglycans combine with water to form a proteoglycan aggregate.

Water makes up 60 to 70% of the total connective tissue content. GAG, which has an enormous water-binding capacity, is considered partially responsible for this high level of water content. According to Viidik, Danielsen, and Oxlund (1982), the importance of the hyaluronate molecule in this regard cannot be underestimated because it takes up a hydrodynamic volume 1,000 times the space occupied by the chain itself in an unhydrated state.

Hyaluronic acid and its attached or entrapped water is the principal fibrous connective tissue lubricant. Specifically, hyaluronic acid with water is thought to serve as a lubricant between the collagen fibers or fibrils. The lubricant appears to maintain a critical distance between the fibers and fibrils, thereby permitting free gliding of the fibers and fibrils past each other and perhaps preventing excessive cross-linking.

The Effects of Aging on Collagen

As collagen ages, specific physical and biochemical changes take place. Ultimately, these changes reflect a loss of the minimal extensibility that existed earlier, and reflects an increased rigidity. For instance, aging increases the diameter of the collagen fibers in various tissues. Also, with the passage of time the fibrils become more crystalline. This increase in crystallinity or orientation strengthens the intermolecular bonds and increases resistance to further deformation. Furthermore, aging is believed to be associated with an increased number of intra- and intermolecular cross-links. These increased cross-links apparently restrict the ability of collagen molecules to slip past each other. Dehydration also occurs with the aging process. The amount of water (i.e, hydration) associated with connective tissues such as tendon declines with age. Although the degree of dehydration varies from source to source, decreases in tendon from approximately 80 or 85% in babies to 70% in adults appear constant (Elliott, 1965).

The Ultrastructural Basis of Elongation and the Physiological Limit of Elongation

Unlike a sarcomere, a collagen fiber is comparatively inextensible. The collagen fiber is so inelastic that a weight of 10,000 times its own weight will not stretch it (Verzar, 1963). Research indicates that microscopic fibers can be stretched to a maximum of only about 10% of their original length before they break. However, at the molecular level, the protofibrils undergo an extension of only about 3% (Ramachandran, 1967). Under a microscope, collagen displays with elongation progressive alteration in intrafibril periodicity and lateral dimensions. One study (Cowan, McGavin, & North, 1955) found that stretching increased the repeated axial interval from 2.86 to 3.1 angstroms or more.

Such an extension is believed to occur through a straightening out of the fibers and/or a gradual slip of one fiber relative to the next. Ultimately, this results in an increase in crystallinity or orientation that strengthens the intermolecular bond and increases resistance to further elongation. This process can be compared to the spinning from a ball of cotton: With an increase in crystallinity there is an increase of the intermeshing of the adjacent molecules. Consequently, there is an increased regularity in packing and enhanced interchain forces which permits increased resistance to deforming forces. Thus, simply stated, collagenous fibers allow elongation until the slack of their wavy bundles is taken up. However, if stretch continues, a point will be reached where all intermolecular forces are exceeded and the tissue parts (Holland, 1968; Laban, 1962; Weiss & Greer, 1977).

Elastic Tissue

Elastic tissue may refer to a connective tissue which has elastic fibers as its principal component. Elastic tissue totally devoid of collagenous and other tissue is called *elastica*. Thus elastic tissue or elastic fiber has a structural connotation while elastin refers to the biochemical character of elastic fibers.

Elastic tissue is a primary structural component of living tissue, and is found in various quantities throughout the body. Electron microphotographs have shown that there is a large amount of elastic tissue in the sarcolemma of the muscle fiber (the connective tissue that surrounds the sarcomere). Thus elastic tissue plays a major role in determining the possible range of extensibility of muscle cells. In certain locations, rather large amounts of almost pure elastic fibers can be found, particularly in the ligaments of the vertebral column. Here too, elastic tissue determines to a major extent the possible ranges of motion.

Elastic fibers perform a variety of functions, including disseminating stresses that originate at isolated points, enhancing coordination of the rhythmic motions of the body parts, conserving energy by maintaining tone during relaxation of muscle elements, providing a defense against excessive forces and assisting organs in returning to their undeformed configuration once all forces have been removed (Jenkins & Little, 1974).

The Composition of Elastic Fibers

Unfortunately, elastic fibers have not been studied as extensively as collagen fibers, and are therefore less understood. Elastic fibers are usually compared with collagen fibers because the two are very closely associated anatomically, morphologically, biochemically, and physiologically. In fact, elastic fibers may have collagen fibers interwoven with their principal components. Usually, elastic fibers are dominated by collagen fibers.

Elastic fibers are optically homogenous. Hence, they are highly refractile and almost isotropic. Under an electron microscope, each fiber appears to consist of a fused mass of fibrils twisted in rope-like fashion. Unlike collagenous fibers, elastic fibers display a complete lack of periodical structure (i.e., banding or striation structure).

Cross-Links

Elastic fibers are thought to be composed of a network of randomly coiled chains, which are probably joined by covalent cross-links. However, the noncovalent interchain forces are considered weak, and the cross-links themselves are believed to be widely spaced (Weiss & Greer, 1977). Consequently, elastic cross-links do not weld the building blocks (the molecules) into a strong rope-like unit similar to collagen. The significance of this difference will be discussed later.

Elastin

Elastin is a complex structure with a mechanical property of elasticity due both to its biochemical composition and to the physical arrangement of its individual molecules. Elastin is also composed of *amino acids*. Unlike collagen, however, elastin is composed mostly of nonpolar hydropholic amino acids, and it has little hydroxyproline and no hydroxylysine. Also, elastin is unique in that it contains *desmosine* and *isodesmosine,* which function as covalent cross-links in and between the polypeptide chains. Similar to collagen, about one-third of the residues of elastin are *glycine* and about 11% are *proline.*

The Relationship Between Collagen and Elastin

As mentioned earlier, elastic fibers are almost always found in close association with collagenous tissues. Furthermore, their performance is dependent upon these tissues, and is thus a combined result of a blending and integrating of two distinctly different mechanical systems. First, there are the elastic fibers themselves, which are typically responsible for what may be called reverse extensibility (the ability of a stretched material to return to its original resting state). Second, there is the collagen meshwork, which provides the rigid constraints that limit the deformations of the elastic elements and are largely responsible for the ultimate properties (tensile strength and relative inextensibility) of those composite structures. Logically, where collagenous fibers dominate, rigidity, stability, tensile strength, and a restricted range of movement will prevail (Eldren, 1968; Gosline, 1976).

The Effects of Aging on Elastic Fibers

Elastic fibers display specific physical and biochemical changes as a result of aging. They lose their resiliency and undergo various other alterations, including fragmentation, fraying, calcification and other mineralizations, and an increased number of cross-linkages. Biochemically, there is an increase in amino acids containing polar groups as well; for example, the content of desmosine, isodesmosine, and lysinonorlencine all increase as elastin ages. Other changes are an increase in the proportion of chrondroitin sulfate B and keratosulphate. Altogether, these alterations appear to be responsible for age-related loss of resiliency and increased rigidity (Bick, 1961; Gosline, 1976; Schubert & Hamerman, 1968; Yu & Blumenthal, 1967).

The Ultrastructural Basis and the Physiological Limit of Elongation

Elastic fibers yield easily to stretching. However, when released they return virtually to their former length. Only when elastic fibers are stretched to about 150% of their original length do they reach their breaking point; a force of only 20 to 30 kg/cm² is necessary to bring this about (Bloom & Fawcett, 1975).

Elastic fibers yield so easily to stretching because, as previously explained, they are composed of a network of randomly coiled chains joined by covalent cross-links. These cross-links impose a restriction on the elastic fibers such that, upon stretching, the individual chains are constrained and cannot slip past one another (Franzblau & Faru, 1981). However, the covalent interchain forces are weak and the cross-links widely spaced. As a result, minimal unidirectional force can produce extensive elongation of chains before the cross-links begin to restrict movement. Thus, similar to the collagenous fibers, elastic fibers allow extensibility until the slack and spacing between the chains are taken up. This concept is best exemplified by the fiber weave in the Chinese finger trap (Akeson, Amiel, & Woo, 1980; Donatelli & Owens-Burkhart, 1981).

Tissues Composed of Connective Tissue

The human body contains numerous structures composed of connective tissue, including tendons, ligaments, and fascia, the three structures that are of greatest concern to us here, and which are analyzed and discussed in this section.

Tendons

Muscles are attached to bones by tough cords called tendons, whose function is to transfer tension to the bones. Consequently, tendons are extremely important in determining one's quality of movement. Verzar (1964) vividly describes this concept:

> The importance of inextensibility, from a physiological point of view, is that the smallest muscular contraction can be transmitted without loss to the articulations. If tendons, i.e., collagen fibers, were only slightly extensible, the finest movements, such as those of the fingers of a violinist or pianist, or the exact movements of the eye, would be impossible. The microscopic helical structure cannot be an expression of morphological waves; otherwise an incipient muscular contraction could not lead to the precise immediate effect on the con-

traction and movement in the articulation. For this the tendon must be inextensible. (p. 255)

The chief constituents of tendons are thick, closely packed, parallel collagenous bundles that vary in length and thickness. They show a distinct longitudinal striation and in many places fuse with one another. The fibrils making up the tendon are virtually all oriented in one direction, that is, toward the long axis, which is also the direction of normal physiological stress. The tendon is thus especially adapted to resist movement in any one direction. Therefore, the greater the proportion of collagen to elastic fibers, and the greater the number of fibers that are oriented in the direction of stress, and the greater the cross-sectional area, or width of the tendon the stronger the tendon.

A study by Johns and Wright (1962) determined that tendons provide about 10% of the total resistance to movement. In the tendon, a stress of 4% is regarded as especially significant and corresponds to the limit of reversibility, and therefore of elasticity (Crisp, 1972). At this point, the tendon's surface waviness disappears, and if the stretch continues, injury may result.

Ligaments

Ligaments bind bone to bone. Consequently, unlike tendons, they attach (insert) to bones at both ends. Their function is primarily to support a joint (the place where two or more bones meet) by holding the bones in place. Ligaments are similar to tendons, except that the elements are less regularly arranged. Like tendons, they are composed mainly of bundles of collagenous fibers placed parallel to, or closely interlaced with, one another. Ligaments are found in different shapes, such as cords, bands, or sheets. However, they lack the glistening whiteness of tendon because there is a greater admixture of elastic and fine collagenous fibers woven among the parallel bundles. Consequently, they are pliant and flexible so as to allow perfect freedom of movement, but strong, tough, and inextensible so as not to yield readily to applied forces.

A biochemical analysis will reveal that ligament contains mostly collagenous tissue. The exceptions to this are the ligamentum flava and ligamentum nuchae which connect the laminae of adjacent vertebrae. These ligaments are made up almost entirely of elastic fibers and are quite elastic.

The ligaments and joint capsule contribute about 47% of the total resistance to movement (Johns & Wright, 1962). Consequently, they are extremely significant in determining the ultimate range of movement of a joint.

Fascia

The word *fascia*, meaning a band or bandage, is taken from the Latin. Technically, fascia is a term used in gross anatomy to designate all fibrous connective structures not otherwise specifically named. Similar to other previously mentioned tissues, fascia varies in thickness and density according to functional demands, and is usually in the form of membraneous sheets.

The fascia that envelops and binds down the muscle into separate groups is named according to where it is found. The sheaths of connective tissue that encase the entire muscle are called the *epimysium*. Next, the *perimysium* encases the bundles of muscle fibers known as fasciculi. Within the perimysium, as many as 150 individual fibers may be found. Then, surrounding each fiber is the *endomysium*. Lastly, there is the *sarcolemma*, the connective tissue that covers the functional unit of the muscle, the sarcomere. It is from the meshwork of these connective tissues that the resting elasticity or resistance to stretch in muscle originates. Thus when the muscle is stretched, the connective tissues become progressively taut. Exactly the same effect can be seen when a knitted stocking is stretched (Carlson & Wilkie, 1974).

The connective tissue makes up as much as 30% of muscle mass. This tissue allows the muscle to change in length. During passive motion, the sum of the muscle's fascia accounts for 41% of the total resistance to movement (Johns & Wright, 1962). Hence the fascia represents the second most important factor limiting the range of motion (see Table 3.2).

Table 3.2 Comparison of the Relative Contribution of Soft-Tissue Structures to Joint Resistance

Structure	Resistance to flexibility
Joint capsule	47%
Muscle (Fascia)	41%
Tendon	10%
Skin	2%

Note. Adapted from "The Relative Importance of Various Tissues in Joint Stiffness" by R.J. Johns and V. Wright, 1962, *Journal of Applied Physiology*, **17**(5), pp. 824-828.

The Effects of Immobilization on Connective Tissues

When joints are immobilized for any length of time, the connective tissue elements of the capsules, ligaments, tendons, muscles, and fascia lose their property of extensibility. In addition, immobilization is associated with a concomitant 40% decrease in hyaluronic acid, 30% decrease in chrondroitin-4- and chrondroitin-6-sulfate, and 4.4% loss of water (Akeson, Amiel, & LaViolette, 1967; Akeson et al., 1977; Akeson, Amiel, & Woo, 1980; Donatelli & Owens-Burkhart, 1981; Woo, Matthews, Akeson, Amiel, & Convery, 1975). If we assume that distances between fibers must be reduced when GAG and water volumes are decreased, then this loss of GAG and water will result in a reduction of the critical fiber distance between collagen fibers. Consequently, the connective tissue fibers will come into contact and eventually stick, thereby encouraging the formation of abnormal cross-linking. The result is the loss of extensibility and an increase in tissue stiffness (see Figures 3.3 and 3.4) (Akeson, Amiel, & Woo, 1980; Donatelli & Owens-Burkhart, 1981; McDonough, 1981).

In addressing the significance of immobilization and mobilization, Donatelli and Owens-Burkhart (1981) succinctly point out:

> If movement is the major stimulus for biological activity, then the amount, the duration, the frequency, the rate, and the time of initiation of the movement are all important in producing the desired therapeutic effects on connective tissue structures. These factors must be determined before we can comprehend the optimal benefits of mobilization. (p. 72)

Summary

Connective tissue plays a significant role in determining one's range of movement. Fibrous connective tissue consists predominantly of collagen, while elastic connective tissue is composed principally of elastic fibers. Range of motion is the combined result of a blending and integrating of these two tissues. Where collagenous fibers dominate, a restricted range of motion will prevail. Conversely, where elastic fibers dominate, range of motion is greater. The properties of these tissues reflect their chemical and physical arrangements.

Collagenous tissues are comprised of progressively smaller units. The largest units, in order of decreasing size, are (a) the tendons, ligaments, and various fascia (e.g., the epimysium, perimysium, and endomysium), (b) collagen fascicle, and (c) bundles of fibrils. Each fibril is composed of smaller units called subfibrils. The subfibrils can be further resolved into

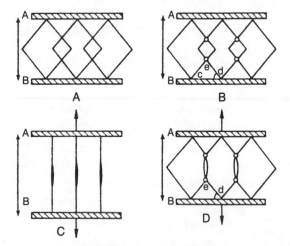

Figure 3.3. The idealized weave pattern of collagen fibers. It can be demonstrated that fixed contact at strategic sites (e.g., points d and e) can severely restrict the extension of this collagen weave. A: collagen fiber arrangement; B: collagen fiber cross-links; C: normal stretch; and D: restricted stretch due to cross-link. *Note.* From "Immobility Effects on Synovial Joints the Pathomechanics of Joint Contracture" by W.H. Akeson, D. Amiel, and S. Woo, in *Biorheology* (Vol. 17, No. 1/2, p. 101), New York: Pergamon Press. Copyright 1980 by Pergamon Press Ltd. Reprinted by permission.

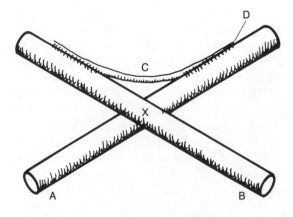

Figure 3.4. An idealized model demonstrating the collagen cross-links interaction at the molecular level. A and B represent the prexisting fibers; C represents the newly synthesized fibril; D represents the cross-links created as the fibril becomes incorporated into the fiber; and X represents the nodal point at which adjacent fibers are normally freely movable past one another. *Note.* From "Immobility Effects on Synovial Joints the Pathomechanics of Joint Contracture" by W.H. Akeson, D. Amiel, and S. Woo, in *Biorheology* (Vol. 17, No. 1/2, p. 104), New York: Pergamon Press. Copyright 1980 by Pergamon Press Ltd. Reprinted by permission.

collagen microfibrils (or filaments). Under high magnification the microfibril is seen to consist of a repeating series of light and dark patterns known as the collagen molecule (the term *tropocollagen* is now considered obsolete). The collagen molecule is the functional unit of a filament, and is composed of three intertwining amino acid chains coiled in a unique type of rigid helical structure.

There are several reasons for the strength of collagen according to current hypothesis. First, the presence of the amino acids proline and hydroxyproline keeps the rope-like packing arrangement of collagen stable and resistant to stretching. The tensile strength, however, is due mostly to the formation of the covalent cross-links. These are the intramolecular cross-links that bind chains from the same molecule and intermolecular cross-links that weld collagen fibrils, filaments, and fibers together. Furthermore, all other things being equal, the greater the proportion of collagen to elastic fibers, and the greater the number of fibers that are oriented in the direction of stress, and the greater the cross-sectional area, the greater will be the strength of the tissues. In contrast, elastic tissues yield easily to stretching, due partially to their unique combination of amino acids and partially to the presence of weak covalent cross-links, which are believed to be widely spaced.

Aging and immobilization of collagenous and elastic fibers contribute to a loss of flexibility. Aging is associated with calcification, dehydration, fragmentation, increased crystallinity, and an increased number of intra- and intermolecular cross-links. Immobilization is thought responsible for the loss of GAG and water, which reduces the critical distance between connective tissue fibers. Consequently, the fibers come into contact with one another and eventually stick, thereby encouraging the formation of abnormal cross-linking. Current hypothesis suggests that exercise can delay the loss of flexibility due to aging and immobilization.

Lastly, total resistance of movement has been determined to be 10% in tendon, 47% in ligament, and 41% in fascia. Fascia gives muscle the ability to change length. Because the connective tissues are the most influential components in limiting range of motion, they must be fully stretched, with the muscle relaxed, for flexibility to be optimally developed.

Review Questions

1. Draw a diagram and label the parts of the organizational structure of collagen.

2. Explain why proper nutrition is essential for collagen synthesis.

3. Explain the relationship of cross-links and tissue elasticity.

4. Proponents of yoga contend that stretching can retard the aging process, and in particular, the loss of flexibility. Analyze this view in the light of scientific information.

5. Explain the statement, ''Muscles (i.e., the contractile components) do not really limit one's flexibility.''

6. Explain the effects of immobilization on connective tissue.

7. Identify the percentage of resistance to movement provided by tendon, ligament, and fascia.

8. Explain the statement, ''I would rather break a bone than tear a ligament.''

9. Explain the danger associated with overstretching a ligament.

10. Explain to a group of high school athletes the physiological benefits pertaining to flexibility that are associated with exercise.

Answers

1. See Figure 3.2. Identify the following structures of collagen: (a) amino acids, (b) triple helix, (c) collagen molecule, and (d) collagen fibrils/filaments.

2. Proper nutrition is essential for collagen synthesis because collagen synthesis requires the presence of a wide variety of substances (e.g., amino acids, enzymes, etc.). Without these ''materials'' gained from proper nutrition, the synthesis of collagen would be like the building of a skyscraper without the use of cement, plastic, steel, wood, aluminum, and glass.

3. Cross-links add tensile strength to collagenous structures and in a sense act as ''welding blocks.'' The closer the links, the higher the elasticity or resistance to stretch of the tissue.

4. Research indicates that movement (including stretching, as in yoga) is the major stimulus for maintaining the critical distance between fibers. Immobilization, on the other

hand, results in a loss of flexibility due to certain physiological adaptations, and in a reduction of the critical fiber distance between fibers.

5. Muscles are capable of increasing over 50% in length and still maintaining one cross-bridge. The true limiting factors of one's range of motion are connective tissue, muscle tension due to the stretch reflex, and joint structure.

6. Immobilization results in a loss of GAGs and water. Consequently, the connective tissue fibers come into contact with one another and eventually stick, thereby encouraging the formation of abnormal cross-linking.

7. Resistance to movement is 10% in tendon, 47% in ligament, and 41% in fascia.

8. Ligament damage causes the loss of flexibility due to the development of adhesion and loss of strength in the tissues.

9. Overstretching a ligament results in an injury to those tissues where the intermolecular forces are exceeded and the tissues part. (Injury, however, can take place even without the tearing of tissues.)

10. Stretching exercises result in physiological adaptations that enhance the development of range of motion. As a consequence, performance can be improved and the chances of injury reduced.

Recommended Readings

Balazs, E.A. (1968). Viscoelastic properties of hyaluronic acid and biological lubrication. *University of Michigan Medical Center Journal* (special issue), 255-259.

Balazs, E.A., Seppala, P.O., Gibbs, D.A., Duff, E.F., & Merrill, E.W. (1967). Effect of aging on the viscoelastic and chemical properties of human synovial fluid. *Arthritic Rheumatology,* **10**(3), 264.

Betsch, D.F., & Baer, E. (1980). Structure and mechanical properties of rat tail tendon. *Biorheology,* **17**(1/2), 83-94.

Diament, J., Keller, A., Baer, E., Litt, M., & Arridge, R.G. (1972). Collagen: Ultrastructure and its relation to mechanical properties as a function of aging. *Proceedings of the Royal Society of London,* B, 180, 293.

Enneking, W.F., & Horowitz, M. (1972). The intra-articular effects of immobilization on the human knee. *Journal of Bone and Joint Surgery,* **54-A**(5), 973-985.

Gibbs, D.A., Merrill, E.W., Smith, K.A., & Balazs, E.A. (1968). Rheology of hyaluronic acid. *Biopolymers,* **6**(6), 777-791.

LaVigne, A., & Watkins, R.P. (1973). Preliminary results on immobilization-induced stiffness of monkey knee joints and posterior capsule. In R. Kenedi (Ed.), *Perspectives in biomedical engineering* (pp. 177-179). Baltimore: University Park Press.

Nimni, M.E. (1980). The molecular organization of collagen and its role in determining the biophysical properties of the connective tissues. *Biorheology,* **17**(1/2), 51-82.

Rydell, N., & Balazs, E.A. (1971). Effect of intra-articular injection of hyaluronic acid on the clinical symptoms of osteoarthritis and on granulative tissue formation. *Clinical Orthopedics and Related Research,* **80**, 25-32.

Swann, D., Radin, E., & Nazimiec, M. (1974). Role of hyaluronic acid in joint lubrication. *Annals of the Rheumatic Diseases,* **33**, 318-326.

Viidak, A. (1973). Functional properties of collagenous tissues. In D. A. Hall & D. S. Jackson (Eds.), *International review of connective tissue research* (Vol. 6, pp. 127-215). New York: Academic Press.

Viidak, A., & Ekholm, R. (1968). Light and electron microscopic studies of collagen fibers under strain. *Zeitschrift fur anatomic und entwicklungsgeshichte,* **127**, 154-164.

Walker, J.M. (1981). Development, maturation and aging of human joints: A review. *Physiotherapy Canada,* **33**(3), 153-160.

Williams, P.L., & Warwick, R. (1980). *Gray's anatomy* (36th British ed.). Philadelphia: W. B. Saunders.

Woo, S., Gomez, M.A., Woo, Y.K., & Akeson, W.H. (1982). Mechanical properties of tendons and ligaments. *Biorheology,* **19**(3), 397-408.

Mechanical and Dynamic Properties of Soft Tissues

Within the past 20 years, a great deal of scientific research has been directed toward identifying the mechanical properties of muscle and connective tissue. *Biophysics* is the science that deals with the study of biological structure and processes with reference to principles and phenomena of physics. A knowledge of biophysics can help one to distinguish between fact and fallacy, cause and effect, and the possible and impossible. Understanding the biophysics of muscle and connective tissue under tensile stress is therefore essential for determining the optimal means of increasing range of motion.

Definitions and Terminology

Before we begin our examination of biophysics, you should understand some of its basic terminology and concepts. At times you will find several different terms used for essentially the same thing (distensibility, extensibility, or stretchability) and some words with definitions not commonly known or accepted (e.g., elasticity, sprain, or strain). The terminology in this book is not unique; it has been adopted because it precisely describes what it is meant to describe.

Deformations

When ever a body or material is subjected to a *force* (i.e., a push or a pull), a change in the shape or size of the body can occur. This is, of course, dependent upon several variables: the body or material, the amount of force, the duration of the force, and the temperature of the body or material, to name a few. These changes are called *deformations*. A body subjected to a compressive force, for instance, shortens in length, and this decrease in length is its deformation. An example is the contraction of a muscle. But when a tensile or horizontal force is applied to a body, the length is increased, and therefore, the lengthening is its deformation. In layman's terms, *stretching* refers to the process of elongation and *stretch* refers to the elongation itself.

Elasticity

A material's resistance to distortion—that property that enables it to return to its original shape or size when a force is removed—is called *elasticity*. Elasticity is measured as the amount of counterforce within the material itself. Since elastic stretch represents spring-like behavior, it's often symbolized pictorially by a spring.

Stress

When a force acts on a body or material, resisting forces within the body react. These resisting forces are called *stresses*. A stress is an internal resistance to an external force. Stress is measured by the force applied per unit area which produces or tends to produce deformation in a body. It is expressed in units as lb/ft²; nt/m²; and dynes/cm². Thus:

$$\text{STRESS} = \frac{\text{Force}}{\text{Area of Surface on Which Force Acts}}$$

$$= \frac{F}{A}$$

Strain

The ratio of length after stress is applied, to original length, is defined as a *strain*. Because it is a ratio of length, strain has no dimensions or units. Thus, strain is a pure number:

$$\text{Longitudinal Strain} = \frac{\text{Change in Length}}{\text{Initial Length}} = \frac{\Delta 1}{\ell}$$

The amount of strain produced by a stress is basically determined by the forces between the material's atoms. The stronger these forces are, the greater stress will have to be before producing a given amount of strain. Mathews, Stacy, and Hoover (1964) have clearly described this concept. The molecules of a material are held together by attractive forces. When there is no external force applied, the length of a material is determined by a balance of attractive forces and repulsive forces between molecules. When a material is lengthened, the molecules become farther apart; the attractive forces then grow stronger while the repulsive forces grow weaker. "Therefore, there is a force generated within the molecules of the material itself which tends to pull the ends of the sample back toward the unstressed condition. This is the elastic force" (p. 69).

Hooke's Law and the Modulus of Elasticity

The numerical relationship between stress and strain was first discovered by Robert Hooke. *Hooke's Law* states that there is a constant or proportional arithmetical relationship between force and elongation. One unit of force will produce one unit of elongation, two units of force will produce two units of elongation and so forth. Within the context of Hooke's Law, the body is perfectly elastic.

The constant in Hooke's Law is the body material's *modulus of elasticity*. The modulus of elasticity is the ratio of the unit stress to the unit of deformation or strain where Y is the proportional constant. Thus the Modulus of Elasticity = stress required to produce one unit strain.

$$Y = \frac{\text{LONGITUDINAL STRESS}}{\text{LONGITUDINAL STRAIN}} = \frac{F/A}{\Delta\ell/\ell} = \frac{F\ell}{A\Delta\ell}$$

Because the strain is a dimensionless ratio, the units of Y are identical with those of stress, namely, force/length^2. Thus Y may be expressed in lb/in^2, nt/mt^2, or dynes/cm^2. The value of Y differs for different materials and does not depend on the material's dimensions.

Elastic Limit, Permanent Set or Sprain, Yield Point, and Ultimate Strength

In materials that are not perfectly elastic, the arithmetical relationship between force and elongation reaches a value known as the *elastic limit*. The elastic limit is the smallest value of stress required to produce permanent strain in the body. Below the elastic limit, materials return to their original length when the deforming force is removed. However, the result of applying a force beyond the elastic limit is that the stressed material will not return to its original length when the force is removed. The difference between the original length and the new length is called the amount of *permanent set* or *sprain*. This nonrecoverable or permanent elongation is also called *plastic stretch*.

When stress is applied beyond the elastic limit, deformation and force are no longer arithmetically proportional. The material elongates much further for each unit of force above the elastic limit than it did below it.

At a stress slightly beyond the elastic limit a deformation occurs without additional stress. This is called the YIELD POINT. As increased forces are applied at this point, the curve tends to flatten, and the maximum stress recorded—that is, the unit stress that occurs just at or before rupture—is called the *ultimate strength* of the material.

Soft Tissues

Tissues may be divided into two categories: hard and soft. The former are those of bone for the most part, although they also include teeth, nails, and hair. Soft tissues include tendons, ligaments, muscles, skin, and most of the other tissues (Mathews, Stacy, & Hoover, 1964), and are divided into two groups: contractile and noncontractile.

Properties of Soft Tissues

Soft tissues vary in quality and in physical and mechanical characteristics. Both contractile and noncontractile tissues are distensible and elastic, but contractile tissues are also contractible. *Contractility* is the ability of a muscle to shorten and develop tension along its length. *Distensibility* (commonly known as *extensibility* or *stretchability*) is the ability of muscle tissue to stretch in response to an externally applied force. The weaker the forces generated within the muscle, the greater will be the amount of stretch. Elasticity, on the other hand, is *resistance* to distortion, and is the opposite of distensibility. Elasticity refers to the property of a tissue to return to its unstrained length after having been deformed.

The Relationship and Significance of the Mechanical Properties of Soft Tissues to Stretching

The greater the elasticity of a soft tissue, the greater the force must be that can produce an elongation. A tissue of low elasticity cannot resist a stretching force as well as a tissue that is highly elastic, and will need a slighter force than the more elastic tissue to produce the same degree of deformation. Therefore, soft tissues with high elasticity are less susceptible to injuries such as sprains (which involve ligamentous or inert tissue) and strains (which involve contractile tissue or muscle).

Soft tissues are not perfectly elastic. Beyond their elastic limit, they cannot return to their original length once the stretching force is removed. The difference between the original length and the new length is called the amount of *permanent set*, and is analogous to a minor sprain or strain. Thus when one suffers a minor sprain or strain, the soft tissues do not return to their original length after the excessive stress is removed.

A natural question arises, then: For flexibility to be developed, should one stretch up to the elastic limit or slightly beyond it? Most authorities recommend stretching to the point of ''discomfort'' or ''tension'' (but not pain!). In turn, this raises another question: Is the point of discomfort below, at, or beyond the elastic limit? Although the literature is not conclusive on this subject, research indicates that factors such as (a) the type of force, (b) the duration of the force, and (c) the temperature of the tissue during and after stretching will determine whether the elongation is recoverable or permanent. Further discussion of these factors follows.

Mechanical Components/ Elements of Muscle

We know a great deal about the various mechanical properties of muscle, as for decades they have been among the favorite topics of researchers. There are several reasons why we should study the mechanical properties of muscle. One is so that we may comprehend the mechanical responses of a whole muscle; another is to help us understand the mechanical properties of the contractile components themselves (Zierler, 1974). Yet for our needs here, the most important reason for studying the mechanical properties of muscle is so that we may understand and determine: (a) the factors that limit flexibility, and (b) the best means of increasing flexibility.

Muscle is composed of three independent mechanical components or elements, which may be classified as either *elastic* or *viscous*. These mechanical components are important because they resist deformation, and therefore play a major role in determining one's flexibility. Elastic components exert a force in response to a change in length. Viscous components exert a force in response to the rate of a change in length. The three mechanical components are

1. the parallel elastic component (PEC),
2. the series elastic component (SEC),
3. the contractile component (CC).

Of the three, the CC is probably the most studied and best understood. Despite the fact that researchers have made many efforts to simulate the mechanical responses of muscles with mechanical models (Zierler, 1974), the precise anatomic counterparts of the two noncontractile components are not completely defined and are still a matter of dispute.

The Parallel Elastic Component (PEC)

If a muscle is removed from a body, it will naturally shorten to about 10% of its original, intact (in situ) length. This shortening is independent of contraction. The length of the isolated, uncontracted muscle is called its *equilibrium length*. This means that muscles are under tension at their intact length. The intact or in situ length of an uncontracted or unstretched muscle is called its *resting length*, symbolized as *Rl* or *Lo*. Resting muscle is elastic and resists lengthening.

The component responsible for passive or resting tensions is the PEC. The parallel elastic component lies parallel to the contractile mechanism, and is thought to consist of the sarcolemma, sarcoplasm, and elastic fibers of the epimysium, perimysium, and endomysium. However, it is possible that the PEC is made up of two other structures: the contractile components themselves and a hypothetical structure called the *S-filament*, whose existence is still open to question. The S-filament is a possible connection between the ends of the secondary myofilaments across the H-zone. Such a connection has been described by Huxley and Hanson (1954).

The volume of muscle fiber remains constant even when muscle is stretched. The cross-sectional area of a muscle, however, must decrease as well as the side spacing between the actin and myosin myofilaments as they move closer to each other. However, because a mutual electrostatic repulsive force exists between the myofilaments, work must be done to move them closer together; that is, some force must exist that maintains the myofilaments in a regular array. That force necessary to move the myofilaments closer against the electrostatic repulsion will appear as the resting tension or the "parallel" resistance to stretch (Davson, 1970; Huxley, 1967).

At lengths less than equilibrium length (.90 Rl) there is no resting tension and the PEC is slack. However, when an unstimulated muscle is stretched, it develops tension in a nonlinear fashion. That is, little tension is developed with initial stretch, and increasingly more tension is developed as stretch continues. As was stated earlier, the same effect can be seen when a knitted stocking is stretched (Carlson & Wilkie, 1974).

The Series Elastic Component (SEC)

The *series elastic component* (SEC) is so named because the elastic components occur directly in line with the contractile components. The SEC has the important function of smoothing out rapid changes in muscle tension. The anatomic counterparts making up the SEC are thought to consist of tendon and/or the Z-line. When muscle is stretched, the CC, PEC, and SEC all contribute to the development of tension.

The Contractile Component (CC)

The muscle's ability to increase tension is called the *contractile component*. The CC of muscle may be regarded as a tension generator. It consists of the myofilaments and their cross-bridges. If tension is proportional to the number of chemical links established between the two myofilaments, then the greater the overlap the greater the tension developed, and vice versa. Maximal contractile tension is assumed to be developed when sarcomere lengths are such that maximal single overlap of actin and myosin myofilaments exists. At greater length, the number of cross-links diminishes as overlap decreases, resulting in reduced tension. As the

stretch continues, the tension developed becomes smaller until, finally, the tension developed during the stretch is no greater than that in a passive muscle. This can be explained by the fact that at such lengths, actin and myosin myofilaments no longer interdigitate. Thus they can develop little or no tension (see Figure 4.1).

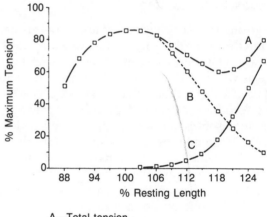

A—Total tension
B—Tension due to active contraction
C—Passive tension due to stretch

Figure 4.1. Length-tension diagram of the total and passive tension. Length-tension diagram for passive stretch of an unstimulated muscle is shown in lower Curve C. Curve A, showing total isometric tension when the muscle was stimulated at various lengths from maximal stretch through moderate shortening, represents the summation of active contraction plus tension due to the stretch. Active tension due solely to muscular contraction is obtained by subtracting passive tension, C, from total tension, A, and is represented by Curve B. Normal resting length is 100%. *Note.* From ''Effect of Stimulation-Length Sequence on Shape of Length-Tension Diagram'' by B.A. Schottelius and L.C. Senay, 1956, *American Journal of Physiology,* **186,** p. 128. Copyright 1956 by the American Physiological Society. Adapted by permission.

Total Tension of Active Muscle During Stretch

Total tension during contraction represents the sum of the PEC and the developed tension of the CC. Thus:

TOTAL ACTIVE TENSION = PEC + CC

In general, the maximum total active tension is found at about 1.2 to 1.3 times the muscle's original or rest length. At greater lengths, total active tension diminishes until the muscle is at about 1.5 times the muscle's rest length. This is because at lengths beyond 1.3 Lo, the number of cross-links diminishes as overlap decreases, resulting in reduced tensions. Furthermore, although the PEC is increasing in its output, its total does not match the corresponding decline in the contractile components. Consequently, total active tension decreases.

The Force-Length Relationship

The length of a tissue depends on the relation of the internal force developed by the tissue to the external force exerted by the resistance or load. If the internal force exceeds the external force, the tissue shortens. Conversely, if the external force exceeds the internal force, the tissue lengthens.

Stress-Relaxation and Creep During Passive Tension

Living tissues are characterized by the presence of time-dependent mechanical properties. These properties include creep and stress-relaxation. When a resting muscle is suddenly stretched and held at a constant length, after a period of time there is a slow loss of tension. This is called *stress-relaxation* (see Figure 4.2). In contrast, the lengthening which occurs when a constant force or load is applied is called *creep* (Mathews, Stacy, & Hoover, 1964).

Stretches Applied During Contraction at and Beyond 1.5 *Lo*

When tissues are stretched, they develop tension. This tension is known as the *stretch response*, which is independent of the central nervous system (CNS) and is a property of the tissues stretched. On the other hand, the *stretch reflex* is a response mediated by the CNS that causes the stretched muscle to contract (Gowitzke & Milner, 1980).

One of the major arguments against the use of ballistic stretching (i.e., bobbing or bouncing) is that it initiates a stretch reflex. However, if one were to initiate such stretching beyond the length of 1.5 *Lo*, the stretch reflex should not result in any increase of tension in the CC because the myofilaments are no longer capable at such lengths of interdigitating and developing tension. This reasoning would be true *if* all sarcomeres in the muscle fiber stretched to the same extent.

However, not all sarcomeres stretch to the same extent. That is, when a muscle is stretched, the stretch is not uniform along its entire length. Sarcomeres near tendons stretch to a much lesser extent than sarcomeres in the middle of a muscle. Hence sarcomeres at the end of the muscle may still have considerable overlap while those in the middle are stretched beyond the point of overlap (Davson, 1970). Therefore, the sarcomeres near tendons can still develop tension and influence the degree of extension. Furthermore, it seems reasonable to argue that the resistance to continued movement arises either from the reattachment of cross-bridges previously broken, or from the attachment of additional cross-bridges to sites on the actin myofilament that are not available initially, but which become accessible as a result of the movement (Flintney & Hirst, 1978). Thus activation of the stretch reflex, even when the muscle fiber is beyond 1.5 *Lo*, will probably result in some additional tension being produced by the CC.

Research Findings

With a basic knowledge of the biophysics of connective tissues and muscles, we are now ready to examine the research findings. When a tensile force is applied to connective tissue or muscle, the original length increases and its cross-section (i.e., width) decreases. Are there different types of

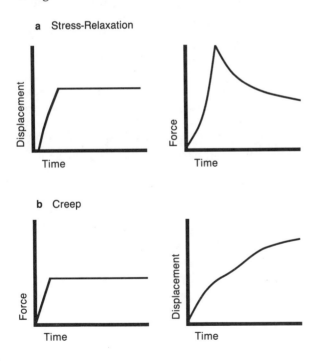

Figure 4.2. Response of tissues to applied force. a. Stress-relaxation results when there is a reduction in force that occurs when a tissue is held at a constant length. b. Creep is the lengthening that occurs over a period of time when a constant force is applied.

forces, then, and/or conditions under which a force can be applied, that will create an optimal change in connective tissue and muscle? Sapega, Quedenfeld, Moyer, and Butler (1981) addressed these questions in an article titled "Biophysical Factors in Range-of-Motion Exercise" that appeared in *The Physician and Sportsmedicine*. Since Sapega et al. have already written a clear and succinct analysis, it would be presumptuous to do other than quote directly from their excellent paper.

When tensile forces are continously applied to an organized connective tissue model (tendon), the time required to stretch the tissue a specific amount varies inversely with the forces used (Warren, Lehmann, & Koblanski, 1971 & 1976). Therefore, a low-force stretching method requires more time to produce the same amount of elongation as a higher-force method. However, the proportion of tissue lengthening that remains after tensile stress is removed is greater for the low-force, long-duration method (Warren et al. 1971 & 1976; LaBan, 1962). Higher-force, short-duration stretching favors recoverable, elastic tissue deformation, whereas low-force, long-duration stretching enhances permanent, plastic deformation (Warren et al. 1971 & 1976; LaBan, 1962). This principle does not necessarily rule out combining higher forces with a prolonged duration of stretch, but in the clinical setting, high-force application has a greater risk of causing pain and possibly tissue rupture. In addition, laboratory studies have shown that when connective tissue structures are permanently elongated, some degree of mechanical weakening takes place, even though outright rupture has not occurred (Warren et al. 1971 & 1976; Rigby, Hirai, Spikes, & Eyring, 1959). The amount of weakening depends on the way the tissue is stretched as well as how much it is stretched. Of particular interest is that for the same amount of tissue elongation, a high-force stretching method produces more structural weakening than a slower, low-force method (Warren et al. 1971 & 1976).

Temperature has a significant influence on the mechanical behavior of connective tissue under tensile stress. As tissue temperature rises, stiffness decreases and extensibility increases (LaBan, 1962; Rigby, 1964). Raising the temperature of tendon samples above 103 F increases the amount of permanent elongation that results from a given amount of initial stretching (LaBan, 1962; Lehmann, Masock, Warren, & Koblanski, 1970). At about 104 F a thermal transition in the microstructure of collagen occurs, which significantly enhances the viscous stress relaxation of collagenous tissue, allowing greater plastic deformation when it is stretched (Mason & Rigby, 1963; Rigby, 1964; Rigby et al. 1959). The mechanism behind this thermal transition is still uncertain, but it is thought that intermolecular bonding becomes partially destabilized, enhancing the viscous flow properties of the collagenous tissue (Rigby, 1964; Rigby et al. 1959).

When connective tissue is stretched at an elevated temperature, the conditions under which the tissue is allowed to cool can significantly affect the amount of elongation that remains after the tensile stress is removed. After the heated tissue has been stretched, maintaining tensile force during tissue cooling has been shown to significantly increase the relative proportion of plastic deformation compared with unloading the tissue while its temperature is still elevated (Lehmann et al. 1970). Cooling the tissue before releasing the tension apparently allows the collagenous microstructure to restabilize more toward its new stretched length (Lehmann et al. 1970).

When stretching connective tissue at temperatures within the usual therapeutic range (102° to 110 °F), the amount of structural weakening produced by a given amount of tissue elongation varies inversely with the temperature (Warren et al. 1971 & 1976). This is apparently related to the progressive increase in the viscous flow properties of the collagen as it is heated. It is possible that thermal destabilization of intermolecular bonding allows elongation to occur with less structural damage.

The factors influencing the viscoelastic behavior of connective tissue can be summarized by stating that elastic or recoverable deformation is most favored by high-force, short-duration stretching at normal or colder tissue temperature, whereas plastic or permanent lengthening is most favored by lower-force, longer-duration stretching at elevated temperatures, but allowing the tissue to cool before releasing the tension. In addition, the structural weakening produced by permanent tissue deformation is minimized when prolonged, low-force application is combined with high therapeutic temperatures, and it is maximal when higher forces and lower temperatures are used. (p. 59-61)[1]

Tables 4.1, 4.2, and 4.3 summarize these factors.

Table 4.1 Summary of Factors That Influence the Proportion of Plastic and Elastic Stretch

Elastic stretch vs plastic stretch

Influential factors:
1. Amount of applied force
2. Duration of applied force
3. Tissue temperature

Table 4.2 Summary of Factors That Influence the Viscoelastic Behavior of Connective Tissue

Elastic deformation	Viscous (plastic) deformation
High-force short-duration stretching	Low-force long-duration stretching
Normal or colder tissue temperatures	Elevated temperatures with cooling before release of tension

Table 4.3 Summary of Factors That Influence Tissue Weakening Due to Deformation

Minimal structural weakening	Maximal structural weakening
Lower forces	Higher forces
Higher temperatures	Lower temperatures

From ''Biophysical Factors in Range-of-Motion Exercise'' by A.A. Sapega, T.C. Quedenfeld, R.A. Moyer, and R.A. Butler, 1981, *The Physician and Sportsmedicine*, **9**(12), pp. 59-60. Copyright 1981. Reprinted by permission of *The Physician and Sportsmedicine*, a McGraw-Hill Publication.

---

[1]From ''Biophysical Factors of Range-of-Motion Exercise'' by A.A. Sapega, T.C. Quedenfeld, R.A. Moyer, and R.A. Butler (1981), *The Physician and Sportsmedicine*, **9**(12), pp. 57-65. Copyright 1981 by McGraw-Hill. Reprinted by permission.

Research by others (Becker, 1979; Glazer, 1980; Jackman, 1963; Kottke, Pauley, & Ptak, 1966; Light, Nuzik, Personius, & Barstrom, 1984) has also demonstrated that stretching at low to moderate tension levels is effective. However, other than the clinical successes of Sapega et al. (1981), no additional studies have been reported that combine tissue temperature manipulation and therapeutic stretching.

One of the most interesting aspects of research is that it raises more questions than it answers, for we are still in the dark about many aspects of flexibility and stretching. We remain uncertain, for instance, about the exact mechanism by which tissues actually develop elasticity. We still do not fully understand what structural or chemical changes occur in tissues as a result of stretching. It is far too early to promise any panacea for those who desire to increase their flexibility in a short period of time. The exciting possibility of applying new and powerful techniques may lie in the future, but such techniques will need to be investigated vigorously at the clinical as well as the experimental level. In the meantime, there are no shortcuts for diligent and hard practice.

An Analysis of the Factors Affecting the Mechanical Properties of Connective Tissues and Muscles

The behavior of connective tissues (collagenous or elastic) and muscle under stress is influenced by a number of related factors. Among these are:

1. The alignment or orientation of the fibers
2. The influence of different interweaving patterns of fibers within specific tissues
3. The influence of different interweaving patterns of collagen molecules within each fibril
4. The presence of interfibrillar substances
5. The number of fibers and fibrils
6. The cross-sectional area of the fibers
7. The proportion of collagen and elastin
8. The chemical composition of the tissues
9. The degree of hydration
10. The degree of relaxation of the contractile components
11. The tissue temperature before and during the applied force
12. The amount of applied force (load)
13. The duration of the applied force (time)

14. The type of applied force (ballistic vs. static)
15. The tissue temperature before releasing the applied force

Summary

All tissues undergo predictable changes when force is applied. The elastic limit is the smallest value of stress required to produce a permanent set or sprain. Until this point is reached, tissues will return to their original nonstretched length. Consequently, with a sprained ankle, the tissues have been so overstretched that they do not return to their original length. If stretch continues, tissues ultimately rupture.

Muscle is composed of three mechanical components: (a) parallel elastic component (PEC), (b) series elastic component (SEC), and (c) contractile component (CC). Mechanical components are important because they resist stress. In combination, these three components will ultimately determine to a major extent the quality and quantity of range of motion.

Research has demonstrated that elastic or recoverable elongation is most favored by high-force, short-duration stretching at normal or colder than normal tissue temperatures. Plastic or permanent lengthening is most favored by low-force, long-duration stretching at elevated temperatures, if the tissue is allowed to cool before releasing the tension. In addition, minimal structural weakening is associated with low-force stretching combined with high-therapeutic temperatures, whereas maximal structural weakening is associated with higher forces and lower temperatures.

Review Questions

1. Define the terms: *deformation, elasticity, stress, strain, elastic limit, sprain,* and *ultimate strength.*
2. Explain the statement, ''Elasticity is more important than flexibility.''
3. Which is more desirable when working to improve flexibility: stress-relaxation or creep? Explain your response.
4. Explain the advantages of static stretching.
5. Identify three factors that will determine whether or not an elongation is recoverable.
6. Cite a case where it would be appropriate to use a stretching procedure that produces maximal structural weakening.
7. Make a list of ten factors that influence the behavior of connective tissues and muscle under stress.
8. Explain the statement, ''One cannot sprain a muscle.''

Answers

1. *Deformation*: a change in the shape or size of a body; changes in dimensions.
   Elasticity: the property of a material that enables it to return to its original shape or size when the load to which it has been subjected is removed; resistance to distortion.
   Stress: the internal resistance to an external force.
   Strain: the ratio of the change in length that is caused by application of a stress to the original length of the object.
   Elastic limit: the smallest value of stress required to produce permanent strain in the body.
   Sprain: the difference between the original length and the new length.
   Ultimate strength: the unit stress that occurs just at or before rupture.

2. Elasticity is more important than flexibility because the latter deals only with the range of motion that is permitted, while the former relates to the ability of the material to return to its original length.

3. Both are important for the development of flexibility. First, stress-relaxation results in a decrease in muscle spindle activity thereby reducing active tension and allowing further stretch to be employed. However, creep is the ultimate goal when the static stretch procedure is used, because the result is the actual lengthening of tissues.

4. Static stretching is advantageous because (a) it reduces the chance of muscle soreness, (b) it reduces the chance of initiating the stretch reflex via the muscle spindles, and (c) it allows for stress-relaxation and creep to take place.

5. The three factors are: the degree of force, the duration of the force, and the temperature of the tissues during the application of the force.

6. Such a case would be where there is the presence of excessive adhesions and cross-linkages.

7. See page 39: An Analysis of the Factors Affecting the Mechanical Properties of Connective Tissues and Muscles.

8. The term *sprain* refers to ligamentous or inert tissues; *strains* involve contractile tissue or muscle.

Recommended Readings

Ciullo, J. V., & Zarins, B. (1983). Biomechanics of the musculotendinous unit: Relation to athletic performance and injury. In B. Zarins (Ed.), *Clinics in sports medicine:* Vol. 2(1), (pp. 70-85). Philadelphia: W. B. Saunders.

Frankel, V. H., & Hang, Y. S. (1975). Recent advances in the biomechanics of sport injuries. *Acta Orthopaedica Scandinavica, 46*(3), 484-497.

Parker, H. (1977). *Simplified mechanics and strengths of materials.* New York: John Wiley & Sons.

Stanish, W. D. (1984). Overuse injuries in athletes: A perspective. *Medicine and Science in Sports and Exercise, 16*(1), 1-7.

Zarins, B. (1982). Soft tissue injury and repair-biomechanical aspects. *International Journal of Sports Medicine, 3*(Suppl. 1), 9-11.

CHAPTER 5

The Neurophysiology of Flexibility: Neural Anatomy and Neural Transmission

The structural and functional unit of the nervous system is the *neuron*. Knowledge of how the neuron functions is basic to the understanding of the nervous system. Neurons, like all of the body's cells, are structurally designed in ways that are appropriate to their primary function, which is receiving and transmitting electric impulses.

For a nervous system response to occur three things are necessary. First, there must be a means of detecting a stimulus, or a change in the environment (such as stretching). Structures called *receptors* perform this function. Second, the stimulus, after it is received, must be transmitted. This is accomplished by the nervous system's conductors—the *neurons*. Finally, responding organs must carry out the appropriate responses to the stimulus. This function is accomplished by the *effectors*.

In the structural make-up of neurons, we find three distinct parts: the cell body, one or more dendrites, and a single axon (see Figure 5.1). The cell body, or soma, contains a nucleus and protoplasm. Protoplasm is all the living substance within a cell. The nucleus is responsible for controlling the various processes of the cell. .

The *dendrite* is one type of nerve fiber extending from the cell body. The term *dendrite* comes from the Greek word *dendron*, meaning tree. Its function is to receive and convey impulses toward the cell body, and is thus known as the *afferent process*.

The long part of a neuron leading away from the cell body is the *axon*, and most axons conduct impulses away from the cell body. They can, however, transmit impulses in either direction. Axons are known as the *efferent system*.

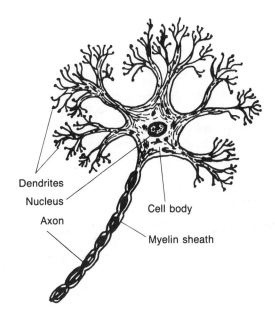

Figure 5.1. Basic components of a motor neuron.

Nerves

Bundles of neuron fibers are called *nerves*. These bundles are bound together by connective tissue sheaths, called myelin sheaths, which provide strength and protection for the neuron. Nearly all nerves are mixed nerves (i.e., they contain both afferent and efferent fibers). Afferent fibers conduct impulses toward the central nervous system (CNS). In contrast, efferent fibers conduct impulses away from the CNS and toward the muscles and glands.

Resting Potential

Neurons are *polarized*. That is, they have an unequal number of different types of ions outside and inside the membrane. An *ion* is an atom which has gained or lost one or more of its electrons and moves through a fluid in response to an electric field.

When a neuron is at rest, there are more sodium ions (Na^+) on the outside of the membrane than there are on the inside, and more potassium ions (K^+) on the inside of the membrane than there are on the outside. The large sodium ions cannot pass inward through the semipermeable membrane in a resting state. Sodium ions can, however, be transported outward through the membrane by an active transport mechanism called the *sodium pump*. A continuous expenditure of energy is necessary to maintain the resting membrane potential in this way. Potassium ions can pass through the membrane by passive transport. Therefore, some of them diffuse out of the cell.

The differences in ionic concentrations are basic to the establishment of a potential difference across the cell membrane, a *membrane potential*. In resting cells, the outside is positively charged, and the inside is negatively charged. However, the membrane is not at zero. Instead, it registers a fraction of a volt. Therefore, the neuron can be considered analogous to a battery, with its negative terminal on the inside.

When an axon is stimulated, changes occur. A stimulus alters the permeability of the nerve membrane. The exact nature of this increased permeability is unknown. With stimulation, the membrane becomes permeable to sodium ions (Na^+). As a result, sodium ions diffuse quickly into the nerve fiber. This inward movement of sodium ions causes a reversal of the membrane's resting potential. That is, the outside of the nerve fiber becomes negative in relation to the inside. Consequently, the nerve's polarity is reversed. The nerve fiber *depolarizes*. When depolarization reaches a critical level, an *action potential* is generated. Thus action potential and depolarization are related, but are not synonymous. Depolarization is the flow of ions across the membrane that pulls the impulse along the fiber. Action potential is the term given to the electrical impulses carried along the nerve fiber.

Depolarization takes place along the entire length of the nerve fiber. At the peak of depolarization, entry of sodium ions into the cell slows down, and the membrane becomes impermeable to sodium.

At this time, another cell membrane permeability change occurs. After a brief interval, the membrane becomes highly permeable to potassium (K^+). The potassium is able to diffuse with great ease because of the high concentration on the inside. Consequently, potassium ions begin to leave the cell carrying positive charges with them. The outflow of the potassium ions restores the original negative charge of the interior of the membrane. Thus the membrane voltage returns to normal. This brings the action potential to an end. This process is called *repolarization*.

In order for the membrane to return to its original resting potential, the sodium ions must be returned to the outside and the potassium ions must be returned to the inside of the membrane. The sodium pump is the active transport mechanism that returns them to the outside of the membrane. The resulting electronegativity inside the membrane then pulls the potassium ions back to the inside. Thus the original potential of the membrane is restored (see Figure 5.2).

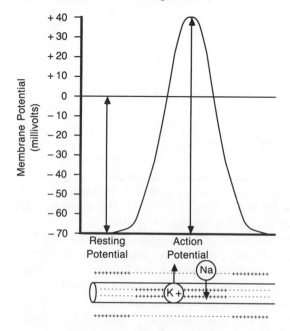

Figure 5.2. The action potential. Ionic movements across the nerve fiber membrane (below) coincide with changes in electric potential (above). As sodium ions must rush into the axon the membrane potential becomes positively charged. Movement of potassium ions to the outside of the fiber follows. At the point of the action potential, the potential across the membrane is reversed about +40 millivolts.

The All-or-None Law

If the stimulus (e.g., stretch) is strong enough to initiate a nerve impulse in the axon, it causes the entire fiber to fire. This is known as the *All-or-None Law*, which can be compared to the process of shooting a gun. As soon as a pull on the trigger is strong enough to drop the firing pin, the gun fires. This is called the *threshold phase*. A harder pull on the trigger will not change the velocity of the bullet, because it is the powder charge in the bullet, and not the pull on the trigger, that causes the response (Sage, 1971). Therefore, either a stimulus is strong enough to stimulate the fiber or it is not. Stronger stimulations do *not* result in larger action potentials.

CNS Feedback on Intensity of Stretching

How, then, does the nerve differentiate between various intensities of stretching? The nerve has two means by which it can transmit information on stretching of different intensities: First, it can transmit stretching sensation simultaneously over varying numbers of nerve fibers. Therefore, a greater intensity of stretching sensation can bring more nerve fibers into action. This is called *spatial summation*. Consequently, intensity of stretch can be increased by increasing the recruitment of receptor organs. For example, a weak stretching stimulus activates only those stretch receptors with the lowest thresholds. However, as intensity is increased, a greater number of less irritable stretch receptors are also activated, thereby involving more sensory units.

Second, the nerve can transmit different numbers of stretch impulses per unit of time over the same fiber. Thus changes in intensity of stretch may be reflected in different frequencies of firing (i.e., rate of discharge) of nerve impulses in single fibers: The more intense the stretch stimuli, the greater the frequency of the stretch impulse. This is called *temporal summation*.

In summary, the stronger the stretching stimulus, the greater the number of active sensory neurons, and the greater the impulse frequency in each. Consequently, the bombardment of the cortical centers of the brain will be more intense, and the sensation will be stronger.

Sensory Adaptation

If a stimulus is applied to a sensory receptor and maintained at a steady strength, the receptor usually responds with an initially high rate of discharge. The generator potential is at first proportional to the stimulus intensity. With time, however, the rate of discharge grows progressively slower until a plateau rate of discharge is struck and maintained. Thus the generator potential declines gradually during the steady stimulation. This phenomenon is known as *adaptation*. If, however, the stimulus is even momentarily stopped and then reapplied, an initial burst of impulse activity will reoccur and the process will be repeated.

Stretch receptors can be categorized as either fast or slow adapting. *Fast-adapting* units show a more rapidly decreasing rate of discharge with maintained stretch. In addition, a faster fall is found with generator potentials in the fast-adapting units. Conversely, *slow-adapting* units display a continued rate of discharge with sustained stimulation. Slow-adapting receptors display long-maintained generator potentials. The terms *phasic* and *tonic* are interchangeably used for fast- and slow-adapting receptors respectively (see Figure 5.3).

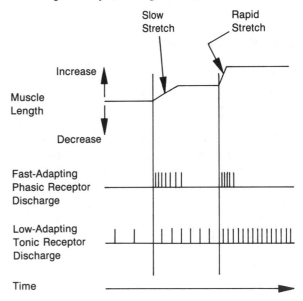

Figure 5.3. Phasic and Tonic receptor discharges. Fast-adapting or Phasic receptors are characterized by a more rapidly decreasing rate of discharge with maintained stretch. Hence, their frequency of discharge is proportional to the rate of change. In contrast, slow-adapting or Tonic receptors display a continued rate of discharge with sustained stimulation.

Research has demonstrated that fast-adapting receptors such as the pacinian corpuscles (which are joint receptors) have mechanical high-pass filters. These filters are thought to be composed of both viscous and elastic components. When a force is delivered to the viscous components of a sufficiently rapid time course, it is then transmitted directly to the central core. The time course of this dynamic component parallels that of the receptor potential of the intact corpuscle. This declines rapidly regardless of the duration of the applied stimulus. The force stored in the stretched elastic components is then transmitted with a marked reduction to the central core. As a result, no steady generator potential results.

In contrast, slow-adapting receptors, such as muscle spindles, have no mechanical high-pass filter at the nerve endings. Consequently, steady generator potentials are produced by steady stretch. The degree of adaptation that does occur from the initial high-frequency discharge to the following steady state (the newly adapted state of discharge) is thought to be due to the presence of viscous components in series within the spindle itself (Mountcastle, 1974). This possibility will be discussed later.

Muscle Spindles

The primary stretch receptors in muscle are the muscle spindles. They are located in varying numbers in most skeletal muscles of the body. Muscle spindles are particularly numerous in the small, delicate muscles of the hand. Because muscle spindles are encased in a fusiform, connective tissue capsule, they are referred to as intrafusal fibers, in contrast to the extrafusal fibers, which are the regular contractile units of the muscle. The spindles attach at both ends to the extrafusal fibers and are therefore parallel to those fibers.

There are two types of intrafusal fibers: the nuclear bag fiber and the nuclear chain fiber. The former contains an abundance of sarcoplasm and cell nuclei in a dilated, or swollen, bag-like structure. This noncontractile structure is located in the center, or equatorial, region of the intrafusal fiber. Hence its name *nuclear bag intrafusal fiber*. At the distal, or polar, end of the nuclear bag fiber are striated contractile myofilaments, where the spindles attach to the extrafusal fibers. In recent years it has been speculated that there are really two types of nuclear bag fiber (termed BAG_1 and BAG_2).

The second type of intrafusal fiber is the nuclear chain intrafusal fiber, which is thinner and shorter than the nuclear bag. Furthermore, it contains only a single row of nuclei through the noncontractile equatorial region, which are spread out in a chain-like structure. The polar ends of the nuclear chain fiber are also composed of striated contractile myofilaments. They often connect to the nuclear bag fibers, which in turn attach to the endomysium of extrafusal fibers.

There are two types of sensory (afferent) endings in each spindle. These are the primary, or annulospiral, endings and the secondary, or flower-spray,

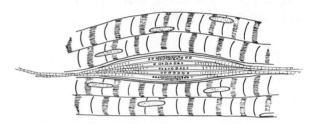

Figure 5.4. The neuromuscular spindle. A muscle spindle containing two nuclear bag intrafusal fibers and three nuclear chain fibers, shown as it lies parallel with the contractile (extrafusal) fibers of the muscle. Innervation is omitted. *Note.* From "Proprioceptive Reflexes and Their Participation in Motor Skills" by E.B. Gardner, 1969, *Quest,* **12,** p. 4. Copyright 1969 by *Quest* Board. Reprinted by permission.

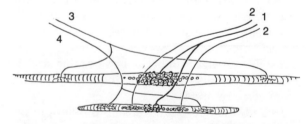

Figure 5.5. Innervation of intrafusal fibers. The upper drawing represents a nuclear bag intrafusal fiber and the lower drawing represents a nuclear chain fiber. The single large primary afferent neuron (1) ends in coiled terminals (annulospiral endings) on the nuclear region of each intrafusal fiber. In contrast, the smaller secondary afferents (2) have branched endings (flower-sprays) located on the outer part of the nuclear region and appear only on the chain intrafusals. Numbers (3) and (4) represent two types of gamma efferent (fusimotor) neurons. Note differences in the form and location of the various endings as distributed to the intrafusal fibers. *Note.* From "Proprioceptive Reflexes and Their Participation in Motor Skills" by E.B. Gardner, 1969, *Quest,* **12,** p. 5. Copyright 1969 by *Quest* Board. Reprinted by permission.

endings. The primary endings terminate as a spiral wrap around the central region of a nuclear bag fiber as a side branch to a nuclear chain fiber. Axons of primary afferents belong to the large Group I fibers, known as Ia (see Figures 5.4 and 5.5).

Primary endings have a very low threshold to stretch, and are thus easily excited. Their response may be either phasic or tonic. A phasic response measures the rate or velocity of the stretch by changing the impulse frequency during the stretch. Specifically, the frequency of discharge increases rapidly with the initial stretch. Then, when the stretching ceases, the frequency of discharge drops to a constant level appropriate to the new tonic length. Hence, a tonic response measures the length of a muscle. In other words, the primary endings measure length plus velocity of stretch.

Secondary endings form spirals or flower-spray-like endings. They are restricted almost entirely to the polar segment of the nuclear chain fiber. However, there is some disagreement among authorities regarding the completeness of the limitation of secondary endings to the chain intrafusal fibers (Gowitzke & Milner, 1980). Axons of the secondary afferents belong to the smaller Group II fiber. In contrast to the primary endings, secondary endings measure tonic length alone. Thus they measure *mainly length alone*.

The Process of Muscle Spindle Excitation

As a general rule, the process of excitation of a muscle spindle may be outlined as follows: First, a minimal stretching stimulus is applied to a muscle spindle. Second, there develops a change in the permeability of the sensory cell. This results in the production of a generator current—a transfer of charge across the nerve terminal membrane. In turn, this produces a depolarization called the generator potential. With a slightly greater degree of stretch, the muscle spindle evokes a generator potential of greater amplitude. When depolarization reaches threshold, a conducted action potential results. If the stretch is even stronger, this can lead to a train of conducted nerve impulses. The difference in the rates of adaptation to steadily applied stretch is thought to be due to the presence of viscous components in series within the spindle itself (Mountcastle, 1974). The steps in muscle spindle excitation could be summarized as follows:

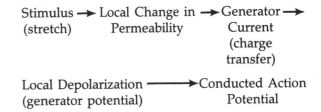

The Myotatic or Stretch Reflex

Whenever a muscle is stretched, the stretch reflex mechanism is initiated. Stretching a muscle lengthens both the muscle fibers (i.e., extrafusal fibers) and the muscle spindles (i.e., the intrafusal fibers). The consequent deformation within the muscle spindles results in the firing of the stretch reflex, which contracts the muscle. This stretch effect can be divided into two components: phasic and tonic.

The classic example of the phasic type of stretch reflex is the knee jerk or patellar reflex. For example, when the patellar tendon is given a light tap, the muscle spindles located in parallel with the muscle fibers are stretched, creating a deformation in the muscle spindles. As a result, the firing of the primary muscle spindle afferents is increased. The message is then sent to the spinal cord (via the dorsal root) and brain. Completing the reflex arc, the spinal cord sends an efferent impulse to the quadriceps and causes them to contract, thus shortening the muscle and taking the tension off the muscle spindles.

Another type of stretch reflex is the static, or tonic, stretch reflex. With this type of reflex the response to maintained stretch results in part from the effect of the secondary afferents. A common tonic response may be found in the postural reaction to stretch, exemplified by the contracting of the gastrocnemius (i.e., calf) to correct an excess shifting of one's center of gravity while standing.

Reciprocal Innervation

Muscles usually operate in pairs so that when one set of muscles, the *agonistic*, are contracting, the opposing *antagonistic* muscles are relaxing. This grouping of coordinated and opposing agonist and antagonist muscles is called *reciprocal innervation*. For example, when the arm is flexed at the elbow by action of the biceps contracting, the triceps muscle, which normally extends the arm at the elbow must relax. If not, the two muscles would be pulling against each other and no movement would occur.

In summary, when one muscle receives an impulse to contract, the other relaxes, because it does not receive an impulse to contract. It is therefore *inhibited* at the same instant that its antagonist contracts. Reflex inhibition is controlled by inhibitory discharge on the motor neurons innervating the antagonistic muscle of the reciprocal pair. If the opposite muscle were similarly stretched, the other muscle would show inhibition by the same process. Without this reciprocal innervation, coordinated muscular activity would be impossible.

The Golgi Tendon Organs

The sensory receptor that is responsible for detecting tension on a tendon is called the *Golgi tendon* *organ* (GTO). Its location is in the tendon near the ends of the muscle fiber. Because these organs lie directly in line with the transmission of force from muscle to the insertion on bone, they are said to be in series with the muscle, rather than in parallel as we found the spindle to be. Consequently, they are stimulated by both passive stretch and contraction of the muscle. Originally, the GTOs were thought to function only as high threshold stretch or tension receptors, but this has been disproven. The GTO is now known to be a tension receptor capable of monitoring all thresholds of muscle tension (Moore, 1984). However, GTOs are most sensitive to tension forces generated by muscle contraction. The GTOs function as *inhibitory* mechanisms. The GTOs, then, are an inhibitory afferent system, whereas the muscle spindle afferents are *excitatory* (see Figure 5.6).

A. Muscle in relaxed state

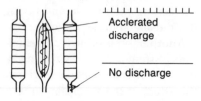

B. Muscle with mild passive stretch

C. Muscle under extensive passive stretch

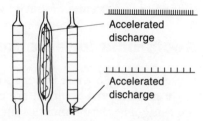

D. Muscle actively contracted

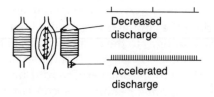

E. Muscle actively contracted, with intrafusal muscle fiber "reset" by contraction at its polar ends, stretching its equatorial region

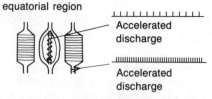

	Relative tension on	
	TO Receptors	AS Receptors
A.	O	+
B.	+ +	+ +
C.	+ + +	+ + +
D.	+ + +	+
E.	+ + +	+ +

Figure 5.6. Simplified scheme of possible variations in afferent discharge from Golgi tendon organs (TO) and from muscle spindle primary or annulospiral receptors (AS) under various conditions of extrafusal relaxation, stretch, and contraction. Both TO and AS receptors are sensitive to passive stretching, although TO receptors have a higher threshold (A, B, and C). The TO receptors respond indiscriminately to extensive stretch (C) and to active extrafusal contraction (D and E). Active contraction relieves the tension on AS receptors (D), unless gamma efferent activity "resets" the tension within the intrafusal fiber (E). Intrafusal secondary or flower-spray receptors have been omitted here, although in actuality they add still another variable factor to the array of afferent information. *Note.* From *Kinesiology and Applied Anatomy* by P.J. Rasch and R.K. Burke, 1978, Philadelphia: Lea and Febiger. Copyright 1978 by Lea and Febiger. Reprinted by permission.

The GTOs operate in the following manner: When the muscle fibers contract, tension is produced. In turn, this tension pulls on the tendon. If the tension is strong enough, it will activate the GTOs. Then an impulse is transmitted to the spinal cord to inhibit nerve transmission in the anterior motor neurons. GTOs have a much higher threshold than muscle spindle receptors. Therefore, ordinarily regular or moderate degrees of tension on the tendon do not stimulate the Golgi receptors. In contrast to contraction, the degree of stimulation by passive stretch is not great because the more elastic muscle fibers take up much of the stretch. That is why it takes a strong stretch to elicit an inhibitory impulse.

The Inverse Myotatic Reflex or the Autogenic Inhibition

If, however, the intensity of the contraction or stretch on the tendon exceeds a certain critical point, an immediate reflex occurs to inhibit the anterior motor neurons that innervate the muscle. As a result, the muscle immediately relaxes, and the excessive tension is removed. This reaction is possible only because the impulse of the GTOs is powerful enough to override the excitatory impulses from the muscle spindles. This relaxation response to a strong stretch is called an *inverse myotatic reflex* or *autogenic inhibition,* and is a protective mechanism—a safety device to prevent injury to tendons and muscles. It prevents muscles and/or tendons from tearing away from their attachments. This may explain an interesting phenomenon that occurs when one is attempting to maintain a stretching position that develops maximal tension: that is, a point is suddenly reached where the tension dissipates and the muscle can be stretched even further.

Another function—the "clasped-knife" reflex—was once believed to be one of the primary actions of the GTO. But this reflex—the sudden "giving away" response of a passively stretched group—is now believed to be the result of afferent input from Group II fibers coming from the muscle spindles and perhaps thinly mylinated C fibers subserving pain (Moore, 1984).

Summary

The structural and functional unit of the nervous system is the neuron. Bundles of neuron fibers are called nerves. They conduct impulses both away and to the CNS, muscles, and glands. According to the All-or-None Law, a stimulus is either strong enough to stimulate a firing or it is not. Stronger stimulations (or stretches) do not result in more powerful firings. However, there are two methods by which stretching intensity can be differentiated. With spatial summation, the stronger the stretching stimulus, the greater will be the number of fibers brought into action. With temporal stimulation the stronger the stretching stimulus, the greater the number of impulses per unit of time are fired.

When a stretch is initially applied, the receptors usually respond with a high rate of discharge. However, if this stimulus is maintained, the rate of discharge grows progressively weaker until a plateau rate of discharge is reached. This phenomenon is called adaptation. Fast-adapting units are characterized by a rapidly decreasing rate of discharge with maintained stretch. Conversely, slow-adapting units display a continued rate of discharge with sustained stimulation.

The primary stretch receptor in muscle is the muscle spindle. It is composed of two types of sensory receptors. The primary endings are sensitive to length plus velocity of the stretch. In contrast, the secondary endings are sensitive to the change in length. Thus with initial stretch, both endings fire. However, when the stretch is held, the secondary endings mainly fire. When muscle spindles fire, they initiate a stretch reflex. This causes the stretched muscle to contract and take tension off the muscle spindles. As a result, the muscle spindles slow down their rate of discharge and the muscle relaxes once again.

The Golgi tendon organ (GTO) is the sensory receptor which is responsible for detecting tension on a tendon. Golgi tendon organs fire when excessive tension (either by contraction or elongation) is placed on the tendon. When this happens, an inhibitory impulse is sent to the muscle causing it to relax, and thereby remove the excessive tension. This is known as the inverse myotatic reflex or autogenic inhibition.

Review Questions

1. Diagram and label and organizational structure of a neuron.

2. Explain why the All-or-None Law is not analogous to the shooting of an arrow.

3. Draw a diagram illustrating the concept of spatial and temporal summation.

4. Explain to a group of young athletes why ballistic stretching is less desirable than static stretching from a neurophysiological viewpoint.

5. Explain why it might be appropriate to contract the quadriceps while stretching the hamstrings.

6. Explain how the Golgi tendon organs and muscle spindles operate when performing a bench press with a maximal weight.

7. Explain why contracting a muscle in a stretched position might actually enhance the development of flexibility.

8. Explain to a group of young pitchers how a wind-up facilitates throwing a ball from a neurophysiological viewpoint.

Answers

1. See Figure 5.1. The following structures of a neuron should be identified: (a) the cell body, (b) the nucleus, (c) the dendrite, and (d) the axon.

2. The farther a bow is pulled back, the greater is the potential force behind the arrow. In the All-or-None Law, however, stronger stimulations do not result in larger action potentials.

3. See Figure 5.5.

4. Ballistic stretching is less desirable because it initiates both the primary and secondary endings, and because it does not permit adequate time for adaptation.

5. Contracting the quadriceps might be appropriate because reciprocal innervation will induce relaxation of the hamstrings.

6. When the bar is at its lowest point the tension on the triceps will be maximal, thereby initiating the stretch reflex. This will result in a stronger contraction of the triceps. However, if the weight is too great, the Golgi tendons will fire and inhibit the triceps. Under such situations, a spotter will need to assist in lifting the bar off the lifter's chest.

7. The Golgi tendons might fire initiating autogenic inhibition. Thus the contracting muscle will actually relax.

8. A wind-up stretches numerous muscles that are involved in the throwing process. As a consequence, the muscle spindles in these muscles will fire and the result is a stronger contraction.

Recommended Readings

Baker, P.F. (1966). The nerve axon. *Scientific American*, **214**(3), 74-82.

Eccles, J. (1965). The synapse. *Scientific American*, **212**(1), 56-66.

Gowitzke, B.A., & Milner, M. (1980). *Understanding the scientific basis of human movement* (2nd ed.). Baltimore: Williams and Wilkins.

Granit, R. (1970). *The basis of motor control*. New York: Academic Press.

Guyton, A.C. (1981). *Basic human neurophysiology* (3rd ed.). Philadelphia: W. B. Saunders.

Shephard, R.J. (1982). *Physiology and biochemistry of exercise*. Praeger Publishers.

Stanish, W.D. (1981). Neurophysiology of stretching. In R. D'Ambrosia & D. Drez (Eds.), *Prevention and treatment of running injuries* (pp. 135-145). Thorfare, NJ: Charles B. Slack.

Williams, P.L., & Warwick, R. (1980). *Gray's Anatomy* (36th British ed.). Philadelphia: W. B. Saunders.

Osteology and Arthrology

Ultimately, range of movement at a joint is restricted by both bone and joint structure. Consequently, some knowledge in the disciplines of *osteology*, the study of bones and *arthrology*, the classification of the major joints and the movement potential of each joint, would appear prudent. However, it should be noted that conventional stretching procedures will generally not be effective in cases where loss of motion is due to abnormal bone and joint structure.

Structural Limitations and Joint Range of Motion

Just as the railroad or subway track determines the route available to the train, so the shape and contour of the joint surfaces ultimately determine the movement pathways available to bones (Steindler, 1977). Obviously, too, these pathways are further influenced by cartilage, ligaments, tendons, and other connective tissues that frequently serve as restraining factors. However, here we will limit our discussion only to the structure of joints.

Classification of Joints and Their Influence on Motion

The junction of two or more bones is an *articulation*, but is commonly known as a *joint*. Joints may be classified in two ways: according to the amount of movement of which they are capable, and according to their structural composition. The simpler form of classification is based on the amount of gross movement that is available at the joint. There are three such classifications of joints:

1. *synarthroses*, or immovable joints,
2. *amphiarthroses*, or slightly movable joints, and
3. *diarthroses*, or freely movable joints.

There are six different classifications of joints according to structural composition (see Figure 6.1a-f).

Plane or gliding joints: As the name implies, this type of joint permits gliding movements only. The vertebrae of the spine are good examples. With this type of joint, the articular surfaces are nearly flat, or one may be slightly convex and the other slightly concave.

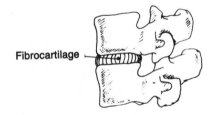

Figure 6.1a. Plane joint.

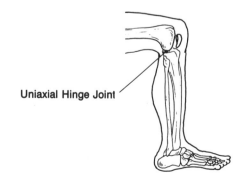

Figure 6.1b. Hinge joint.

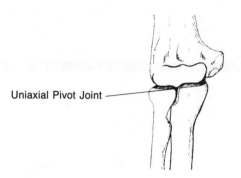

Figure 6.1c. Pivot joint.

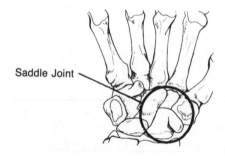

Figure 6.1d. Condyloid joint.

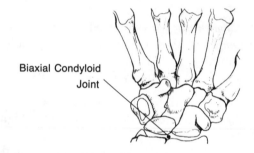

Figure 6.1e. Saddle joint.

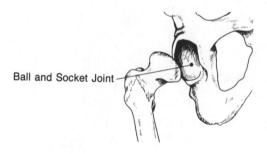

Figure 6.1f. Ball and socket joint.

Hinge joints: This type of joint allows angular movement in only one direction. This movement is similar to a door on a hinge, hence the origin of its name. Examples of hinge joints are the ankles, elbows, and knees.

Pivot joints: These are joints with a rotary movement in one axis. In this form, a ring rotates around a pivot, or a pivotlike process rotates within a ring that is formed of bone and connective tissue. Examples of this kind of joint are the atlas and axis of the vertebrae, and the elbow, where pronation and supination take place.

Condyloid joints: In this type of joint, movement is permitted in two directions. The surface of the articulation is oval shaped, with the bone received into an elliptical cavity. Such an example is the wrist joint.

Saddle joints: This joint exhibits a saddle-like surface as its name implies. That is, the surface of one bone is concave, while the other is convex. This joint allows movement in two directions. The wrist joint is an example.

Ball and socket joints: These provide the freest movement and the greatest range of motion. Specifically, movement can take place in three directions. In this form of joint, a bone with a more or less rounded head lies in a cuplike cavity or bowl-shaped socket. An example of this joint is the hip.

Types of Motion

There are seven primary types of movement (see Figure 6.2) that a body segment can pass through. Most clearly depend on rotary motion. At this point, you will need to understand the proper terminology used to describe different types of motion.

Flexion is a movement that generally decreases an angle. Flexion involves bending and folding movements, or what may be thought of as "withdrawing" movements. Examples are bending the arms at the elbow, bending the head forward as when praying, or raising the heel toward the buttocks (Figure 6.2a).

Extension refers to lengthening or stretching to a greater length. Therefore, whereas bending movements are flexions, straightening movements are extensions. Consequently, extension movements return a part from the flexed position to its former, anatomical position, thus increasing the angle formed between the two segments. When extension continues beyond the anatomical position, it is called *hyperextension* (Figure 6.2b).

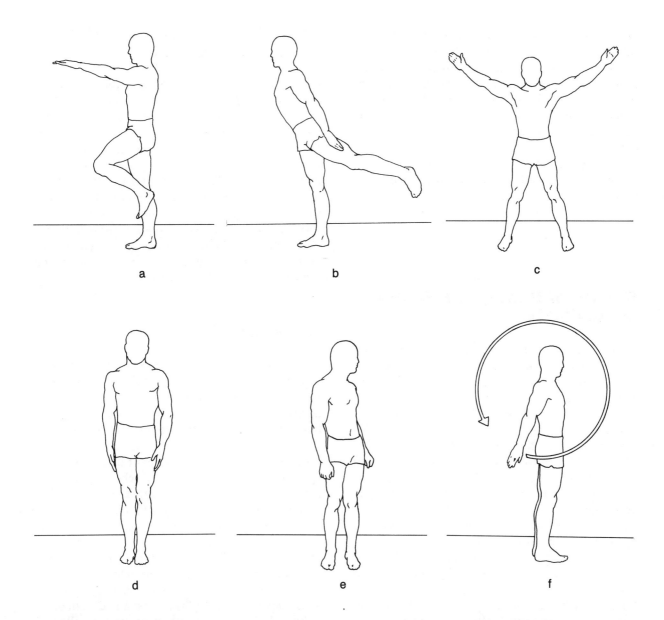

Figure 6.2. Examples of the seven primary types of movements. (a) Flexion of the knee. (b) Hyperextension of the hip. (c) Abduction of the arms and legs. (d) Adduction of the arms and legs. (e) Rotation of the head and upper torso. (f) Circumduction of the arm.

Abduction refers to the movement of a body segment away from the midline of the body or body part to which it is attached (i.e., away from the median plane of the body). Examples of abduction are the moving of the arms or legs straight out to the sides (e.g., a jumping jack; Figure 6.2c).

Adduction is the opposite of abduction. It refers to the movement of a body segment toward the midline of the body or body part to which it is attached. An example of adduction is bringing the arms back to the sides (Figure 6.2d).

Rotation is the pivoting or moving of a body segment around its own axis. An example is the hold-

ing of the head in an upright position and turning it from side to side (Figure 6.2e).

Circumduction refers to movement that allows the end of the segment to describe or trace a circle. Circumduction is often a combination of flexion, abduction, extension, and adduction movements. An example is circling the arms (Figure 6.2f).

Special movements: There are several special terms that have been developed to describe certain types of movements. *Supination* refers to the outward rotation of the forearm. Thus this movement is associated with turning the palm forward. In contrast, *pronation* is the inward rotation of the forearm. This movement is used when a tennis player follows through with a top spin swing.

Another type of unique movement is *inversion*. Inversion is the turning of the sole of the foot inward, which is what often happens when a person sprains an ankle. In contrast, *eversion* involves the outward rotation of the sole of the foot.

The last two types of special movement are *protraction* and *retroaction*. The former involves moving a part forward, while the latter involves pulling a part backward.

Growth of Bones as a Factor of Flexibility

Longitudinal growth occurs in the bones, along with the soft tissues such as the muscle and tendon. However, during periods of rapid growth there can be an increase in muscle-tendon tightness about the joints and a loss of flexibility due to the bones growing much faster than the muscles stretch (Kendall & Kendall, 1948; Leard, 1984; Micheli, 1983; Sutro, 1947). Consequently, Leard recommends that children perform stretching exercises consistently to maintain flexibility and prevent injuries.

There is also a possibility that the relative rate of growth of the bones and their attachments be disproportionate—a situation that is a likely cause of hypermobility (Sutro, 1947). That is, in certain stages of development of the skeleton, the rate of bone growth may not be parallel to that of the ligamentous and capsular tissues. Thus an excess of ligament could lead to hypermobility, and an insufficiency of ligament to rigidity of the bones comprising the joints.

Close-Packing as a Limiting Factor of Flexibility

Close-packing is defined as the final position where "the joint surfaces become fully congruent, their area of contact is maximal, and they are tightly compressed having in a sense been 'screwed-home,' while the fibrous capsule and ligaments are maximally spiralized and tense, and no movement is possible" (Williams & Warwick, 1980). Close-packed joint surfaces can be described as having their articulating bones temporarily locked together, as if there were no joint between them. When the articulating surfaces are not congruent and some parts of the articular capsule are lax, the joint is said to be *loose-packed*.

Osteoporosis

Osteoporosis is known as the "bone-robbing" disease. It primarily affects small-boned white women who have never been active. People who have osteoporosis usually show no symptoms until their bones become so brittle that an otherwise minor fall or stumble results in a fractured or broken bone. For those under treatment by a physician, special care must be employed when a stretching program is undertaken. Overzealous stretching may induce a fracture (Hickok, 1976).

Another related disease is *osteoarthritis*. This disease is defined as an idiopathic, slowly progressive disease of diarthrodial synovial-lined joints. Osteoarthritis is the most common musculoskeletal problem in the elderly (Stevens & Wigley, 1984). This disease's symptoms are usually described as a dull ache, with intermittent sharpness, followed by localized stiffness. Many patients do well with a series of common-sense "limbering-up" exercises (Stevens & Wigley, 1984). Ideally, the joint

Table 6.1 Close-Packed Versus Loose-Packed Positions

Joint	Close-packed position	Loose-packed position
Ankle	dorsiflexion	neutral
Knee	full extension	semiflexion
Hip	extension + medial rotation	semiflexion
Vertebral	dorsiflexion	neutral
Shoulder	abduction + lateral rotation	semiabduction
Wrist	dorsiflexion	semiflexion

or joints affected should be moved through a full range of motion several times daily to prevent capsular contraction (Turek, 1977). However, excessive or extreme motion will result in dangerously high compression of the joint surfaces and must be avoided (Turek, 1977).

Summary

Ultimately, range of motion at a joint is restricted by both bone and joint structure. There are numerous methods of classifying or describing joints and their motions, and basic knowledge of such terminology is essential if one wishes to describe a given movement with accuracy and precision.

Joint motion is restricted when the joint is in a close-packed position. This position is best exemplified when the joint surfaces are in full congruence. Conversely, when the articulating surface is not congruent, and parts of the articular capsule are lax, the joint is said to be loosely-packed.

Lastly, when certain diseases are present, i.e., osteoporosis and osteoarthritis, special consideration must be taken to ensure the maximum safety of the individual, particularly when exercising and stretching.

Review Questions

1. Explain the statement, "Just as the railroad or subway track determines the route available to the train, so the shape and contour of the joint surfaces ultimately determine the movement pathways available to bones."

2. Draw a diagram and label the seven primary types of movement.

3. Analyze the movements involved in a straddle jump.

4. Describe two skills that require a close-packed position.

5. You are teaching a stretching class at the home of the aged. What considerations and precautions must you take?

Answers

1. The structure of a particular joint limits joint motion due to the impingement of articulat-

ing surfaces. Similarly, the tracks of a railroad or subway and the wheels are the impinging factors in the applied metaphor.

2. Refer to Figure 6.2.

3. Keeping the upper body erect, simultaneously flex the knees and swing the arms backward (hyperextension). At the low point, swing the arms upward (flexion) and spring upward from the floor. As the feet leave the floor straddle the legs (abduction) with the ankles in plantarflexion and move the arms sideways (abduction) to touch the toes. Bring the legs back together (adduction) and land on the floor with the knees slightly flexed.

4. An iron cross in gymnastics and a pointe position in ballet require a close-packed position.

5. Considerations:
   (A) The specific ends of the class
   (B) The specific means of the class
   (C) The physical condition of the participants
   Precautions:
   (A) Consult with medical officials who work at the facility
   (B) Investigate the condition of the participants
   (C) Provide a brief pre-class discussion
   (D) Provide clear and concise instructions
   (E) Avoid ballistic movements

Recommended Readings

Barnett, C. H. (1969). Factors limiting joint mobility. *Journal of Anatomy*, **105**(1), 185.

Basmajian, J. V. (1979). *Muscles alive—their functions revealed by electromyography* (4th ed.). Baltimore: Williams and Wilkins.

Hollinshead, W. F., & Jenkins, D. B. (1981). *Functional anatomy of the limbs and back* (5th ed.). Philadelphia: W. B. Saunders.

Kapandji, I. A. (1974). *The physiology of joints* (Vols. 1-3). Edinburgh: Churchill Livingston.

Luttgens, K., & Wells, K. (1982). *Kinesiology: Scientific basis of human motion* (6th ed.). Philadelphia: W.B. Saunders.

CHAPTER 7

Social Facilitation and Psychology in Relation to Stretching

The discipline of *psychology* is associated with attempts to describe, explain, and predict behavior. The field of *social psychology* is concerned with how and why the behavior of any person affects the behavior of another (Sage, 1971). No matter how much an athlete tells you that he or she does not hear the audience or teammates, there are times when that athlete cannot escape their influence.

Many athletes are, for all practical purposes, on their own and in a sense loners, such as those athletes who perform in gymnastics, swimming, and track and field. Nevertheless, these sports still involve dynamic social relationships, because they involve interaction with teammates, opponents, and frequently with fans and spectators. For those people involved in activities such as cheerleading, dancing, or team sports, the interactions with one's comrades and the audience are obvious. These things may well affect the development of flexibility, and ultimately the performance itself.

Because the people in these situations—friends, parents, peers, strangers, authority figures—vary in their relationship to the individual, they also vary in their potential for affecting the individual's behavior and psychological state. They may be perceived as *positive*, *neutral*, or *negative elements*, depending upon the individual's past associations and experiences with them. These possibilities and their ramifications are discussed in the following section.

The Effect of an Audience on Developing Flexibility

The audience or crowd can be passive and do nothing to encourage or discourage the performer or it can be active and verbal, giving either encouraging or razzing remarks. Research involving the effects of a passive audience on individual performance has yielded contradictory results. In some studies performance was impaired, and in others improved. In general, research has found that performance is facilitated, and learning is impaired, by the presence of spectators (Sage, 1971; Zajonc, 1965).

The motivational effects induced by spectators may be learned, for they are likely a function of positive or negative experiences associated with being observed or evaluated. The anxiety level of the individual must also be considered in such instances. Research indicates that the level of a person's anxiety is parallel to the level of perceived stress in a given situation, and again, certain performing situations may be regarded as stressful because of past experiences with spectators.

How, then, does social facilitation of an audience affect the potential development of flexibility and suppleness? One example is the general attitude of society toward males becoming involved in classical ballet or modern dance. Children are very impressionable. They learn that conformity to group standards is the price that one must pay to be accepted by one's peers. They learn to read the cues, acquire social sensitivity, and behave in ways endorsed by their peer group. Unfortunately, the consequences of this socialization can be quite negative.

Over the years, there have evolved certain misconceptions and stereotypes regarding the development and/or presence of extreme flexibility in males. The ability of a male to perform a split, for instance, or some other skill of extreme suppleness, has nothing to do with either manliness or lack of it—but that has little bearing on certain stereotypes that have become entrenched in the minds of some people.

For very young and impressionable children, such a situation may present a very real conflict and a source of potential anxiety and psychological stress. If, as Toufexis (1974) sadly points out, male dancers do indeed have the reputation of being homosexual, at least in the U.S. and England, then male children who wish to participate in such activities as classical ballet and dance face a real problem. Needless to say, many boys who might otherwise have been interested in such creative arts are probably often discouraged instead. The key question is, to what extent does the individual value peer approval over desired goals? Under such circumstances, it may be appropriate to conduct practice sessions during the early stages of learning in privacy. In this way, peer pressure from either an active or a passive audience can be eliminated. It might also be appropriate for the instructor to explain those factors that determine one's flexibility, thereby eliminating the influence of "negative misconceptions."

The Effect of Coaction on Developing Flexibility

Coaction with teammates—that is, engaging in the same activity or task while in view of one another (Sage, 1971)—is most common during the stretching and/or warm-up period just before a practice session or performance. Coaction is a definite aid in the development of flexibility. When teammates (or coactors) stretch and warm up together, they often provide each other with learning clues, and thus serve as guides or models for one another. That is, they can reinforce the dominant, and correct, responses to achieve maximum flexibility and warm-up.

However, coaction can also elicit the desired response (or action) through negative means. Social pressure may be imposed on one to produce

in practice, or else be ostracized. Such an example is illustrated by Councilman's (1968) concept of the *hurt-pain-agony approach*. Although not entirely practical in the development of flexibility, this concept is still somewhat plausible. Essentially it suggests that unless one is willing to pay the price of the highest levels of discomfort, one is not likely to excel in sports. Pride is fostered when swimmers push themselves hard during the agony phase of exertion; furthermore, other team members will develop contempt for a laggard or one who does not "put out" in practice.

If suffering pain or discomfort becomes an everyday experience, shared by all members of the team, the aversion to it tends to subside. Consequently, the more the athletes engage in unemotional talk about their discomfort and pain, the more acceptable their discomfort becomes. Thus they develop mental as well as physical callousness to pain. In short, the solution lies in accepting some degree of pain as a natural and necessary part of attaining one's goal. Such an approach is practical for competitive swimming and running, but definitely *not* ideal for developing flexibility.

A more fitting and safe approach for the development of flexibility is *stretching to the edge* and the *wall strategy*. As described by its proponents (Fanning & Fanning, 1978; Jackson, 1975), a point exists in stretching at which it becomes painful to proceed. You can find that point very easily for any muscle or muscle group. Initially, the stretch feels warm and good, but if the stretch is continued, it becomes unpleasant and even painful.

As a practical example, let's analyze a stretch for the hamstrings—the modified hurdler's stretch. Sit upright on the floor, keeping one leg straight. Flex the other leg and slide the heel toward the buttocks. Next, lower the outer side of the thigh and calf onto the floor and place the heel against the inner side of the extended thigh. Now, exhale and bend gradually forward until you feel a mild resistance or tension. Try to identify where the tension is and how it feels. Relax and hold the stretch for a few breathing cycles. If you do this properly, the feeling of resistance or tension will subside, which can be likened to a "second wind" for a runner. At this point, stress-relaxation, creep, and adaptation of the muscles and muscle spindles are taking place. However, if you cannot catch your "second wind," slow down, ease off slightly, and find the degree of tension that is comfortable. Remember, you are not competing with anyone.

After catching your "second wind," exhale again, and continue bending forward until you again feel a mild resistance or tension. This stretch has been called the *developmental stretch* (Anderson, 1980), and has been described as a fine-tuning of the muscles. At this point, hold the stretch 30 to 60 seconds and visualize the tissues oozing and stretching out. As before, the muscles and spindles will adapt and the tension should diminish. This can be likened to a "second second wind." If the strain is too great, slow down and ease off. Remember, this is not a hurt-pain-agony approach to developing flexibility.

Now, if the stretching continues, you may notice that the pleasant warmth will turn into a burning sensation or some other form of discomfort. In some instances, the muscle may actually begin to quiver. You have just gone over the edge for the muscles that are being stretched. This point has been called *drastic stretch* (Anderson, 1980), and, besides being painful, is thought to cause physical damage due to microscopic tearing of muscle fibers. At this point, then, you need to prevent the possibility of injury.

When you have reached this edge, there are three possible approaches you can adopt. You can quit—but then you will not progress. You can, with one sudden thrust, break through the wall—but you run the distinct risk of injury by doing so. Or you can "play" the edge instead of trying to break through it. To do this, imagine that the edge is like a wall across a path. Explore the wall and play with it. Just be careful not to fall off! Remember, you have to find your own edge; do not attempt to compete with anyone else. You can determine the edge for each muscle group you stretch by the way it feels. Just remember that your edge will move from hour to hour, day to day, and week to week—this will depend on you.

Another psychological approach to the development of flexibility is the *cybernetic stretch*, a technique developed by Bates (1976), but which is actually a direct adaptation from Dr. Maxwell Maltz's highly recommended book *Psycho-Cybernetics* (1970). The basic approach here is "mind over matter." In the preface, Maltz states: "The 'self image' sets the boundaries of individual accomplishment. It defines what you can and cannot do. Expand the self image and you expand the area of the possible." (p. ix). Following are some of the more important principles to remember about this technique:

1. The word *cybernetics* comes from the Greek word meaning "steersman."
2. Psycho-cybernetics does not argue that man is machine, but rather that man has a machine which he uses.

3. The human brain, nervous system, and muscular system are together a highly complex "servo-mechanism" used and directed by the mind.
4. When *you* select the goal and trigger the action towards achieving it, an automatic mechanism takes over (you are the operator of the machine).
5. The automatic creative mechanism within you can operate in only one way. It must have a target to shoot for—you must clearly see a thing in your mind before you can do it.
6. Hold a picture of yourself long and steadily enough in your mind and you will be drawn toward it.
7. The important thing is to make these pictures as *vivid* and as *detailed* as possible—to make your mental pictures approximate actual experience as much as possible.
8. Rational thought, to be effective in changing belief and behavior, must be accompanied by deep feeling and desire.
9. The automatic mechanism must be given true facts about the environment.
10. Experiencing success is the key to functioning successfully.
11. Confidence is built upon experience of success.
12. When we first begin any undertaking, we are likely to have little confidence because we have not yet learned from experience that we can succeed.
13. Fortunately, for individuals who have no successful experiences to call upon, the nervous system cannot tell the difference between an *imagined experience* and a *real experience*. In either case, it reacts automatically to information which you give to it from your midbrain.
14. The method itself consists in learning, practicing, and experiencing new habits of thinking, imaging, remembering, and acting in order to bring success and happiness in achieving particular goals.
15. It usually requires a minimum of about twenty-one days to effect any perceptible change in mental image.

As described by Bates (1976), cybernetic stretch consists of two steps: the direct practice step, and the mental practice step. Following Maltz's guidelines, the first task is to select and trigger a specific goal/target. To facilitate this, true facts must be provided. "Physiologically, a 50 percent increase in muscle length is possible if no inhibitions to stretch are operative; therefore your goal of 'making it flat' in the side split exists.'' Of course, this assumes the absence of any structural limitations. Remember, it is essential to know that your goal is attainable and practical.

Next, by the use of imagination, you can set up mental images that your servo-mechanism will work to fulfill. To do this properly, a mental practice period of thirty minutes each day is recommended. The setting should be quiet, comfortable, and relaxing. As elaborated earlier, the key to the mental practice step is making the image as real and as vivid an experience as possible. As Bates points out, ''It is most important that you see yourself successfully and ideally completing the flexibility action.''

The final step is the direct practice step. As for this step Bates (1976) writes:

> Skill learning of any kind is accomplished by trial and error, mentally correcting aim after an error, until a successful motion is achieved. Your servo-mechanism achieves its goal in the same manner, it remembers the successful responses and forgets the past errors. Stretch slowly, keeping spindle firing to a minimum, up to the point of pain; ease off slightly, causing spindles to stop firing briefly and allowing the muscle to relax. The servo-mechanism remembers that position and the absence of muscle contraction that opposes holding that relaxed position, if you are supplying it with the ''end result'' or goal.

> Relax while you maintain your held position; you must allow your servo-mechanism to work rather than force it to work. Connections exist on both alpha and gamma motor neurons from higher centers such that sensory information to these motor neurons may be offset by information from the higher brain centers. While relaxing, your servo-mechanism is finding the pathway and the degree of inhibition to maintain in order to achieve your goal.

> Proceed further forward when you have learned to reduce the tension at your present level. As increased stretch positions are achieved it is helpful to have a partner maintain your position, after you have eased off slightly. Initially, this aids in allowing the subject to relax, that is, concentrate on one thing at a time. In fact, it is often advisable in the very beginning for the partner to passively as-

sist in increasing the range of motion, allowing for the easing off, and then maintain the subject's position. (pp. 240-41)

Summary

The mind sets the boundaries of individual accomplishment and defines what you can and cannot do. Accordingly, if one can expand the self-image and mind, one can expand the ''area of the possible.'' However, being social in nature, we are all affected by the presence of those around us. This presence may be perceived as being positive, neutral, or negative.

To avoid any negative effects of an audience, practice sessions in the early stages of learning should be held in privacy. Teammates can also significantly affect the development of flexibility. They can serve as models to reinforce correct responses, and can also impose social pressure on those who are not ''paying the price.'' This idea of pressuring an individual to pay the price of the highest levels of discomfort has *no* basis in flexibility development. Stretching, rather, should be done in a relaxed, noncompetitive manner, and tailored to one's needs.

Review Questions

1. What effect do spectators have on learning and performance?

2. You are the coach of a football team. Design a program that utilizes coaction to facilitate the development of flexibility.

3. Describe a situation where coaction would be detrimental to the development of flexibility.

4. What unusual problems might be encountered during a stretching period of a coed physical education class? What are some potential solutions?

5. You are talking to an athlete who has very ''tight'' hamstrings. Explain to the athlete the relationship between ''physiological limitation'' and ''psychological limitation'' as they pertain to working for a split.

6. Briefly explain stretching to the edge and the wall strategy.

7. Why is stretching to the edge and the wall strategy more practical for developing flexibility than the hurt-pain-agony approach?

8. Explain the psycho-cybernetic stretch technique to master a straddle split.

Answers

1. Generally speaking, performance is facilitated and learning impaired by the presence of spectators.

2. Squad leaders are appointed to lead warm-up and stretching exercises. These leaders have the responsibility of making sure that those individuals under their charge are optimally performing the desired skills. The leaders can set examples, provide camaraderie, and encourage collective action.

3. Such a situation would be one in which squad leaders openly criticize and razz those who cannot keep up with the members of the team.

4. The members of the class may not be suitably attired thereby creating a degree of ''distraction.'' Here the solution is to require the class to wear appropriate clothing (i.e., a warm-up suit). Another problem might be the attempt of class members to compete against one another. Here the remedy is to explain to the class that comparing and competing are meaningless. No two people are alike. Furthermore, females are generally more flexible than males.

5. A split is possible assuming there are no structural limitations. The problem is usually that the mind gives in before the body does.

Remember, each sarcomere has the ability to increase 50%, assuming there are no inhibitions to stretch.

6. Assume the stretch position and feel the tension. Take a few breaths, exhale, and stretch a bit further. When tension reoccurs, repeat the process. At each point of tension, imagine that you are at a wall. Play the edge of the wall. However, do not try to break through it with a sudden thrust.

7. The hurt-pain-agony approach is not the practical course to follow. It's painful, and may result in an impairment in learning/performance. In contrast, stretching to the edge and the wall strategy are safe, effective, enjoyable, and more likely to be used every day.

8. First, imagine that you are capable of, and are executing, a straddle split.
Second, spend 30 minutes each day concentrating on a mental image that is real and vivid.
Third, by trial and error, mentally correct yourself after any error—that is, having the muscle spindles fire.
Fourth, hold the stretch and concentrate on relaxing.
Fifth, as your tissues and spindles adapt, exhale and stretch further repeating the process.

Recommended Readings

Singer, R. N. (1975). *Motor learning and human performance* (2nd ed.). New York: Macmillan.

Tutko, T. A., & Richards, J. W. (1971). *Psychology of coaching*. Boston: Allyn and Bacon.

Potpourri

Besides the factors we have already discussed, there are a number of additional factors that can affect one's potential degree of flexibility and suppleness. A few examples of these are age, sex, and body build, all of which are analyzed in the following section.

Age and Flexibility Development

Conflicting data exist concerning the relationship between age and flexibility, especially concerning the increase or decrease of flexibility during the growing years. However, research does seem to indicate that small children are quite supple, and that during the school years flexibility increases. With adolescence, however, flexibility tends to level off, and then begin to decrease.

According to Sermeev (1966), flexibility is not developed identically in various age periods and not equally for various movements. Nonetheless, Harris (1969a) is of the opinion that one age is as good as another to study the structure of flexibility as long as the study is kept within a limited age range. However, Corbin and Noble (1980) suggest that when evaluating the flexibility of children and adolescents, growth (especially individual differences in growth) should be considered.

One's desired degree of flexibility clearly depends upon a multitude of interacting factors. In the area of athletics, flexibility should relate to the level of sports preparation (Nelson, Johnson, & Smith, 1983; Sermeev, 1966). As would be expected, the higher the qualification requirements for many sports and events, the greater the mobility of the athlete. For lay persons, the quality and quantity of one's activities, both occupationally and avocationally, would be of chief importance.

Critical Periods of Flexibility Development

Is there a critical period during which stretching is most effective in developing flexibility? A *critical period* is the period of time following the age when one becomes capable of performing a given act effectively, such as touching the floor with the palms of the hands while the legs remain straight. It can also be defined as the period of time in an individual's life when changes are most likely to occur at rapid or optimum rates. It is true that flexibility can be developed at any age given the appropriate training; however, the rate of improvement will not be the same at every age nor will the potential for improvement.

Sermeev's research on the mobility of the hip joint of 1,440 sportsmen and 3,000 children and adults not participating in sports demonstrated that mobility in the hip joint is not developed identically in various age periods and not equally for various movements. Specifically, he observed that the greatest growth occurs between the ages of 7 and 11. However, by 15 years of age the indices of mobility in the hip joint achieve a maximum amount; in later years that amount decreases. By 50 years of age there is a significant drop in mobility in the hip joint, and an even sharper drop after 60 to 70 years of age. Similarly, a review of the literature by Corbin and Noble (1980) reveals that flexibility increases during the school years until early adolescence, when a leveling off or decrease begins.

All of this does not mean that a stretching program has no effect after the critical period has passed or that one critical period determines all potential. The question, then, that must be asked is, "Can the effects of the lack of stretching and consequent tightness during the critical period (i.e., the growing years) be counteracted by engaging in stretching programs *after* the critical period has passed?'' This question is relevant for those in their late adolescence or those entering adulthood.

As mentioned previously, evidence so far indicates that flexibility can be developed at any age given the appropriate training. However, the rate of improvement will not be the same at every age, nor will the potential for improvement. There is evidence that even senior adults benefit from flexibility training (Bell & Hoshizaki, 1981; Dummer, Vaccaro, & Clarke, 1985; Germain & Blair, 1983). In general, it is safe to conclude that the longer one waits to start on some type of flexibility program after adolescence, the less likely there will be an absolute improvement.

Sex Differences in Flexibility

Evidence suggests that, as a general rule, females are more flexible than males. Although conclusive evidence to this effect is lacking, there appear to be several anatomical differences that may account for the differences in flexibility between the sexes. The female is designed for a greater range of flexibility, especially in the pelvic region, which makes her better adapted to pregnancy and child-bearing. Specifically, because females have broader hips, they have a greater potential for ROM. Furthermore, females tend to have lighter and smaller bone composition (see Figure 8.1).

Flexibility is also affected by pregnancy itself (Abramson, Roberts, & Wilson, 1934; Bird, Calguneri, & Wright, 1981; Brewer & Hinson, 1978). During pregnancy, the pelvic joints and ligaments are relaxed and capable of greater extension, which renders the locking mechanism of the sacroiliac joint less restrictive, permitting greater rotation. According to Beighton, Grahame, and Bird (1983), the changes in the pelvic joint during late pregnancy may arise from both local and systemic causes. The former would include the weight of the uterus upon the pelvic brim; the latter are presumably circulating hormones. The hormone most commonly thought to be responsible for this change is *relaxin*. After childbirth, the production of relaxin decreases, and the ligaments tighten up again. However, Beighton et al. point out that whether these changes should be attributed to relaxin, progestogens and oestrogens, or altered steroid metabolism remains undetermined.

Corbin (1973) also suggests that girls have greater potential for flexibility after puberty in such areas as trunk flexion because of their lower center of gravity and shorter leg length. Corbin and Noble (1980) suggest that regular activity differences between the sexes may also account for the flexibility differences between the sexes.

Body Build and Flexibility

Numerous attempts have been made to relate flexibility to different factors such as body proportions, body surface area, skinfold, and weight. However, the results of such research have been inconsistent. What is almost unanimously agreed upon is that flexibility is specific (Dickenson, 1968; Harris, 1969a, 1969b). That is, the amount or degree of range of motion is specific to each joint. Therefore, range of motion in the shoulder does not ensure range of motion in the hip, and range of motion in one hip or shoulder may not be highly related to range of motion in the other. This concept of the specificity of flexibility is based on the fact that different musculature, bone structure, and connective tissue are involved in different movements of a joint. Consequently, flexibility is not merely specific to the joints of the body, but is also specific to individual joint movements. There is no evidence, therefore, that flexibility exists as a single general characteristic of the human body. Thus no one composite test or joint action measure can give a satisfactory index of the flexibility characteristics of an individual (Harris, 1969a, 1969b).

Following is a brief summary of studies pertaining to the relationship between body build and flexibility. Several investigators have found that body build as determined by segmental length is nonsignificantly correlated with toe-touch flexibility (Broer & Gales, 1958; Harvey & Scott, 1967; Mathews, Shaw, & Bohnen, 1957; Mathews, Shaw, & Woods, 1959). In direct contrast, Wear (1963) found for those persons with extreme body types that the relationship of trunk-plus-arm length to leg length was a significant factor in the performance of the toe-touch test. Specifically, those persons with a longer trunk-plus-arm measurement and relatively short legs have an advantage over those persons with long legs and relatively short trunk-plus-arm measurements (Broer & Gales, 1958). It has also been contended that the ability to touch the toes with the finger tips may be considered normal for young children and adults;

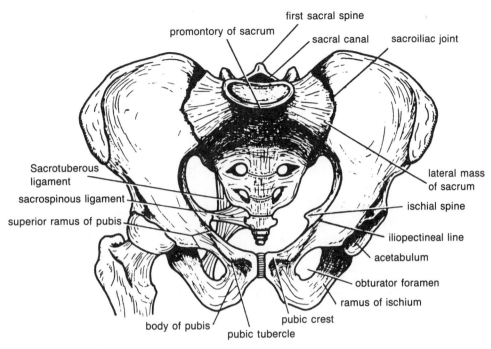

Figure 8.1a. The male pelvis.

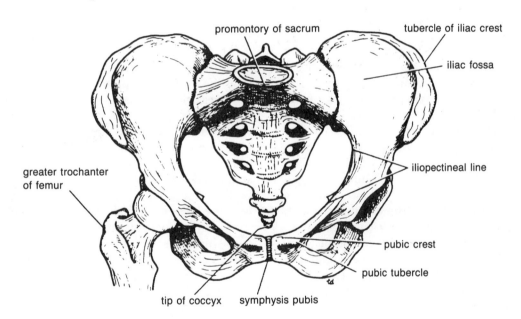

Figure 8.1b.   The female pelvis. *Note*. From *Clinical Anatomy for Medical Students* (3rd ed., p. 304) by R.S. Snell, 1986, Boston: Little, Brown and Company. Copyright 1986 by Little, Brown and Company. Reprinted by permission.

however, between the ages of 11 and 14, many young adolescents who show no signs of muscle or joint tightness are unable to complete this movement. Thus, as shown in Figure 8.2, apparently limited flexibility occurs gradually over the period of years that the legs become proportionally longer in relation to the trunk (Kendall & Kendall, 1948;

Kendall, Kendall, & Boynton, 1970; Kendall, Kendall, & Wadsworth, 1971). However, in a previously cited investigation, Harvey and Scott (1969) found that no significant difference existed between means of the best bend-and-reach scores and excess length (T + A − L) or the ratio of the trunk-plus-arm length to leg length (T + A)/ L. When

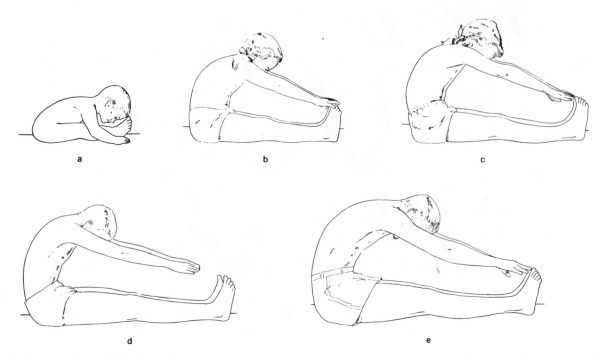

Figure 8.2. Normal flexibility according to age level. *Note*. From *Muscles Testing and Function* (2nd ed., p. 233) by H.O. Kendall, F.P. Kendall, and G.E. Wadsworth, 1971, Baltimore: Williams and Wilkins. Copyright 1971 by Williams and Wilkins. Reprinted by permission.

prone back extension and supine back extension was correlated to trunk length, no significant correlation was found (Wear, 1963).

Weight, body somatotype, skinfold, and body surface area have all been investigated in terms of their relationship to flexibility. McCue (1963) found very few significant relationships between overweight and underweight subjects and flexibility. In a similar study, Tyrance (1958) found few significant relationships between flexibility and three extremes in body build: thinnest-underweight; fattest-overweight; and most muscular. Measurements between flexibility and somatotype were also generally found to be insignificant (Laubach & McConville, 1966a, 1966b). In terms of lean body mass as calculated by skinfold measurements, flexibility measurements were again found to be insignificant (Laubach & McConville, 1966b). Lastly, an attempt was made to find a relationship between body surface area and flexibility. The results of the study by Krahenbuhl and Martin (1977) were significantly negative-related or not related at all depending upon the body parts tested.

Viscosity's Effect on Flexibility

Viscosity is defined as resistance to flow, or an apparent force that prevents fluids from flowing easily. Connective tissue and muscle viscosity might be partially responsible for restricting movement (Leighton, 1960). First, we know that temperature has an inverse effect upon viscosity; that is, as the temperature of the body tissues increases, fluid viscosity decreases, and vice versa. Second, this reduced viscosity significantly enhances the viscous relaxation of collagenous tissues (Sapega et al., 1981). The mechanism behind this thermal transition is still unknown. However, it has been suggested (Mason & Rigby, 1963; Rigby, Hirai, Spikes, & Eyring, 1959) that the intermolecular bonding becomes partially destabilized, enhancing the viscous flow properties of the collagenous tissue. Third, this in turn provides less resistance to movement and results in an increase in flexibility.

Probably the most common method used to elevate body temperature and reduce tissue viscosity is the use of warm-up exercises. Other methods include the use of heat packs, hot showers, diathermy, ultrasound, and massage. Viscosity has no long-term effect on the improvement of one's flexibility. Rather, its effects are relative to various physiological factors that exist at the moment when stretch is being developed (Aten & Knight, 1978).

Warming Up and Cooling Down (Warming Down)

Warm-up may be defined as a group of exercises performed immediately before an activity that provides the body with a period of adjustment from rest to exercise. Warm-up is designed to improve performance and reduce the chance of injury by mobilizing the individual mentally as well as physically.

Warm-up may be divided into two types: formal and general. The formal type includes movements that either mimic, or are employed in, the actual performance activity. For example, a baseball player will throw a ball or swing a bat to warm up. In contrast, the general type of warm-up may consist of various movements not directly related to those employed in the activity itself. These movements may include light calisthenics, jogging, or stationary bicycling. Obviously, the nature of the warm-up will depend upon the individual's needs, but should generally be intense enough to increase the body temperature and cause some sweating, but not so intense as to cause fatigue (Kulund & Töttössy, 1983). The effects of warm-up will ultimately wear off. How soon will depend upon a number of factors such as the level of intensity and specificity of the warm-up.

An important distinction should be made here between warm-up exercises and flexibility exercises. Flexibility exercises are those exercises that are used to increase the range of motion of a joint or set of joints progressively and permanently. Flexibility exercises should always be preceded by a mild set of warm-up exercises, because the increase in the tissue temperature produced by the muscular exercise will make the stretching both safer and more productive (Sapega et al., 1981). However, an increase of temperature also involves a reduction in tensile strength of connective tissue, and thus more ruptures might be expected after warming up. Increased temperature, however, seems to involve at the same time an increase in extensibility, and this greater extensibility is a plausible explanation for the fact that warming up does indeed prevent ruptures (Troels, 1973).

Among the benefits associated with warming up are:

1. Increases in the body and tissue temperature
2. Increases in blood flow through active muscles by reducing vascular bed viscosity (or resistance)
3. Increases in the heart rate, which will prepare the cardiovascular system for work
4. Increases in the rate of the metabolic processes
5. Increases in the Bohr effect, which facilitates the exchange of oxygen from hemoglobin
6. Increases in the speed at which nerve impulses travel and thereby facilitate body movements

7. Increases in the efficiency process of reciprocal innervation (thus allowing muscles to contract and relax faster and more efficiently)
8. Increases in the physical working capacity
9. Decreases in the viscosity (or resistance) of connective tissue and muscle
10. Decreases in muscular tension
11. Enhanced connective tissue and muscular extensibility
12. Enhanced psychological performance of the individual

Analogous to warm-up is cool-down (also called warm-down). *Cool-down* may be defined as a group of exercises performed immediately after an activity that provides the body a period of adjustment from exercise to rest. Although cool-down may serve as an additional effort to improve flexibility, its main objective is to facilitate muscular relaxation, promote the removal of waste products, and reduce muscle soreness. It is recommended that stretching be incorporated immediately after the main part of a workout and cool-down period, because tissue temperatures will be highest (Sapega et al., 1981).

Strength Training

Many misconceptions and stereotypes still exist regarding the relationship between strength training and flexibility. Simply stated, the belief that weight training causes a muscle-bound condition is false. Why do such beliefs persist? Jones (1975) points out several possible reasons, along with a brief rebuttal of the idea: (a) It is true that certain individuals with large muscles do lack a degree of flexibility; (b) it is also true that large muscles can be developed while doing absolutely nothing in the way of improving one's flexibility; and (c) it is even true that activities that build large muscles can produce a loss of flexibility. However, the size of a person's muscle has very little or nothing to do with flexibility, and in fact, if strength training is properly conducted, it can actually help to increase flexibility. This last point deserves special attention. The research of several investigators (Leighton, 1956; Massey & Chaudet, 1956; Wickstrom, 1963; Wilmore et al. 1978) demonstrates that weight training does not decrease flexibility, and in some instances actually improves it. Thus, with proper training, one can improve overall strength and flexibility—as long as the training is technically correct.

There are two key principles to remember in developing flexibility with resistance techniques.

First, the entire muscle or muscle group must be worked through its full range of motion. Second, there must be a gradual emphasis on the negative phase of work. *Negative work* or *eccentric contraction* takes place when a muscle is stretched (i.e., elongated) while it is contracting. This is associated with the lowering phase of a resistance.

During negative work, the number of contracting muscle fibers decreases. Since the workload is shared by a smaller number of cellular components (i.e, contractile components), the tension increases. Consequently, the excessive stress and tension produces a greater stretch on the respective fibers, resulting in enhanced flexibility. One should remember, however, that eccentric training is also associated with muscle soreness.

Summary

There are a number of factors that can affect and determine one's potential degree of flexibility and suppleness. Flexibility can be developed at any age given the appropriate training; however, the rate of development will not be the same at every age, nor will the potential for improvement. The longer one waits to start on some type of flexibility program after adolescence, the less likely is an absolute improvement.

Attempts to correlate flexibility to body proportions, body surface area, skinfold, and weight have yielded inconsistent results. Research does agree, however, that flexibility is specific to each joint. Empirical evidence indicates that females are more flexible than males, especially in the area of the pelvic region where greater flexibility makes women better adapted to pregnancy and childbearing.

Warm-up should always precede a stretching program because the increase in tissue temperature, along with other benefits, will make stretching both safer and more productive. Cool-down and stretching after exercises are also strongly recommended.

Flexibility can be significantly enhanced even while participating in a resistance or weight training program. To develop range of motion while working with resistance requires: (a) exercising the entire muscle or muscle group through its full range, and (b) gradually emphasizing the negative phase of the work. If strength training is improperly conducted, there may be an actual decrease in flexibility.

Review Questions

1. Explain the relationship between age and flexibility.

2. Define the term *critical period*.

3. Explain the relationship between critical periods and the development of flexibility.

4. Draw a diagram of a female and male pelvis illustrating a potentially greater range of motion in the former.

5. Design a warm-up program for a physical education class.

6. Prepare a general and a formal warm-up program for a Little League baseball team.

7. Design a cool-down program for a track team.

8. You are conducting a weight training class. Explain to your students two basic principles to enhance the development of flexibility.

9. Explain several misconceptions regarding strength training and flexibility.

10. Although many textbooks provide values for normal ranges of motion, standardization norm tables according to age, sex, and body build have not been established. Explain why.

Answers

1. With age there is a decrease in flexibility after adolescence.

2. A critical period is the period of time following the age when one becomes capable of performing a given act effectively, or a period when changes are most likely to occur at rapid or optimum rates.

3. Flexibility can be developed at any age given the appropriate training. However, the rate of improvement will not be the same at every age, nor will the potential for improvement.

4. See Figure 8.1a and b.

5. (A) Sit on the floor and perform 10 foot rotations.
   (B) Stand up and perform 10 jumping jacks on the four count.

(C) Stand up and perform 10 hip and trunk rotations both clockwise and counter-clockwise.

(D) Lie on your back and peform 30 seconds of bicycling.

(E) Perform 15 bent-leg sit-ups.

6. General warm-up
   (A) Jogging in place
   (B) Jumping jacks
   (C) Sit-ups
   (D) Hip and trunk rotations
   Formal warm-up
   (A) Swinging a weighted bat
   (B) Throwing a weighted ball
   (C) Mimic picking up a ball and throwing off balance to first base

7. (A) Light jogging
   (B) Hip and trunk rotation
   (C) Standing, alternating toe-touch

8. Work through the full range of motion and emphasize the negative phase of the exercise.

9. Weight training causes a muscle-bound condition and cannot enhance the development of flexibility.

10. Joint ranges of motion defy the definition "average" because so many factors are involved that correlations are almost impossible to find.

Recommended Readings

Adrian, M.J. (1981). Flexibility in the aging adult. In E.L. Smith & R.C. Serfass (Eds.), *Exercise and aging: The scientific basis.* Hillside, NJ: Enslow.

Bloomfield, J., & Blanksby, B.A. (1971). Strength, flexibility and anthropometric measurements: A comparison of highly successful male university swimmers and normal university students. *The Australian Journal of Sports Medicine, 3*(10), 8-15.

Crosman, L.J., Chateauvert, S.R., & Weisberg, J. (1984). The effects of massage to the hamstring muscle group on range of motion. *The Journal of Orthopaedic and Sports Physical Therapy, 6*(3), 168-172.

Gutmann, E. (1977). Muscle. In C.E. Finch & L. Hayflick (Eds.), *Handbook of the biology of aging* (pp. 445-469). New York: Van Nostrand Reinhold.

Haywood, K.M. (1980). Strength and flexibility in gymnasts before and after menarche. *The British Journal of Sports Medicine, 14*(4), 189-192.

Kirby, R.L., Simms, F.C., Symington, V.J., & Garner, J.B. (1981). Flexibility and musculo-skeletal symptomatology in female gymnasts and age-matched controls. *The American Journal of Sports Medicine, 9*(3), 160-164.

Lonnerblad, L. (1984). Exercises to promote independent living in older patients. *Geriatrics, 39*(2), 93-100.

Nelson, J.K., Johnson, B.L., & Smith, G.C. (1983). Physical characteristics, hip flexibility and arm strength of female gymnasts classified by intensity of training across age. *The Journal of Sports Medicine and Physical Fitness, 23*(1), 95-101.

Shellock, F.G., & Prentice, W.E. (1985). Warming-up and stretching for improved physical performance and prevention of sports-related injuries. *Sports Medicine, 2*(4), 267-278.

Stevens, M.B., & Wigley, F.M. (1984). Osteoarthritis: Practical management in older patients. *Geriatrics, 39*(3), 101-120.

Taunton, J.E. (1982). Pre-game warm-up and flexibility. *The New Zealand Journal of Sports Medicine, 10*(1), 14-18.

Vallbona, C., & Baker, S.B. (1984). Physical fitness in the elderly. *Archives of Physical Medicine and Rehabilitation, 65*(4), 194-200.

Wiktorsson-Möller, M., Öberg, B., Ekstrand, J., & Gillquist, J. (1983). Effects of warm-up, massage, and stretching on range of motion and muscle strength in the lower extremity. *The American Journal of Sports Medicine, 11*(4), 249-251.

CHAPTER 9

Relaxation

A multitude of articles and books has been written on the topic of relaxation. What is relaxation and why is it so important? We must first define the term before addressing these questions.

Defining Relaxation

Relaxation may be defined in several ways. In the discipline of motor learning, it is "the ability to control muscle activity such that muscles not specifically required for a task are quiet, and those which are required are fired at the minimal level needed to achieve the desired results" (Coville, 1979, p. 178). Accordingly, relaxation "can be considered as a motor skill in itself because the ability to reduce muscle fire is as important to motor control as is generation of firing" (Coville, 1979, p. 177). Consequently, relaxation may be regarded as a factor that determines optimum performance.

In skilled performance, movement is characterized by an appearance of ease, smoothness of movement, coordination, grace, self-control, and complete and total freedom. It may also be characterized by beauty, harmony, precision, and virtuosity. Thus in motor learning the term applies to the absence of anxiety, inhibition, tension, or extraneous motion.

Relaxation is economical energy consumption and resistance to fatigue. It is a minimal expenditure of energy consistent with the desired ends (Basmajian, 1975). When more muscle fibers than necessary are activated, an inefficient energy expenditure results (Coville, 1979). To compensate for the shortfall of oxygen and energy in such an instance, the cardiovascular system is taxed that much more. This unnecessary expenditure of energy may actually interfere with the execution of the task at hand and more significantly, may help to bring on fatigue more quickly (Coville, 1979).

Relaxation can help reduce the risk of injury. If one is relaxed, there is an economical expenditure of energy, and thus there is resistance to fatigue. When one is less fatigued, one is less prone to injury. Furthermore, because awkward movements and psychological tensions are potential factors in accidents, relaxation of tension in general should reduce the frequency of accidents (Rathbone, 1971).

Although muscular relaxation is important for all of these reasons, our concern here is with flexibility (i.e., range of motion) and stretching. How does relaxation affect flexibility and why should a muscle be relaxed prior to stretching? Ideally, stretching should begin when a muscle is in a completely relaxed state. That is, there should be a minimal amount of tension developed by the contractile components. As a result of this reduced internal tension, the individual can most effectively and efficiently work on stretching out the connective tissue that truly limits extensibility. Remember, each muscle cell is capable of at least a 50% increase in length accomplished by the displacement of the actin and myosin myofilaments with at least one cross-bridge maintained. Usually, this phase (the stretching phase) is performed constantly and/or slowly, thus eliminating the likelihood of activating the stretch reflex, and ultimately the contractile components.

Methodologies of Muscular Relaxation

There are numerous physical and psychological methods of producing a state of relaxation. The question that arises is, "What is the most cost-effective and efficient plan of action?" Among the factors to consider are: (a) the safety of the plan; (b) necessary special assistance or instruction; (c) the need for special equipment and ergogenic aids (i.e., anything that enhances performance); (d) the amount of time required; and (e) the financial cost. Whatever method you choose, it can probably be classified into one of three categories:

1. The use of special stretching techniques
2. The use of special modalities, drugs, or aids
3. The use of mind-controlling techniques

Stretching

Stretching can be used to facilitate relaxation. The theoretical basis for this idea is founded primarily on spinal reflex physiology. The two strategies employed to induce relaxation are the static stretch and proprioceptive neuromuscular facilitation.

The Static Stretch.   Static stretching involves stretching the muscle to the point where further movement is limited and prevented by its own tension. At this point, the stretch is held and maintained for an extended period of time, during which relaxation and reduction of tension take place. This phenomenon has three possible explanations: First, the muscle's stretch receptors (i.e., muscle spindles) become desensitized and subsequently adapt to stretch. Hence, the stretch reflex is neutralized. Second, if the tension from the stretch is great enough, the autogenic inhibition reflex can be initiated. In turn, this will inhibit the muscle under stretch. Consequently, the muscle's tension will decrease, thereby facilitating relaxation. The third and last explanation is based on the fact that muscle and connective tissue possess time-dependent mechanical properties. That is, when a constant force is applied, creep or a progressive change in length occurs, along with stress relaxation, a progressive reduction in tension. Accompanying this change, too, would be a decrease in the discharge of the muscles spindle's firings.

Proprioceptive Neuromuscular Facilitation (PNF).
Proprioceptive neuromuscular facilitation (PNF) is a strategy that can induce relaxation of a muscle. Its operation is based on the physiology of the GTOs. Using the *hold-relax* technique, a limb or muscle is stretched to the point where further motion in the desired direction is prevented by the tension in the antagonist muscle (i.e., the muscle being stretched). At this point, a maximal isometric contraction for five to ten seconds is applied by the muscle being stretched. This will cause the GTOs to fire, consequently initiating the autogenic inhibition.

Special Modalities, Drugs, or Aids

In the following section, a variety of methods to induce relaxation will be discussed, ranging from the simple to the complex and from the safe to the dangerous. Regardless of the technique employed, increased knowledge will make the goal more effective, efficient, and safe.

Heat.   Probably one of the oldest and most common methods to achieve relief of pain and muscular tension is the use of heat. Its therapeutic effects have been recognized for centuries. However, as far as we are concerned here, heat is important because it can facilitate relaxation either as an analgesic or as a sedative. The exact mechanisms and effects of heat in these two areas, however, are poorly understood.

Two natural questions arise: First, what method of heating is to be employed? Second, in what dosage should it be used? Ideally, the advice of a physician, therapist, or athletic trainer will help answer these questions because they are potentially a matter of clinical judgment. If professional advice is not sought, common sense, as an absolute minimum, must be employed. However, what is common sense for one may not be common sense for another.

One of the most common methods of applying heat is the application of hot water, including the use of special bottles or wet packs. Agitated water baths may also be used. These stir heated water in a whirlpool or jacuzzi-type device. Because the temperature usually ranges from 40 to 43 °C (104 to 110 °F), caution must be used not to burn oneself, induce mild fever, or fall asleep while in the bath or tub. In most instances, however, a simple hot shower should more than adequately fulfill one's needs.

Electric heating pads offer another simple method of applying heat to a given area. The advantages of a heating pad are its different levels of intensity and its steadily maintained temperature. Because the temperature is maintained, however, one is more likely to be burned if not careful. Wrapping an electric heating pad around a wet hot pack must obviously be avoided to prevent the danger of electrical shock.

Diathermy.   Another method to induce relaxation and facilitate stretching is the use of diathermy modalities. For our purposes here, *diathermy* will be defined as deep heating (Lehmann & DeLateur,

1982). Generally, three types of diathermy modalities are used for therapeutic purposes.

Short wave diathermy works on the principle that energy is transferred into deep tissue layers by a frequency current. Such currents have frequencies greater than a million cycles per second (Hz or cps). Another high frequency current is *microwave*, which employs the use of energy generated by means of electromagnetic radiation. Microwaves have a shorter wave length than short waves. The third type of diathermy is *ultrasound*. Ultrasound utilizes a high frequency vibration capable of penetrating into the deeper tissue layers. Here, too, high frequency currents in the neighborhood of a million Hz are used to produce mechanical vibration.

No matter what form of diathermy is used, its immediate effect is purely physical: a rise in temperature in the heated tissue. The degree and extent of treatment will vary in relation to the source of heating, its intensity, and the length of application (Lehmann & DeLateur, 1982). Such heating can act as either a sedative or an irritative condition on sensory and motor nerves. This explains the relief given by diathermy, which is thought to someway lessen nerve sensibility. Among other effects associated with deep heating diathermy are (a) increased blood flow; (b) an initial increase in tissue metabolism; (c) a decrease in muscle spindle sensitivity to stretch; (d) muscular relaxation; and (e) tissue that yields more readily to stretch.

Common sense indicates that diathermy is not a toy. Each modality must be prescribed by a physician, physical therapist, or athletic trainer who selects it for a precise purpose. Lastly, diathermy should be used intelligently, effectively, and safely only by a qualified and trained person (Shriber, 1975).

Cold. *Cryotherapy* is the therapeutic use of cold. In recent years, it has become increasingly popular (Nielsen, 1981; Travell & Simons, 1983). The major advantages of cryotherapy are similar to heat in that it acts as an anesthesia and can effectively promote muscular relaxation. Cryotherapy should be used only: (a) when the therapeutic goal is to tear connective tissue (such as adhesions) rather than stretch it; (b) when no other range of motion therapy can be attempted due to the pain; or (c) when muscle spasticity significantly interferes with the proper range of motion therapy (Sapega et al., 1981).

How does cold affect the nerves? Harris (1978) provides the following explanation:

> The relaxing effect of deep cold may be based on the same phenomenon as relaxation obtained through slow stretch, with the difference that slow stretch physiologically desensitizes the stretch receptors, thereby lowering the background level of stretch afferent input, while deep cold (penetrating the muscle mass) produces "cold block" of the receptor excitatory process or of the afferent fibers themselves. The latter is a state resembling blockage of impulse conduction which can be achieved by applying a local anesthetic to the nerve fibers. Just as muscle can be reduced to a state of complete flaccidity by interrupting all dorsal root fibers carrying stretch afferent input to it, muscle tone can be diminished by cold block of conduction in the stretch afferent, which temporarily prevents impulse conduction while leaving the fibers themselves intact. (p. 105)

A study by Prentice (1982) found the use of cold followed by static stretching superior to heat combined with stretching in reducing delayed muscle pain. Cold used to relieve pain is thought to send impulses to the spinal cord that compete with pain-producing impulses conveyed by much slower fibers. Thus it has been argued that cold does not produce anesthesia, but rather counterirritation.

Since cryotherapy is relatively simple, an individual may treat oneself at home under a physician's or trainer's directions. One should be aware of the danger of freezing tissue, which can result in frostbite, but this occurs only if ice is left directly and continuously on the body part. When ice is applied to a surface, the area goes through varying stages of sensations: Initially there is the feeling of cold; subsequently there is the sensation of burning, stinging, or intense aching; and finally, there is the partial loss of sensation and numbness.

Massage. Massage is probably the oldest of all remedies since it is instinctive not only in man, but in lower animals as well. Most cultures, both ancient and modern, have employed this means as a health aid. The term *massage* implies the scientific and systematic manipulation of body tissues for the purpose of affecting the nervous and muscular system and general circulation (Knapp, 1982).

The effects of massage may be classified into two general groups: *reflex effects* and *mechanical effects*. By reflex action, the sensory nerves in the skin act to produce sensations of pleasure or relaxation, which cause the muscles to relax and blood vessels to dilate. Another reflex effect is sedative. This also results in relaxation of the muscles as well as reduction of mental tension. To achieve these results, the massage should be given in a monotonously repetitive manner (Knapp, 1982).

The mechanical effects consist of: (a) stimulating circulation of venous blood and flow of lymph through or from an area; (b) stimulating metabolism in an area, thus increasing absorption of waste or fatigue products; and (c) stretching adhesions between muscle fibers. Furthermore, a recent study by Crosman, Chateauvert, and Weisberg (1984) found that massage is an effective means of increasing range of motion. In contrast, a study by Wiktorsson-Möller, Öberg, Ekstrand, and Gillquist (1983) found that stretching resulted in a significantly increased range of motion in all muscle groups tested, whereas only one muscle group was influenced by massage or warming up, separately or combined.

Basically, there are three types of massage movements. *Stroking* or *effleurage* may be superficial or deep. The movements must be slow, rhythmic, and gentle. The major objective of this technique is to improve the movement of venous blood and lymph flow. *Compression* or *petrissage* includes kneading, squeezing, and friction. This method is used to limit or eliminate adhesions. Finally, *percussion* or *tapotement* employs hacking, clapping, or beating and is used to produce stimulation.

Analgesic/Counterirritant Balms and Liniments.
Analgesics and counterirritants are among the most extensively used aids for the treatment of athletic or everyday muscular aches and sores due to overexertion. The most common ingredients are oil of wintergreen (menthyl salicylate), peppermint (menthol), red pepper, and/or camphor. When applied to the skin, they create a mild irritant that counters or masks the sense of pain. Besides creating a slight degree of local anesthesia, they also cause the muscle fibers surrounding the blood vessels to relax and consequently the blood vessels to dilate. In turn, the increased circulation helps promote the absorption of inflammatory products and brings more blood and nutrients into the applied area.

Muscle Relaxant Drugs.
Muscle relaxants fall into two categories: nonprescription or over the counter drugs, and prescription drugs. The precise mechanism of many of these drugs is not fully understood. In many drugs, the therapeutic action may be related to analgesic or sedative properties. Those drugs are understood either to block nerve impulses to skeletal muscles at the myoneural junction, or to act as general CNS depressants. In many instances, these drugs are indicated as an adjunct to rest, physical therapy, and other measures for the relief of discomfort associated with acute painful musculoskeletal conditions. There are a number of potentially negative side effects associated with some of these drugs, including depression, allergies, dizziness, headaches, irritability, lightheadedness, and nausea. The most recent edition of the *Physicians' Desk Reference* is a helpful source for those who desire more information.

As a rule, prescription drugs should be taken only as a last resort, and must be used carefully, following all recommended directions. Medication should be taken in as limited doses as necessary and eliminated as soon as possible.

Biofeedback.
Biofeedback is a relatively recent scientific technique. It is based upon an integration of physiology and psychology. Certain functions, which are actually under the voluntary control of the brain, are not normally felt or sensed. Prior to the advent of biofeedback, it was not considered possible for one to be able to gain conscious control of individual motor cells. However, today we know that it is possible to fire single motor nerve cells or to produce deliberate changes in the rate of their firing.

What, then, is biofeedback? *Biofeedback* is defined by Basmajian (1981) as ''the technique of using electronic equipment to reveal instantaneously to patients and therapist certain physiological events and to teach the patients to control these otherwise involuntary events by manipulating the displayed signals (usually visual and/or acoustic)'' (p. 469). Thus, given instant and continuous electronic displays of one's internal physiological events, individuals can be taught to manipulate voluntarily those otherwise unsensed events by concentrating on either increasing or decreasing the electronic signals that indicate the level of physiologic activity (Basmajian, 1981). In brief, the proponents of biofeedback believe that by recognizing a biological function, you can gain control of that function.

The psychology of biofeedback is in part based upon B. F. Skinner's theory of *operant conditioning*, which basically states that to obtain a reward, a person must operate upon his or her environment.

Because the reward in biofeedback is relaxation, and the environment is the biofeedback modality being employed, the person must consciously operate upon the equipment to produce the desired effects.

There are several problems associated with biofeedback. For one thing, it is expensive: biofeedback equipment can cost up to $1,000 for the needs of most persons. There is also confusion about the possibility of a "placebo effect." Finally, one might ask: Aren't there more practical methods of achieving muscular relaxation?

Progressive Relaxation.   The concept of *progressive relaxation* was developed by Dr. Edmund Jacobson, one of the earliest and foremost researchers in the field of relaxation. Progressive relaxation seeks to relax the voluntary skeletal muscles by conscious control. The technique is practiced in a quiet setting and with a passive attitude. A muscle is contracted hard and then suddenly relaxed. As a result, the individual becomes aware of the contrast between the feeling of tension and the feeling of relaxation. Then the individual relaxes one muscle group at a time in a systematic order from foot to head or head to foot. Gradually, the entire body is relaxed progressively. With careful and dedicated practice, one can be taught to recognize the most minute contractions and learn to avoid them, thus achieving the deepest degree of relaxation possible (Jacobson, 1938).

The Relaxation Response.   One of the most recent developments in the field of relaxation is the *relaxation response* as discovered and publicized by Dr. Herbert Benson (1980) of the Harvard Medical School. Based upon age-old techniques which have been practiced for thousands of years by numerous cultures and cults, Benson identifies four basic components necessary to bring forth the relaxation response:

1. A *quiet environment*. This will allow one to "turn off" both internal stimuli and external distractions, and can be likened to a mental and emotional decompression chamber.
2. A *mental device*, or an object to dwell on. This should be a constant stimulus. It may involve word repetition (e.g., *relax* or *stretch*); gazing at an object (e.g., mentally trying to reach for one's toes); or concentrating on a particular feeling (e.g., letting the muscles ooze out or feeling the connective tissue untwining).
3. A *passive attitude*. In the opinion of Benson, "this appears to be the most essential factor in eliciting the relaxation response" (p. 111) and is accomplished by emptying all thoughts and distractions from one's mind.
4. A *comfortable position*. The purpose of a comfortable posture is to eliminate any "undue muscular tension" (p. 161) and allow one to remain in the same position for an extended period of time.

Breathing and Imagery.   *Breathing* may be defined as the voluntary or involuntary act of taking air into the lungs and letting it out again. Normal breathing goes through four phases which include:

1. Exhalation or expiration, which results in the emptying of the lungs
2. A suspension of breathing after exhalation when the lungs are relatively empty
3. Inhalation or inspiration, which results in the filling of the lungs
4. A brief period of retention or holding the breath

In summary, the phases of a relaxed breathing rhythm are a tension-reducing, long, slow exhalation, followed by a slight pause of relaxed, relative emptiness until the need for oxygen finally prompts a passive inhalation, followed by another brief pause.

Controlled breathing not only facilitates relaxation, it can also enhance stretching. As explained by Jencks (1977), the appropriate breathing phases coupled with *imagination*—that is, the ability to envision results in vivid images—can be extremely effective in achieving desired outcomes. For example, if the desired effect is a lengthening of the connective tissues and a detaching of the muscle cross-bridges, imagery should be timed to coincide respectively with inhalations and exhalations.

How, then, should breathing, imagery, and stretching be combined to optimize the development of flexibility? First, it must be understood that flexibility is enhanced by exhalation. Second, one must couple the exhalation with the imagery. Third, flexibility must be developed through a slow and static stretch. The following is an example.

Slowly enter into the desired stretch position. When tension or resistance is encountered, stretch very slowly into an intermediate position. Hold this position for a few breathing cycles and adjust to it, especially during the relaxing exhalations. At this point, the stretch should feel good. Then, during subsequent exhalations, stretch a little more until tension or resistance is felt again. During this developmental stretch, exhale through the nose, visualize yourself lengthening further, and proceed to stretch a little again until tension or resistance is felt. Remember, the imagery must be as vivid and detailed as possible. If the strain becomes too great, ease off slightly. Do not forget that your purpose is to stretch while inducing a relaxed state in the mind and muscles. If properly performed, this stretching of the desired tissues will take approximately one minute.

Summary

Muscular relaxation can be induced or facilitated by: (a) using special stretching methodologies (i.e., static or PNF); (b) using special modalities, drugs, or aids (e.g., heat, cold, massage, analgesic rubs, and muscle relaxant drugs); and (c) incorporating the use of mind-over-body techniques (e.g., biofeedback, progressive relaxation, relaxation response, or breathing and imagery). Various factors should be considered before deciding which is the most effective, efficient, and safe means to achieve the desired goal.

Relaxation, or the absence of muscular tension, must exist before stretching is begun. Reduced internal tension can aid in effectively and efficiently stretching out connective tissues, which truly limit extensibility.

Review Questions

1. Explain how a lecture on the topic of relaxation to laypersons would differ from a lecture on the same topic to athletes.

2. Explain why relaxation is essential for the optimal development of flexibility.

3. Explain three methods of static stretching that will facilitate relaxation and a reduction of tension.

4. You are an athletic trainer. Explain under what conditions you would use cryotherapy instead of heat to facilitate relaxation during therapeutic stretching.

5. You are the coach of a high school varsity athletic team. Explain to your athletes the potential dangers of taking drugs to facilitate relaxation.

6. You are an instructor for a progressive relaxation class. Prepare a five-minute tape recording that incorporates proper directions to achieve a state of relaxation.

7. According to Benson, what four elements are necessary to bring forth a relaxation response?

8. Describe the proper integration of breathing and imagery techniques to enhance relaxation when stretching for a split.

Answers

1. A lecture on relaxation to housewives would deal with feeling good, attempting to reduce fatigue, and reducing the chance of developing excessive muscle stiffness. For the athlete, the lecture would include all of this as well as discussion of the enhancement of human performance.

2. With reduced "internal tension" the individual can most effectively and efficiently work on stretching out the connective tissue, which truly limits extensibility.

3. Static stretching can facilitate relaxation and a reduction of tension via (a) adaptation of the muscle spindles, (b) initiation of the autogenic inhibition reflex, and (c) by the development of creep and stress relaxation.

4. Cryotherapy should be used (a) when the therapeutic goal is to tear connective tissue rather than stretch it; (b) when without cold-induced analgesia, no range of motion therapy could be attempted due to the pain; or (c) when muscle spasticity significantly interferes with the proper range of motion therapy.

5. There are numerous potentially negative side effects associated with some drugs. These are not only possibly dangerous, they might also substantially interfere with level of performance.

6. Play the tape for an individual or group and get some feedback on it.

7. The four requisites for Benson's relaxation response are: (a) a quiet environment, (b) a

mental device, (c) a passive attitude, and (d) a comfortable position.

8. Lower to a modified split position. Visualize your connective tissues oozing out and the muscle cross-bridges slowly detaching themselves. At the same time, exhale and hold the stretch position. Continue to see yourself effortlessly holding the split position. As you sense tension, pause and hold the stretch. Take a few light breaths without allowing your lungs to lift up the upper trunk. When the tension subsides, exhale and allow the weight of your upper torso to apply an additional stretch until tension is felt once again. Then repeat the process.

Recommended Readings

Jacobson, E. (1978). *You must relax* (5th ed.). New York: McGraw-Hill.

Maltz, M. (1970). *Psycho-cybernetics*. New York: Simon & Schuster.

CHAPTER 10

Muscular Soreness: Its Etiology and Consequences

Exercise and stretching may result in varying degrees of discomfort, soreness, stiffness, or pain of two general kinds: that which occurs during and immediately after the exercise or stretching and which may persist for several hours, and that which usually does not appear until 24 to 48 hours later.

There are four basic hypotheses that attempt to explain the nature of muscular soreness:

1. The torn tissue hypothesis
2. The connective tissue damage hypothesis
3. The osmotic pressure or metabolic accumulation-swelling hypothesis
4. The localized spasm of motor units hypothesis

Although these hypotheses will be reviewed separately, this does not mean that they cannot occur together or that there are no other possible causes for muscular soreness.

The Torn Tissue and Connective Tissue Damage Hypotheses

All tissues have elastic limits beyond which intrinsic damage can occur. When a tissue is stretched beyond certain limits, the injury is known as a *sprain* for collagenous tissues, or a *strain* for muscle tissue. Sprains and strains may vary in degree from mild to severe. In mild cases there may be only a little hemorrhage with disruption of a few fibers and a mild inflammatory reaction, whereas in severe instances there can be considerable intra-muscular hemorrhage with partial or complete tear of the muscle and its connective tissue.

Etiology

Hough (1902) first suggested that muscular soreness results from the microscopic tearing of muscle fibers and/or connective tissues. However, de Vries (1961a, 1961b, 1962, 1966) was originally of the opinion that this probably occurs much less frequently than is thought by athletes, coaches, and laypersons. He argued that this is not a plausible explanation for muscle soreness because ''it is somewhat illogical to postulate that a tissue has been structurally damaged by the very function for which it is specifically differentiated'' (p. 119). Nonetheless, de Vries reminds us that some types of activity are more likely to result in sore muscles than others. Among these are:

1. Vigorous contractions while the muscle is in a shortened position.
2. Muscle contractions involving jerky or uncoordinated movements. In this case, some fibers in the muscle may be temporarily overloaded when a full load is placed on the muscle before a sufficient number of motor units has been recruited.
3. Activity involving repetition of the same movement over a long period of time.
4. Bouncing movements, because at the end of a ballistic motion, the movement is stopped by the muscle and its connective tissues, bringing about reflex contractions at the same time the muscle is being forcefully elongated.

Another explanation of the etiology might relate to the nature of the tension that develops in the tissues during elongation or stretching. When a muscle contracts *concentrically*, the fibers shorten and *positive* work is performed. As the muscle continually shortens, its tension decreases. This compels a greater number of fibers to take part in the contraction and reduces the pull exerted by individual muscle fibers and its connective tissue. The workload is thus shared by a greater mass of cellular components and each is spared excessive stress and tension so that the tissues escape injury.

During elongation of a muscle, individual muscle fibers are capable of contracting. This is called an *eccentric* contraction and produces *negative* work. As in concentric contractions, eccentric contractions produce tension that is transmitted via connective tissues. However, during eccentric contractions muscle fibers lengthen and the number of participating fibers decreases (see Figure 10.1). Since the workload is shared by a smaller number of cellular components, the tension increases. Consequently, the excessive pull (i.e., tension) traumatizes the connective tissue (Asmussen, 1956). Recently several studies (Fridén, Sjöstrom, and Ekblom, 1981; Fridén, 1984; Newham, McPhail, Mills, & Edwards, 1983; Newham, Mills, Quigley, & Edwards, 1983) actually published photographs showing some mechanical disruption of the Z-lines. Their findings indicated that the Z-lines during overloading constitute a potential weak link in the myofibrillar contractile chain. However, they noted that the structural disturbances may also be secondary, resulting from an activation of lysosomal enzymes, bringing about a concomitant inflation. Other researchers such as Abraham (1977, 1979) and Tullson and Armstrong (1968, 1981) also provide additional support for the relationship between muscle soreness and connective tissue irritation or damage. This, too, is based on the idea that the connective tissues are damaged with eccentric contraction due to greater tension (Sutton, 1983).

A popular explanation is that the degree of muscular pain, soreness, or stiffness corresponds to the state of training of the tissues involved. That is, nonexercised and tight persons usually show a markedly higher reactivity when subjected to a variety of physical stresses. Consequently, fibers and connective tissues are more susceptible to strain and rupture. Thus it can be claimed that "stiffness is a disease of the unfit" (Williams & Sperryn, 1976, p. 301).

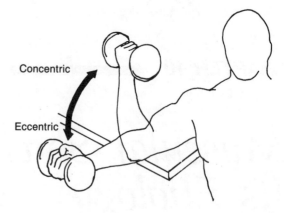

Figure 10.1. Concentric and eccentric contractions. Muscle shortens during concentric contractions and lengthens during eccentric contractions.

Yet another explanation is that of the long-held popular opinion of coaches and athletes that muscle soreness results from failing to warm up before exercising or stretching. According to Mellerowicz and Hansen (1971) poor blood circulation and cold muscles or tendons have a greater tendency to result in strains and ruptures. However, there is currently very little experimental evidence to support this theory. An obvious explanation (de Vries, 1966) is that probably no researcher cares to set up an experiment in which the subjects may be injured. Nonetheless, all that is known of muscle physiology tends to support the need for warm-up as a prudent protective measure.

The Inflammatory Response and Consequences

The initial biologic response in virtually all injuries is inflammation. *Inflammation* is a vascular and cellular response that serves to promote the recovery of damaged tissues. The degree of inflammation present is proportional to the amount or degree of tissue damage. In turn, the extent of damage depends on the amount of force applied to the fibers involved.

The changes in the tissues which constitute inflammation are complicated but predictable. The initial stages of inflammation are characterized by vascular changes. Immediately following injury, there occurs a temporary constriction of the local vasculature lasting five to ten minutes. The vasoconstriction is followed by active vasodilation of all local small vessels and by increased blood flow.

Simultaneously with vasodilation, increased permeability occurs at the level of the small venules. The increased vascular permeability appears to be the result of changes in the venule wall. The vascular changes are thought to be mediated by substances released at the injury site. The most notable substance is *histamine*, which is known to cause vasodilation and increased small-vessel permeability. The increased blood vessel permeability facilitates the removal of cellular debris and injured tissue fragments, an essential part of the injury healing stage. It also allows the passage of plasma proteins into the affected tissues. This may become an important asset to the defense of the tissues. In addition, the blood may also possess a number of antimicrobial substances as well as nutrients vital to the repair of damaged cells.

It is during this time that tissues exhibit the symptoms and signs of warmth, redness, swelling, pain, and loss of function. The increased blood flow to the region causes the warmth and redness. Swelling is a result of the outpouring of fluid into the tissue. Pain is either from direct stimulation of nerve fibers by chemical substances of the damaged cells or from the swelling itself.

During the next stages, scar tissue (sometimes referred to as adhesions) is produced. Scar is an enlarged, dense structure of collagen, whose fibers are randomly oriented. Over a period of time the scar remodels, for example, microscopically the weave or architecture of the collagen fibers change to a more organized pattern. If the damage is relatively severe, there may be considerable scarring. The extent to which a scar remodels varies among individuals and also within the same individual depending on age at the time of injury. Ultimately, the strength and plastic characteristics of scar tissue depends on the formation and density of intermolecular covalent bonds and the orientation and weave of the individual collagen fibers.

Although scarring represents the lesser evil as opposed to having an open or unhealed injury, it also presents potential problems. This is most evident when scarring is extensive as with a severe strain or rupture. In addressing this problem, it must be recognized that muscle regains strength slowly, and the rate for tendon injuries is even slower. In spite of prolonged strength gains, some injuries rarely, if ever, regain their full strength. In addition, strength is not the only important physical parameter of scars. Normal elasticity, so important in tissue function, is lost in scars, which often convert an elastic, pliable tissue to an inelastic, brittle mass (Sabiston, 1972). As Klafs and Arnheim (1977) point out, scarring can produce far more serious consequences for some people, especially athletes, because strains have a tendency to recur due to the already brittle nature of scar tissue. Furthermore, the higher the incidence of strains at a particular muscle site, the greater the amount of scar tissue that is present, and the greater the potential for recurrent injuries. Then, worse yet, the fear of another "pull" may become for some individuals an almost neurotic obsession more handicapping than the injury itself.

Stretching and Scar Tissue

Can stretching affect the remodeling of damaged (scar) tissue? Current hypothesis suggests that exercise can decrease the number of collagen cross-links by increasing the collagen turnover rate (Shephard, 1982). If you recall, the strength of collagen and scar tissue appears to be in part the result of the intramolecular cross-linking between the $alpha_1$ and $alpha_2$ chains of the collagen molecule and the intermolecular cross-linking between the collagen fibrils, filaments, and fibers. Bryant speculates (1977) that modifications of adhesions and scars are probably related to the development or dissolution of cross-links between collagen units. This is a collagen turnover—a continuous and simultaneous collagen production and breakdown. If the rate of breakdown exceeds production, the scar becomes softer and less bulky. If, on the other hand, the rate of production exceeds breakdown, the opposite occurs (debilitating adhesions and scars are thought to be shorter and more compactly organized). Thus if in fact exercise can decrease the number of collagen cross-links by increasing the collagen turnover rate, stretching could possibly determine the ultimate degree of extensibility and elasticity of the remodeled tissues.

However, stretching scar tissue can also be dangerous, because it might tear the vascular bed and result in more bleeding. Consequently, inflammation will increase and rehabilitation will be prolonged. Furthermore, inflammation may result in pain and muscle spasms, thus limiting range of motion (Burkhardt, 1982). At such times, the new collagen has not yet matured with cross-linkages, increased collagen content, or increased fiber diameter, and is thus susceptible to new injury (Booth & Gould, 1975; Ciullo & Zarins, 1983).

The Metabolic Accumulation or Osmotic Pressure and Swelling Hypothesis

One of the more popular explanations of immediate muscle soreness is the accumulation of waste products, especially lactic acid (Committee on the Medical Aspects of Sports of the American Medical Association and the National Federation, 1975; Karpovich & Sinning, 1971; Morehouse & Miller, 1971). Another explanation (Committee on Medical Aspects, 1975) is that the pain is due to the outward passage of potassium across the muscle cell membrane into the tissue space. However, the soreness soon dissipates after the exercise.

There are similar explanations for delayed muscle soreness. These range from the accumulation of lactic acid, to an excessive accumulation of metabolites that causes an increased osmotic pressure inside and outside muscle fibers, to retained excess water causing edema and pressure on sensory nerves (Asmussen, 1956; Karpovich & Sinning, 1971). Yet another explanation is that the swelling of the muscle causes it to become shorter, thicker, and more resistant to stretching. This gives rise to a sensation of stiffness when the muscle is stretched during the contraction of the antagonistic muscles (Morehouse & Miller, 1971).

However, there are several problems with these explanations. Muscle soreness is greater after exercise consisting of eccentric work as opposed to concentric work. But the metabolism of eccentric work is five to seven times smaller than concentric work. Consequently, a greater quantity of lactic acid and metabolites results from concentric work. Furthermore, studies by Schwane, Johnson, Vandenakker, & Armstrong (1981) and Watrous, Armstrong, and Schwane (1981) indicate that lactic acid is not a cause of delayed soreness. Nonetheless, stretching and cool-down after exercise is strongly encouraged to allow the muscles time to promote the removal of accumulated waste products.

The Localized Spasm of Motor Units Hypothesis

As postulated in numerous works by de Vries (1961a, 1961b, 1962, 1966), the delayed localized soreness that occurs after unaccustomed exercise is caused by tonic, localized spasm of motor units whose number varies with the severity of pain. Accordingly:

1. Exercise above a minimal level causes some degree of ischemia (i.e., temporary lack of blood supply) in active muscle.
2. Ischemia causes muscle pain. This pain probably occurs by means of the transfer of P-substance across the muscle cell membrane into the tissue fluid from which it gains access to pain endings.
3. Consequently, the resulting pain brings about a protective, reflex, tonic muscle contraction.
4. Then, the tonic contraction brings about localized areas of ischemia in the muscle tissue and a vicious cycle is born, which results in a local, tonic muscle spasm.

By using specially developed electromyographic equipment, muscular pain has been demonstrated quantitatively by de Vries. That is, EMG found a positive relationship between the severity of accidentally induced pain and the level of muscular electrical activity. More important, de Vries found static stretching to furnish symptomatic relief and also to cause a significant decrease in the electrical activity of the hurting muscles. The GTO may be the basis for this phenomenon. Thus de Vries contends that we may assume some degree of control over the soreness phenomenon, both as to prevention and relief.

However, when Abraham (1977) attempted to duplicate the EMG experiments of de Vries, he was unable to find significant EMG changes as a result of induced muscle soreness. This discrepancy, though, was probably related to the choice of recording electrodes (de Vries, 1980; Francis, 1983). Nonetheless, Francis contends that the spasm theory of delayed muscle soreness is not considered as favorable as the torn tissue and connective tissue damage proposals.

Summary

Two types of muscle soreness sometimes develop after exercise: immediate soreness and delayed localized soreness, which does not appear for 24 to 48 hours after activity. Currently, muscular soreness is explained by four possible mechanisms that may work together or independently of one another: the torn tissue hypothesis, the connective tissue damage hypothesis, the osmotic pressure or metabolic accumulation-swelling hypothesis, and the localized spasm of motor units hypothesis. Regardless of the causes, all that is known of muscle physiology tends to support the need for warm-up, cool-down, and stretching as prudent protective measures.

Review Questions

1. Identify two categories of muscular soreness.

2. Explain why eccentric contractions are associated with an increased likelihood of postexercise soreness.

3. Describe a running program that would most likely induce muscular soreness via accentuating eccentric contractions in the lower limbs.

4. Explain the statement, ''Inflammation is a necessary evil.''

5. Explain how stretching is hypothesized to affect the remodeling of damaged (scar) tissue.

6. Explain the potential risks associated with overzealous stretching during rehabilitation of a pulled hamstring.

7. Given that lactic acid can be produced only in the absence of oxygen, explain how its production can be reduced by training.

8. Explain the localized spasm of motor units hypothesis.

9. Given that you are an athletic trainer, what is the most prudent protective measure to take to help reduce or eliminate the possibility of muscular soreness as a result of exercise?

10. Given that you are an athletic trainer, prescribe measures to help reduce or eliminate muscular soreness as a result of exercise. State specific treatments and dosages where appropriate.

Answers

1. There exist two categories of muscular soreness: (a) that which occurs during and immediately after exercise, and which may persist for several hours, and (b) that which usually does not appear until 24 to 48 hours later (i.e., delayed muscle soreness).

2. Eccentric contractions are associated with an increased likelihood of postexercise soreness because there is a greater amount of mechanical trauma caused by the high tension generated in relatively few active fibers.

3. A common running program that would most likely induce muscular soreness via accentuating eccentric contractions in the lower limbs is one in which athletes run down the aisles of a gymnasium or stadium. This will commonly result with the complaint of shinsplints in the following days.

4. Inflammation is a necessary evil because it serves to promote the recovery of damaged tissues.

5. Stretching is hypothesized to affect the remodeling of damaged tissue by decreasing the number of collagen cross-links and by increasing the collagen turnover rate.

6. Several of the associated risks with overzealous stretching during rehabilitation of a pulled hamstring are: (a) it might result in more bleeding, (b) it might prolong the rehabilitation time, (c) it might induce more pain, (d) it might lead to the production of muscle spasms, and (e) it might damage the new, not yet matured cross-links.

7. Lactic acid production can be reduced by emphasizing training that will develop the cardiorespiratory system and local muscular endurance.

8. The localized spasm of motor units is hypothesized to work as follows: (a) exercise above a minimal level causes some degree of ischemia; (b) ischemia causes pain; (c) the pain brings about a protective, reflex, tonic muscle contraction; and (d) the tonic contraction results in more ischemia and the cycle is repeated.

9. The most prudent protective measure to take to help reduce or eliminate the possibility of muscular soreness as a result of exercise is to incorporate a well-rounded conditioning program.

10. Treatment and dosages will vary according to individual cases. Conservative treatment might include: (a) cryotherapy, (b) massage, (c) whirlpool, (d) medication, and (e) rest.

Recommended Readings

de Vries, H.A. (1980). *Physiology of exercise for physical education and athletics* (3rd ed.). Dubuque, Iowa: Wm. C. Brown Company.

Talag, T.S. (1973). Residual muscular soreness as influenced by concentric, eccentric, and static contractions. *Research Quarterly, 44*(4), 458-469.

CHAPTER 11 ━━━━━━━━━━━━━━━━━

Types and Varieties of Stretching

Coaches of sports and teachers of dance, yoga, and other highly specialized activities have long recognized the need for more than normal flexibility in certain joints or groups of joints. To help the participants under their direction achieve these flexibilities, they have developed special stretching exercises and drills, which can be broadly classified into two categories: ballistic and static.

Traditional Classifications

Ballistic stretching is usually associated with bobbing, bouncing, rebounding, and rhythmic motion. Often the terms *isotonic, dynamic, kinetic,* or *fast stretching* are used to refer to this kind of movement. In contrast, *static* stretching involves the use of a position that is held, and which may or may not be repeated. Static stretching is often associated with isometric, controlled, or slow stretch.

Regardless of the method employed, the possibility of overstretching is dependent upon a variety of factors, including (a) the amount, or intensity, of stretch; (b) the duration of the stretch; (c) the number, or frequency, of movements performed in a given period; and (d) the velocity, or nature, of the stretch.

One of the most controversial topics in sports science is the relative value of static versus ballistic stretching programs for developing flexibility. The controversy is complicated by the lack of research on ballistic flexibility. Ballistic stretching is difficult to assess because of the need for elaborate equipment and technical expertise in measuring the force that is required to move the joint through its range of motion at both fast and slow speeds (Stamford, 1984). What can be stated is that there is a considerable amount of research

indicating that both ballistic and static methods are effective in developing flexibility (Corbin & Noble, 1980; Logan & Egstrom, 1961; Sady, Wortman, & Blanke, 1982; Stamford, 1984).

Arguments Supporting Ballistic Stretching

One of the practical advantages of ballistic stretching is its use during team stretching and warm-up, for it can be easily practiced in unison to a beat or cadence, thus promoting team camaraderie and togetherness. Ballistic stretching also helps to develop dynamic flexibility. Because most activities and movements are ballistic in nature, fast stretching would be appropriate in terms of specificity of training and warm-up. Finally, ballistic stretching can be less boring than static stretching; and, as indicated earlier, research has in fact demonstrated that it is effective in developing flexibility.

Arguments Against Ballistic Stretching

There are four major arguments against ballistic stretching. These arguments involve the following issues: (a) tissue adaptation; (b) soreness resulting from injury; (c) initiation of the stretch reflex; and (d) neurological adaptation.

When muscle and its supporting connective tissues are rapidly stretched, they are not given adequate time to adapt. If you recall, all living tissues are characterized by the presence of time-dependent mechanical properties, including stress-relaxation and creep. If tissues are stretched too rapidly, lasting flexibility cannot be optimally developed. Remember, research has demonstrated that permanent lengthening is most favored by lower force, longer duration stretching at elevated temperatures (Laban, 1962; Light, Nuzik, Personius, & Barstrom, 1984; Warren, Lehmann, & Koblanski, 1971, 1976).

A logical extension of the first argument (concerning tissue adaptation) is the hypothesis that ballistic stretching can result in soreness or injury. Obviously, if a tissue is stretched too fast, it can be strained or ruptured. In either event, the result is pain and/or impairment of ROM. As an example, imagine a 6-inch rubber band rapidly stretched to a length of 10 to 12 inches. Under those conditions, and at such a length, the rubber band will probably break. However, if the rubber band is *slowly* stretched through the same range of movement, it is less likely to tear. The mechanical reason for this is that the rubber band is *not required to absorb the same amount of energy/force per unit of time.* All tissues, if continually stretched, regardless of velocity, will ultimately reach a point of rupture.

Another reason why ballistic stretching should be avoided is that it generates rather large and uncontrollable amounts of angular momentum. This is a direct result of a high moment of inertia coupled with a high angular velocity ($A = I\omega$). Such movements are commonly seen when swinging the arms horizontally in an extended position. Consequently, when the movement reaches its limit and suddenly stops, the angular momentum can often exceed the absorbing capacity of the tissues being stretched.

A third argument against ballistic stretching concerns the stretch reflex. If a sudden stretch is applied to a muscle, a reflex action is set into motion that causes the muscles to contract. As a result, muscular tension will increase, making it more difficult to stretch out the connective tissues. Consequently, this defeats the very purpose of the procedure. For stretching to be most effective, the contractile elements of the muscle must be totally relaxed.

Finally, it can be argued that ballistic stretching does not allow adequate time for neurological adaptation to take place. For example, Walker (1961) found that the amount of tension for a given amount of stretch is more than doubled by a quick stretch as compared to a slow stretch. Similarly, Granit (1962) reported that a pull on a muscle with a given force produced an efferent impulse frequency of more than 100 impulses per second within one second. However, with a slower increase in stretch, until the same force was applied, a peak volley of about 40 impulses/second was produced within six seconds.

Arguments Supporting Static Stretching

There appears to be general agreement that static or slow stretching is preferable to ballistic stretching. Static stretching has been used for centuries by those involved in Hatha Yoga. Furthermore, some argue that static stretching is required for the optimal development of static flexibility (i.e., specificity of training). According to de Vries (1966, 1980), static stretching is preferable because: (a) it requires less energy expenditure than the ballistic method; (b) it will probably result in less muscle soreness; and (c) it can provide more qualitative relief from muscular distress.

Arguments Against Static Stretching

The arguments against static stretching are generally rather weak. Some claim that static stretching is boring. However, the most persuasive argument against static stretching is that it may be practiced exclusively, and at the expense of ballistic exercise (Schultz, 1979). Needless to say, an optimal blending of both stretching methods is the solution to this problem (Corbin & Noble, 1980; Dick, 1980; Schultz, 1979; Stamford, 1984).

Additional Classifications

In addition to these two kinds of stretching, there is a third way to categorize stretching based upon the concept of who or what develops and is responsible for the range of motion. The range of motion of a stretch can be separated into four categories in this way: passive, passive-active, active-assisted, and active.

Passive Stretching

In *passive* stretching, as the name implies the individual makes no contribution or active contraction. Rather, the motion is performed by an outside agent responsible for the stretch. This agent may be either a partner or special equipment such as traction (see Figure 11.1a).

With this technique, forced motion restores the normal ROM when it is limited by the loss of soft tissue extensibility. Its effect on muscle is to lengthen the elastic portion passively. The greater length will then allow greater range of motion of the affected joints. Passive stretching is indicated either because the agonist, or prime mover, is too weak to respond, or because attempts to inhibit the antagonist are unsuccessful.

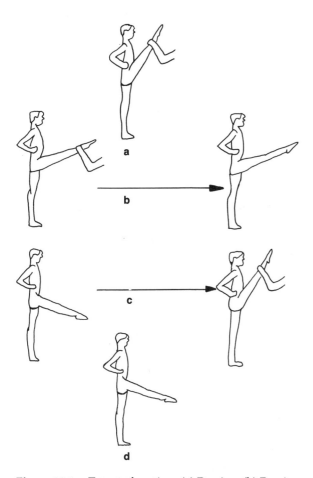

Figure 11.1. Types of motion. (a) Passive. (b) Passive-active. (c) Active-assisted. (d) Active.

According to Dowsing (1978) and Olcott (1980), passive stretching with partners provides several additional benefits:

1. Teammates counting for each other ensure that repetitions are completed. Furthermore, the individual tries harder to complete the repetitions because the partner is always watching.
2. The coach is free to walk around and help with corrections. Once a correction is made, that partner can help future partners avoid the same mistakes.
3. A greater feeling of progress exists when partners can recognize improvement in others and let them know it.
4. Partner exercises tend to promote the teammates' concern for one other.
5. Tandem exercises are more enjoyable.

However, when implementing partner flexibility exercises, both partners need to be totally familiar with each exercise. Because each partner is work-

ing the other's body, each must listen to the other's signal of when to stop and hold the stretch. Obviously, just one mistake by a partner can wipe out all the benefits of a flexibility training program.

However, passive stretching may not be the optimal technique in treating tightness (Cherry, 1980) or in attempting to regain muscular range of motion, especially after injury (Jacobs, 1976). According to Jacobs, there appear to be at least four reasons why passive stretching is contraindicated:

1. Extreme stretch could cause the GTOs to fire.
2. Passive stretching could be painful.
3. There would be no retention of flexibility because the muscular imbalance would not be eradicated by the tendon organ's short-lived inhibitory message. Consequently, there would be no motor learning and no improvement in the capacity for active motion of the tight muscle or its opponent.
4. If passive stretching occurs too rapidly, the muscle spindle complex would be activated, and the resultant stretch reflex would initiate contraction of the muscle, thus defeating the very purpose of the procedure.

Passive-Active Stretching

Passive-active stretching is only slightly different from passive stretching. Initially, the stretch is accomplished by some outside force. Then the individual attempts to hold the position by contracting the muscles isometrically for several seconds (see Figure 11.1b). This approach strengthens the weak, overstretched agonist opposing the tight muscle.

Active-Assisted Stretching

Active-assisted stretching is accomplished by the initial active contraction of the opposing groups of muscles. When the limit of one's ability is reached, the range of motion is then completed by the partner (see Figure 11.1c). The advantage of this method is that it can activate or strengthen the weak, overstretched agonist opposing the tight muscle and help to establish the pattern for coordinated motion.

Active Stretching

Active stretching is accomplished by the activities of one's muscles without aid (see Figure 11.1d).

Research by Iashvili (1983) has verified that: (a) active flexibility values are lower than passive ones, and (b) active flexibility has a higher correlation to the level of sports achievement ($r = 0.81$) than does passive mobility ($r = 0.69$). In addition, Iashvili also found that when using stretching exercises primarily, the coefficient of correlation between active and passive movements varies within the limits 0.61 to 0.73. However, when using strength and combined exercises, the coefficient of correlation increases to 0.91. Therefore, it can be concluded that the relationship between passive and active flexibility is dependent on the training methods (Hardy, 1985; Iashvili, 1983; Tumanyan & Dzhanyan, 1984).

Total range of motion is the combination of active and passive ranges of motion (see Figure 11.1c). If passive stretching exercises are used to develop flexibility, then mainly passive flexibility will be developed. Consequently, there is a reduction of the passive inadequacy zone. However, the greater the difference between the range of active and passive movement in a joint, the greater is the likelihood of an injury (Iashvili, 1983). To avoid such risks, strength exercises in the active inadequacy zone are recommended. Consequently, this will reduce the passive inadequacy and increase the zone of active mobility (see Figure 11.2).

In a recent study Tumanyan and Dzhanyan (1984) compared four training methods. Their study yielded the following results:

1. The control group showed no changes in active or passive flexibility.
2. The second group, which used stretching exercises alone, increased approximately the same amount in active and passive flexi-

bility. However, the difference between the groups remained unchanged.
3. The third group, which used strength exercises alone, increased only in active flexibility.
4. The fourth group, which used both strength and stretching exercises, had the greatest gain in active flexibility. Consequently, the difference between passive and active flexibility decreased.

If active stretching increases active range of motion, does the duration of isometric contraction also affect flexibility? A study by Hardy (1985) found that it did. Larger gains in active flexibility were associated with longer periods of isometric contraction in the active group.

Active stretching can be either ballistic or static. According to Matveyev (1981), ballistic exercises should be performed in series, with a gradual increase of the swing of the movements to maximum. The number of repetitions in a series usually ranges from 8 to 12. Repetitions should cease when amplitude of the movements decreases due to fatigue. Well-trained athletes may perform as many as 40 or more repetitions with maximum amplitude. Static stretching is characterized by a gradual increase in holding time—from a few to dozens of seconds.

Although both active and passive exercises contribute to the improvement of flexibility, their effects upon active and passive flexibility are different. When should one type of exercise be preferred over another? To answer this question, we must start from a point that has already been made. Obviously, passive stretching should be the preference when the elasticity of the muscles to be stretched restricts flexibility; but active stretching should be the preference when the low strength level of those muscles causing the movement restricts flexibility. Therefore, one should know the elasticity of the former and the strength of the latter at the joints in question (Pechtl, 1982).

Proprioceptive Neuromuscular Facilitation (PNF)

Proprioceptive neuromuscular facilitation (PNF) may be defined as a method "promoting or hastening the neuromuscular mechanism through stimulation of the proprioceptors" (Knott & Voss, 1968). PNF was originally formulated and developed as a physical therapy procedure for the rehabilitation of patients. Today, some PNF techniques are used

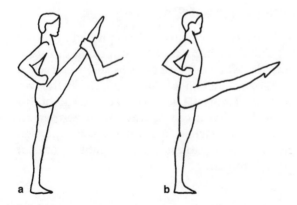

Figure 11.2. Flexibility zones. (a) Zone of passive inadequacy (30 degrees). Zone of passive adequacy (150 degrees). (b) Zone of active inadequacy (80 degrees). Zone of active adequacy (100 degrees).

as new and more advanced methods to develop flexibility.

The Neurophysiological Basis of PNF

PNF is based on several important neurophysiological mechanisms, including facilitation and inhibition, resistance, irradiation, successive induction, and reflexes. *Facilitation* or *faciliatory* actions are those that increase neuron excitability. Examples of faciliatory PNF are any stimuli that decrease the threshold of motorneurons or cause the recruitment of additional motorneurons. In contrast, *inhibitory* PNF actions are those that decrease excitability. That is, they initiate any stimuli that raise the threshold of motorneurons or result in a drop in the number of actively discharging motoneurons (Harris, 1978; Knott & Voss, 1968; Prentice, 1983). Although inhibition is thus the opposite of facilitation, they are inseparable from one another: A technique which promotes facilitation of the agonist, or prime mover, simultaneously promotes relaxation or inhibition of the antagonist, that is, the muscle components with patterns of action exactly opposite those of the agonistic pattern. Thus there is an overlapping effect (Knott & Voss, 1968).

Facilitation and inhibition are produced predominantly by muscular *resistance* (i.e., active contractions). *Maximal resistance* may be defined as the greatest amount of resistance that can be applied to an isotonic or active contraction allowing full range of motion to occur (Knott & Voss, 1968). Maximal resistance provides the means of securing overflow or *irradiation* from more adequate to less adequate patterns of movement. Thus irradiation may be defined as the spread of excitation in the central nervous system that causes contraction of synergist muscles in a specific pattern (Holt, ND; Surburg, 1981). This is commonly achieved via *successive induction* or the contraction of an agonist muscle immediately followed by the activation of an antagonistic muscle (Holt, ND; Surburg, 1981).

The effectiveness of PNF techniques also involves the stretch reflex. As was discussed in chapter 5, the stretch reflex involves two types of receptors: muscle spindles, which are sensitive to a change in length as well as to the rate of change in length of the muscle fiber, and Golgi tendon organs (GTOs), which detect changes in tension. Both receptors help cause muscles to relax under specific conditions.

An isometric contraction of a muscle placed on a slight stretch is followed by relaxation stemming from the autogenic inhibition (Cornelius, 1981; Cornelius & Hinson, 1980; Holt, ND; Prentice, 1983; Tanigawa, 1972). According to Ruch and Patton (1965), autogenic inhibition is "inhibition which is mediated by afferent fibers from a stretched muscle and acting on the alpha motorneurons supplying that muscle, thus causing it to relax" (p. 196). In other words, the muscle being stretched is inhibited and caused to relax. It is hypothesized that the GTOs are involved in this inhibition.

According to several investigators (Åstrand & Rodahl, 1978; Houk & Hennemann, 1967; Moore, 1984), the GTOs are sensitive to both stretch and contraction. During a maximal isometric contraction with the muscles (i.e., the antagonist) in their lengthened range, the combined tension produced may stimulate the GTOs to fire and cause them to reflexively relax. However, another explanation of this relaxation phenomenon is that the isometric contractions somehow alter the manner in which the muscle spindles respond to stretching conditions by decreasing the afferent flow of impulses from these proprioceptors (Holt, ND). Consequently, this decrease in muscle spindle firing would tend to enhance greater ROM by offering less resistance to stretch.

The second method to induce relaxation of the antagonistic muscles is through an isometric contraction of the agonistic muscles. This action facilitates relaxation through the reciprocal inhibition reflex. Thus when motorneurons of the agonist muscle receive excitatory impulses from afferent nerves, the motorneurons that supply the antagonist muscles are inhibited by the afferent impulses (e.g., if the quadriceps contract, the hamstrings must relax).

Advantages and Benefits of PNF Techniques

Those who endorse PNF techniques claim they offer a wider range of advantages and benefits. The particular benefits will be dependent upon the technique employed. As far as ROM is concerned, research by numerous investigators (Moore & Hutton, 1980; Prentice, 1983; Sady, Wortman, & Blanke, 1982; Tanigawa, 1972) found that PNF techniques produced the largest gains. This effectiveness has also been claimed by others (Beaulieu, 1981; Cherry, 1980; Cornelius, 1983; Cornelius & Hinson, 1980; Hartley-O'Brien, 1980; Hatfield, 1982; Holt, Travis, & Okita, 1970; Sullivan, Markos, & Minor, 1982; Surburg, 1983). Among other potential benefits are greater strength, balance of strength, and stability about a joint (Cherry, 1980; Hatfield, 1982; Holt, ND; Knott & Voss, 1968; Sullivan et al. 1982; Surburg, 1981, 1983); improved endurance and blood circulation (Cailliet, 1981a; Knott & Voss, 1968; Sullivan et al. 1982; Surburg, 1981); enhanced coordination (Knott & Voss, 1968; Sullivan et al. 1982; Surburg, 1981); and superior relaxation of the muscles (Cherry, 1980; Holt, ND; Knott & Voss, 1968; Prentice, 1983; Sullivan et al. 1982; Tanigawa, 1972).

Lastly, proponents of certain PNF techniques claim that individuals afterwards experience a greater ease of passive motion. One explanation for this is that the voluntary contraction of the agonists (i.e., the muscles not being stretched) masks the discomfort arising from the stretch of the antagonists (i.e., the muscles being stretched) (Moore & Hutton, 1980). However, there is another possible explanation. During the initial isometric contraction of the muscle in its stretched state, *total tension* is the summation of the contractile component (CC) and the connective tissues. Therefore, the tension is maximal. However, when the muscle no longer contracts, it must relax. Then the only thing contributing to the tension is the connective tissue. As a result, actual tension must decline. Obviously, such reduction in tension will be perceived by the respective proprioceptors. In turn, the individual will sense a reduction of tension. Hence the perceived greater ease.

Arguments and Controversy Against PNF Techniques

Although PNF techniques offer many potential benefits, they also have disadvantages. For instance, Moore and Hutton (1980) found that certain PNF methods are uncomfortable and painful, and most methods require a well-motivated individual (Cornelius, 1983; Moore & Hutton, 1980). Furthermore, they are sometimes more dangerous than static stretching, because PNF stretching actually occurs with more tension in the muscle. PNF procedures therefore need to be more closely monitored if the chance of soft tissue injury is to be minimized. Furthermore, most PNF exercises are designed as partner stretches, and if done incorrectly, can cause injury (Beaulieu, 1981; Cornelius, 1983).

Another disadvantage of PNF techniques is the possibility of the *valsalva phenomenon*, which elevates systolic blood pressure and has obvious implications for hypertensive individuals (Cornelius, 1983; Knott & Voss, 1968). The valsalva phenomenon is defined as an expiratory effort against a closed glottis, and can occur during the performance of an isometric or heavy resistance exercise. The process begins with a deep inspiration followed by closure of the glottis and contraction of the abdominal muscles. Consequently, there is an increase in intrathoracic and intra-abdominal pressures which leads to decreased venous blood flow to the heart. This results in a decreased venous return, which leads to a decreased cardiac output followed by a temporary drop in arterial blood pressure and an increase in the heart rate. Then, when the expiratory effort is released and expiration occurs, an increase in blood pressure follows, which may reach levels of up to 200 mmHg or higher. Finally, there is a rapid venous blood flow into the heart and a subsequent forceful heart contraction.

Those with a history of coronary artery disease or high blood pressure should avoid the possibility of this phenomenon occurring. People in the former group may run an increased risk of cerebral vessel rupture (Jones, 1965). For those in the latter group there is the risk of increased ischemia. Another danger is herniation if a weakness or defect in a muscular or fascial layer of the abdominal wall is present (Jones, 1965). However, one recent review (Fardy, 1981) indicated that the risk of the valsalva phenomenon occurring during isometric exercise is less than has been presumed. Obviously, preventive measures should be incorporated into an exercise program to reduce any potential risks. These measures would include exhaling during heavy resistance exercise and breathing rhythmically during other exercises.

Finally, it should be noted that recent experiments by Eldred, Hutton, and Smith (1976) and Suzuki and Hutton (1976) are now challenging some of the ideas supporting the neurophysiological basis of PNF. Specifically, these studies have found that a static contraction preceding a muscle stretch facilitates contractile activity through a lingering afterdischarge of the same muscle. Furthermore, contrary to traditional views, it has been demonstrated that a muscle is initially more resistant to change in length after a static contraction (Smith, Hutton, & Eldred, 1976). Supposedly, this is because the GTOs are only momentarily depressed following sustained contractions of muscle on stretch.

PNF Techniques

PNF involves a variety of strategies and techniques that promote specific results. They may combine isotonic (i.e., concentric and eccentric) and isometric contractions in different combinations. The following descriptions of PNF techniques are based on the works of Knott and Voss (1968), Sullivan, Markos, and Minor (1982), and Surburg (1981).

Repeated Contractions (RC).   This technique involves repeated contractions until fatigue is evident in the performance of a specific motion. In the less advanced form of RC, only isotonic contractions are used. However, RC may be preceded by an isotonic contraction of the muscles of the stronger antagonistic pattern to facilitate the weakened musculature. The more advanced form of RC is initially performed against resistance with resultant overflow to a weak pivot action. Then, the individual is instructed to hold an isometric contraction to the point where active motion is felt to be lessening in power. When resistance is increased at the weakened pivot, the individual is instructed to pull again, and the isometric contraction becomes an isotonic one. RC helps to develop strength and endurance, and promotes ease of transmission of impulses through the central nervous system pathway (see Figure 11.3a).

Rhythmic Initiation (RI).   Rhythmic initiation involves voluntary relaxation, passive movement, and repeated isotonic contractions of the major components of the agonist pattern. With this technique, passive, active-assisted, active, and resistive exercises are progressively executed. RI is used to improve the ability to initiate movement (see Figure 11.3b).

Slow Reversal (SR).   Slow reversal involves an isotonic contraction of the antagonist, followed by an isotonic contraction of the agonist. This technique may be used to improve action of the agonistic muscles, facilitate normal reversal of antagonistic muscles, and develop strength of antagonistic muscles. Resistance is always graded to allow movement through as much active range as possible (see Figure 11.3c).

Slow Reversal-Hold (SRH).   Slow reversal-hold involves an isotonic contraction of the antagonist, followed by an isometric contraction of the antagonist, followed by the same sequence of contraction of the agonist. It may be applied to the stronger pattern, because it may have a facilitatory effect on the weaker antagonistic musculature. SRH is used to achieve the same beneficial effects as the SR technique (see Figure 11.3d).

Rhythmic Stabilization (RS).   Rhythmic stabilization employs an isometric contraction of an agonistic pattern followed by an isometric contraction of the antagonistic pattern. The strength of the con-

tractions is gradually increased during the entire sequence. RS results in an increase of holding power, relaxation, and an increase in local circulation (see Figure 11.3e).

Contract-Relax (CR).   This technique involves a maximal isotonic contraction of the antagonist from a point of resistance against a partner, followed by a period of relaxation. Next, the partner moves the part passively through as much range as possible to the point where limitation of ROM is again felt to occur. Then the process is repeated. CR is used to improve ROM. According to some, the CR method presents a greater chance of injury because of the gradual increase of tension within the muscle (see Figure 11.3f).

Hold-Relax (HR).   Hold-relax is an isometric technique that is effective when ROM has decreased because of muscle tightness on one side of a joint. This technique employs an isometric contraction of the antagonist followed by a period of relaxation. Then the limb actively moves against minimal resistance through the newly gained range to the new point of limitation (see Figure 11.3g).

Slow Reversal-Hold-Relax (SRHR).   Slow reversal-hold-relax involves an isotonic contraction of the antagonistic pattern, followed by an isometric contraction of the antagonistic pattern, followed by a brief period of voluntary relaxation, followed by an isotonic contraction of the agonistic pattern. SRHR facilitates normal reversal of the antagonistic muscles and develops strength of the antagonistic muscles (see Figure 11.3h).

Agonistic Reversal (AR).   This technique employs movement isotonically through a ROM with resistance to tolerance. At the end of the concentric range, a slow, controlled, rhythmical sequence of eccentric, concentric, and eccentric contractions of the same muscle is repeated a number of times. AR is used to promote both concentric and eccentric contractions of a movement pattern (see Figure 11.3i).

Manipulation

Manipulation is probably the most controversial technique to enhance the development of ROM. Similar to massage, its origins are lost in antiquity. Although commonly associated with the spine, manipulation can be employed on other joints as well. *Dorland's Medical Dictionary* (1981) defines manipulation as "skillful or dextrous treatment by the hand. In physical therapy, the forceful passive

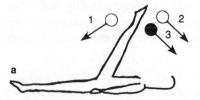

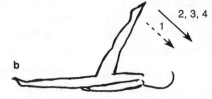

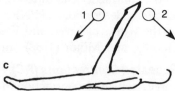

a

1. Isotonic contraction of antagonist.
2. Isotonic contraction of agonist.
3. Isometric contraction of agonist.

b

1. Passive stretch of antagonist.
2. Active-assistive contraction of agonist.
3. Active contraction of agonist.
4. Active-resistive contraction of agonist.

c

1. Isotonic contraction of antagonist.
2. Isotonic contraction of agonist.

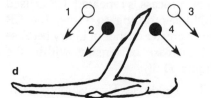

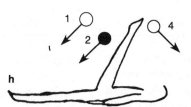

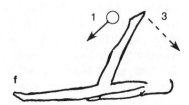

d

1. Isotonic contraction of antagonist.
2. Isotonic contraction of antagonist.
3. Isotonic contraction of agonist.
4. Isometric contraction of agonist.

e

1. Isometric contraction of agonist.
2. Isometric contraction of antagonist.

f

1. Isotonic contraction of antagonist.
2. Relaxation.
3. Passive stretch of antagonist.

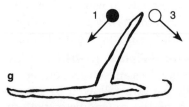

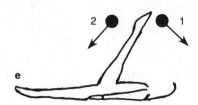

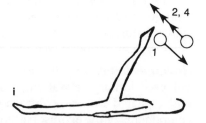

g

1. Isometric contraction of antagonist.
2. Relaxation.
3. Isotonic contraction of agonist against minimal resistance.

h

1. Isotonic contraction of antagonist.
2. Isometric contraction of antagonist.
3. Relaxation.
4. Isotonic contraction of agonist.
5. Relaxation.

i

1. Isotonic contraction of agonist.
2. Eccentric contraction of agonist.
3. Relaxation.
4. Eccentric contraction of agonist.

Figure 11.3. PNF procedures. (Isotonic contraction = open circle; isometric contraction = closed circle; passive stretch = dotted line; active stretch or contraction = solid line; eccentric contraction = line with arrows.) (a) Repeated Contraction (RC). (b) Rhythmic Initiation (RI). (c) Slow Reversal (SR). (d) Slow Reversal-Hold (SRH). (e) Rhythmic Stabilization (RS). (f) Contract-Relax (CR). (g) Hold-Relax (HR). (h) Slow Reversal-Hold Relax (SRHR). (i) Agonistic Reversal (AR).

movement of a joint beyond its active limit of motion.''

Manipulation is practiced by chiropractors, osteopaths, physical therapists, and orthopedic physicians and surgeons. These practitioners are identified by their initials D.C. (for Doctor of Chiropractic and/or Chiropractic Physician), D.O. (for Doctor of Osteopathy), and R.P.T. or L.P.T. (for Registered Physical Therapist or Licensed Physical Therapist). If manipulative treatment is indicated, it should be performed only by a specialist, and used with the greatest care.

The medical and physical therapy professions grow increasingly inclined to accept the technique of manipulation despite the controversies that have surrounded its practice (Paris, 1983). The rejection of this technique is both emotional and rational.

At one level, the term *manipulation* is complicated by the various philosophies of its practitioners who refer to identical techniques by different names. As Paris points out, this difference is due more to philosophy (vertebral adjustment) than to mechanical emphasis (stretch or oscillation). At another level, some forms of manipulation have been charged with being nonspecific, unscientific, and verging on quackery. There is also concern about reported adverse effects of the technique ranging from minor sprains and soreness to serious complications (Consumer Reports, 1975).

The technique of manipulation enhances range of motion in several different ways. These include

1. Stretching shortened muscles, tendons, connective tissues, adhesions, or scars

2. Correcting structural misalignment
3. Improving neural transmission
4. Facilitating relaxation, relieving pain and improving function.

Manipulation can be employed using either *mobilization* or *dynamic thrust*. With the former, one can voluntarily resist—and therefore control—a manipulation that is performed slowly or rhythmically. The advantage of this technique is that one can prevent further movement or advise the therapist if pain is present. The latter involves a sudden maneuver, or thrust, that is neither violent nor forceful, but precise and controlled. As described by Maigne (1980), the manipulation involves passive movement, carrying the element of an articulation beyond the usual ROM to the limit of the anatomical range (see Figure 11.4). Often, an audible crack or snap is heard, although this is not necessary for a successful maneuver. Obviously, every case demands a maneuver particularly adopted to its individual needs. Again, it cannot be overemphasized that manipulation should be performed only by a specialist and only with the greatest of care.

Traction

Traction is a technique in which a tractive force is applied to a part of the body to stretch soft tissues and to separate joint surfaces or bone fragments (Hinterbuchner, 1980). The major purposes of traction are to reduce and immobilize fracture; to correct existing deformities; to regain normal length

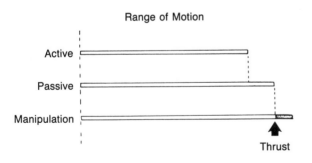

Figure 11.4. Concept of manipulation. A joint has an active range of motion that can passively be physiologically exceeded. When that range is reached, a firm but gentle thrust achieves the desired ''joint play'' that restores motion that frequently is lost. *Note.* From *Low Back Pain Syndrome* (3rd ed., p. 92) by R. Cailliet, 1981, Philadelphia: F.A. Davis. Copyright 1981 by F.A. Davis Company. Reprinted by permission.

and alignment of an injured extremity; to relieve muscle spasm; and to reduce pain. To apply the force needed to overcome the natural force or pull of muscle groups and connective tissues, a system of ropes, pulleys, and weights is commonly used. This force may be either continuous (i.e., 20 to 40 hours), sustained (i.e., 20 minutes to 1 hour), or intermittent. Traction is usually administered in conjunction with heat, massage, immobilization, and/or exercise, and should be administered only by an experienced physician or therapist.

A relatively recent innovation in traction is the use of *gravitonics* or *inversion boots* (a technique that places the subject in an inverted position with gravity providing a tractive force). With this technique, the force of gravity decompresses the spine disks and stretches the back muscles. Research has found that gravity-facilitated traction does in fact produce significant separation of the intervertebral dimensions of the lumbar spine (Kane, Karl, & Swain, 1985). If increases in intervertebral dimensions play a role in the relief of low back syndrome, then gravity-facilitated traction may indeed be an effective way to treat this condition.

However, some researchers express concern that inversion exercises may in fact be potentially harmful (Ballantyne, Reser, Lorenz, & Smidt, 1986; Klatz, Goldman, Pinchuk, Nelson, & Tarr, 1983; Ploucher, 1982). For example, Klatz et al. found that when twenty healthy students at the Chicago College of Osteopathic Medicine were inverted, blood pressure rose from an average of 119 systolic and 74 diastolic to 157/93. Ploucher warns that there may consequently be risk to intracranial circulation and periorbital petechiae (i.e., blood vessels in the eye might rupture). However, proponents of the technique argue that a person's blood pressure rises after any form of exercise. There is further speculation that the use of gravitonics could be dangerous for anyone with glaucoma, hypertension, weakness in a blood vessel, or spinal instability, or with individuals on anticoagulants or aspirin therapy.

Summary

Special stretching exercises and drills have been developed to achieve flexibility. These can be divided into two general classifications: ballistic or static. Ballistic exercises are associated with bouncing movements, whereas static exercises involve the use of slow stretching. Both kinds of exercise are effective in developing flexibility, although static stretching is more often preferred and recommended. Another way to classify flexibility exercises is on the basis of the agent responsible for ROM. These classifications include: passive, passive-active, active-assisted, and active types of stretching. With passive stretching, the individual makes no contribution to the motion, which is controlled solely by an outside agent. Passive-active stretching is initiated by an outside agent, and then the stretch is held by the individual. Active-assisted stretching is initiated by the individual until one's limit is reached, and the range of motion is completed by a partner. With active stretching, the individual is entirely responsible for the stretch. Which strategy to use is entirely dependent upon one's needs.

Proprioceptive neuromuscular facilitation (PNF) is one of the newer and more advanced methods of developing flexibility, and can be employed using a variety of strategies and techniques which will also be dependent upon one's needs. Other methods to increase range of motion include the use of manipulation and traction.

Regardless of the method employed, overstretching may result for several reasons, depending on (a) the amount or intensity of stretch, (b) the duration of the stretch, (c) the frequency of the movements performed in a given period, and (d) the velocity or the nature of the stretch.

Review Questions

1. Compare and contrast the advantages and disadvantages of ballistic and static stretching.

2. Explain the significance of the valsalva phenomenon.

3. Compare and contrast the advantages and disadvantages of passive, active-assisted, passive-active, and active stretching.

4. Prepare a series of exercises that will enhance both flexibility and strength in the hamstrings.

5. Explain the statement, "Active flexibility is more important than passive flexibility."

6. Describe a situation when passive stretching should be the preferred method of stretching; when active stretching should be the preferred method of stretching.

7. Draw a diagram illustrating the hold-relax technique.

8. Identify one situation where manipulation would be contraindicated.

9. You are instructing a stretching class of aged citizens. What is the preferred method of improving their flexibility? What is the most dangerous method? Explain why.

10. You are an instructor at a fitness health club. Identify those groups of people that should be excluded from inversion techniques.

Answers

1. The advantages of ballistic stretching are: (a) it is less boring; (b) it is appropriate in terms of specificity of training; and (c) research indicates it is effective. The disadvantages of ballistic stretching are: (a) it does not allow time for adaptation; (b) it can result in soreness; (c) it initiates the stretch reflex; and (d) it does not allow for neurological adaptation. The advantages of static stretching are: (a) it requires less energy, and (b) it reduces the probability of muscular soreness. The disadvantage of static stretching is that it may be overdone at the expense of ballistic stretching.

2. The valsalva phenomenon is potentially dangerous for those with cardiovascular problems.

3. Passive stretching:
   a. Advantages—increases the ROM; promotes camaraderie.
   b. Disadvantages—no transfer for active stretching; possible injury due to a lack of communication.
   Active-Assisted:
   a. Advantages—strengthens the weak, overstretched agonist.
   b. Disadvantages—possible overstretch by the partner.
   Passive-Active:
   a. Advantages—strengthens the weak, overstretched agonist.
   b. Disadvantages—initial pain in certain cases.

Active:
   a. Advantages—increases the active and passive ROM.
   b. Disadvantages—painful in certain cases.

4. Standing or lying PNF exercises: CR, HR, SRHR. (Modify Exercises #59 & 60.)

5. Active flexibility is more important than passive flexibility because it corresponds to the ability to use a range of joint motion in the performance of physical activities. Furthermore, most athletic performances deal with dynamic situations.

6. Passive stretching is preferred when the elasticity of the muscles to be stretched restricts flexibility. Active stretching is preferred when the low strength level of those muscles causing the movement restricts flexibility.

7. See Figure 11.3g.

8. Each case depends on its specific circumstances. For example, one would not use a ''dynamic thrust'' in the case of a severely sprained ankle.

9. Static stretching is the preferred method. Ballistic stretching would be dangerous because the tissues of older people have lost elasticity and are more susceptible to injury.

10. Those with a history of high blood pressure and spinal instability should be possibly excluded from inversion techniques.

Recommended Readings

Atha, J., & Wheatley, D. W. (1976a). The mobilising effects of repeated measurement on hip flexion. *The British Journal of Sports Medicine*, **10**(1), 22-25.

Atha, J., & Wheatley, D. W. (1976b). Joint mobility changes due to low frequency vibration and stretching exercise. *The British Journal of Sports Medicine*, **10**(1), 26-34.

Corbin, C.B. (1984). Flexibility. In J.A. Nicholas & E.B. Hershman (Eds.), *Clinics in sports medicine* (Vol. 3, pp. 101-117). Philadelphia: W.B. Saunders.

Henricson, A. S., Fredriksson, K., Persson, I., Pereira, R., Rostedt, Y., & Westlin, N. E. (1984). The effect of heat and stretching on the range of hip motion. *The Journal of Orthopaedic and Sports Physical Therapy*, **6**(2), 110-115.

Hogg, J. M. (1978). Flexibility training. *Coaching Review*, **1**(3), 39-44.

Hubley, C. L., Kozey, J. W., & Stanish, W. D. (1984). The effects of static stretching exercises and stationary cycling on range of motion at the hip joint. *The Journal of Orthopaedic and Sports Physical Therapy*, **6**(2), 104-109.

McGlynn, G. H., & Laughlin, N. (1980). The effect of biofeedback and static stretching on muscle pain. *Athletic Training*, **15**(1), 42-45.

Möller, M., Ekstrand, J., Öberg, B., & Gillquist, J. (1985). Duration of stretching effect on range of motion in lower extremities. *The Archives of Physical Medicine and Rehabilitation*, **66**(3), 171-173.

Perez, H. R., & Fusmasoli, S. (1984). Benefit of proprioceptive neuromuscular facilitation on the joint mobility of youth-aged female gymnasts with correlations for rehabilitation. *The American Corrective Therapy Journal*, **38**(6), 142-146.

Stanish, W. D. (1981). Neurophysiology of stretching. In R. A. D'Ambrosia & D. Drez (Eds.), *Prevention and treatment of running injuries* (pp. 135-145). Thorofare, NJ: Charles B. Slack.

CHAPTER 12 ▬▬▬▬▬▬▬▬▬▬▬

Stretching Concepts

In recent years, there has been growing acceptance of the *hurt-pain-agony approach* to training. Not only has this philosophy been widely adopted, it has also been widely proselytized. This is due, however, to a basic lack of knowledge about several things, including normal ROM, causes of restricted motion, and the most effective and efficient methods of increasing flexibility.

Why do people find it so difficult to motivate themselves to stretch regularly? Anderson (1978) addresses this important question by arguing that the painful experience, which many runners believe is the correct approach to stretching, is not the approach that leads to everyday benefits, personal understanding, and enjoyment. Many people lack a basic knowledge about proper stretching and how it should be done. Because many physical educators and coaches teach with the belief that unless stretching hurts, it is not doing any good, few physical educators ever present an approach to stretching that could be useful and enjoyable in everyday life.

Consequently, the task that we face is basically one of reeducation. What needs to be taught is that stretching is both beneficial and potentially enjoyable. It must also be stressed that the *quality* of stretching, not the quantity of stretching, is what ultimately determines the degree of flexibility. If one wishes to obtain optimum development of flexibility, the hurt-pain-agony concept should not be regarded as an end in itself.

Homeostasis

Homeostasis may be defined as the maintenance of a steady state. The internal environment of an organism is, in large measure, a product of the organism and controlled by it. Organisms also have means of maintaining steady states in their external environment. Stressful environmental factors (such as overwork) may alter the steady state of an organism. When an organism's homeostatic ability is exceeded, injury or death may result.

The concept of homeostasis can be extended to the cellular and even subcellular level. Thus, within certain limits, the cell is capable of adjusting to varying demands. However, like the organism as a whole, its adaptive capability may be exceeded and cellular injury or even death may follow.

An individual's response to stress depends, in part, upon one's ability to adapt oneself to new conditions. Following stress, the functioning of the homeostatic mechanism may change, and the individual may enter a new state. This process is called *adaptation*.

Cells adapt to change in their environment just as individuals do. The well-developed muscles of an Olympic weight lifter are an excellent example of cellular adaptation. This type of adaptation is called *hypertrophy*, which is an increase in size. The well-stretched tissues of a ballerina are also an excellent example of cellular adaptation. This type of adaptation is called *elongation*, which is an increase in length. Another speculated adaptation is *sarcomeregenesis*, which is generation of additional sarcomeres within the muscle fiber itself (Fridén, 1984).

Thus the adaptive responses of the ballerina involve both functional and structural changes. Consequently, there can be quantitative as well as qualitative improvement in performance. However, for such changes to occur, one's homeostatic state must be overloaded.

The Overstretching Principle

Doherty (1971) suggests that ''if we accept the word *overloading* as related to building strength in muscles, then, *overstretching* should be acceptable in building flexibility'' (p. 425). The *overstretching principle* may be defined as the physiological principle on which flexibility development depends. It implies that when one is regularly stimulated by an increasingly intense overstretching program, the body will respond with an increased ability to stretch. Therefore, the body adapts to the increasing demands placed on it.

Flexibility is a result of pure and simple stretching. No other factor is more important in its development. Increased flexibility is achieved by implementing a movement that exceeds the momentarily existing range of possible motion (Jones, 1975). Consequently, flexibility is best acquired by stretching up to the edge of discomfort. Needless to say, discomfort is a subjective matter, and will vary from person to person.

Requisites

The methods of stretching employed in the disciplines of athletics, dance, physical therapy, and yoga can vary considerably. However, certain basic principles apply to all. Ideally, a basic knowledge of the normal neuromuscular mechanism, including motor development, anatomy, neurophysiology, and kinesiology would be most helpful, if not essential. Furthermore, whatever the method of stretching used, one should be thoroughly familiar with the structure and function of the joint in question. Therefore, one should know not only the degree of limitation of motion, but also which tissues are responsible for the limitations.

Knowledge of Limitations

Range of motion at a joint, and thus flexibility, is restricted primarily by four conditions:

1. The elasticity of connective tissues in muscles or joints
2. Muscle tension
3. Lack of coordination and strength as in the case of active movement
4. Bone and joint structure

Therefore, to increase ROM at a joint, stretching procedures must do at least one of three things: (a) increase the extensibility of connective tissues in muscles or joints, (b) reduce muscular tension and thus produce relaxation, and (c) increase the coordination of the body segments and the strength of the agonistic muscle group. Generally speaking,

loss of motion due to abnormal bone and joint structure is beyond the scope of traditional stretching procedures (see Table 12.1).

Principles of Stretching

Following are some principles that should be observed when developing flexibility. These principles are not necessarily the final word, but do represent some of the more important points to remember when undertaking a flexibility program.

Safety

Safety always comes first. Although the coach, instructor, or trainer is ultimately responsible for the safety of the participants, participants should also be involved in the prevention of injury. This requires sufficient attitudes, skills, and knowledge about the control of potential hazards. The American Alliance for Health, Physical Education, Recreation, and Dance (1968) advocates a simple four-step approach to safety issues: (a) know the hazards; (b) remove the hazards when feasible; (c) control the hazards that cannot be removed; and (d) create no additional hazards.

Medical Exam

Ideally, a medical examination should be obtained before undertaking any exercise program. Such an examination may reveal that certain types of stretching exercises are contraindicated in cases of hypermobility, inflammation, sprains and strains, fracture, or active painful musculoskeletal, vascular, or skin diseases (Rusk, 1977).

Identifiable Goals

You should define your goals before you begin a flexibility program, and should have an idea of the time it will take to reach your desired degree of flexibility. For example, after six weeks of stretching, you may want to be able to place your palms flat on the floor, with your legs straight. Make sure, whatever your goals may be, that they are realistic.

Individualized Program

All exercises should be designed to fit an individual's specific needs. Often, however, one is expected to fit into a group or team in a flexibility

Table 12.1 Theoretical Model of Approaches and Courses of Action to Improve Range of Motion

Approach	Psychological conditions	Courses of action	
		Physical	Psychological
Decrease resistance of target area	Lengthen connective tissue	(a) Prolonged stretch (b) Contract target area while under stretch	
	Relax myotatic reflex	(a) Reciprocal inhibition (b) Accomodation (c) Heat, ice, massage, exercise fatigue, etc.	(a) Mind-set (Gamma bias) (b) Biofeedback (monitored inhibition) (c) Relaxation training
Increase strength of opposing muscles	Muscle loading of opposing muscles	Strength training (a) Isometric (b) Concentric (c) Eccentric	(a) Motivation
	Facilitation techniques	(a) Successive induction (proprioceptive neuromuscular facilitation)	(b) Learning: recruitment, coordination, synchronization

From "Six Mobilization Exercises for Active Range of Hip Flexion" by S.J. Hartley-O'Brien, 1980, *Research Quarterly for Exercise and Sport*, **51**(4), p. 627. Copyright 1980. Reprinted by permission of the American Alliance for Health, Physical Education, Recreation and Dance, 1900 Association Drive, Reston, Virginia 22091.

program. Thus the question arises, "Should a coach insist that a given stretch be mastered in a specific time, or rather encourage each athlete to sustain the stretch until his or her individual threshold or objective is fulfilled?"

The answer to this question depends upon a number of factors. Ideally, one should have already warmed up and stretched out on one's own before participating in the team stretch. However, this is not always possible, and not even desirable if the individual does not have the knowledge to warm up safely. In most instances, the team approach is the most appropriate course to follow. At least a minimal stretching program is guaranteed to have been carried out if one participates in a group, and such a program fosters camaraderie and team spirit. Then, at the end of the team workout, the individual can concentrate on those areas that need additional stretching.

However, if one is stretching in a class at a fitness or health club, one should listen and tune into one's own body and either participate with the class, or hold the stretch as seen fit. In such a class,

there is a potentially wider range of abilities, and overstretching is a real possibility, especially for beginners. Instructors should educate class members about what exercises should be attempted, and to what degree.

Keep Accurate Records

A well-planned program is also recorded. Records should be kept that include the date and time of exercise, types of exercises performed (intensity, duration, and frequency), and a self-evaluation before, during, and after the program. A number of devices can be used for measuring purposes ranging from the sophisticated and expensive to the simple and inexpensive. These include radiography, photography, schematography, outline tracing, goniometers or protractors, electrogoniometers, tape measures, performance charts, and visual observations. The value of record-keeping may be purely motivational or it may reveal positive or negative patterns in the training program (Uram, 1980).

Gradualism

The development of flexibility takes time; it does not develop overnight. Therefore, be sure that you set realistic goals, remembering that it is necessary to begin with easy exercises and advance to more difficult ones. You should recognize that plateaus, or periods of no apparent progress, are part of the learning process.

Comparing and Competing

Do not attempt to compare yourself to others. Improvement and progress are important, not competition with someone who may in fact be at an entirely different level of ability. No two people are alike: Some may develop flexibility rapidly; others may take a longer period of time to reach the same level (see Figure 12.1).

Clothes and Positioning

Wear loose and comfortable clothes when working out. Because a warmed muscle is believed to be more flexible and pliant, you will often see people wearing sweat suits and woolen socks. You should also be sure to position yourself as comfortably as possible to reduce tension and make the stretching more enjoyable.

Mental Set

A positive mental attitude is important. The mental, physical, and spiritual aspects of life are inseparable from one another. Without a positive mind set, the best of all possible results will never be achieved in a physical training program.

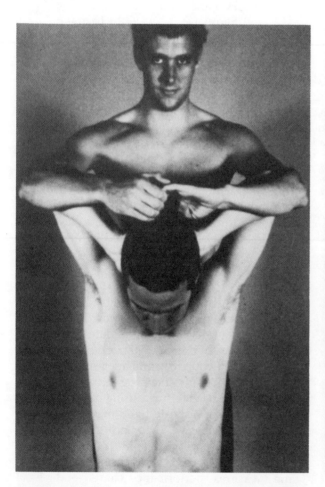 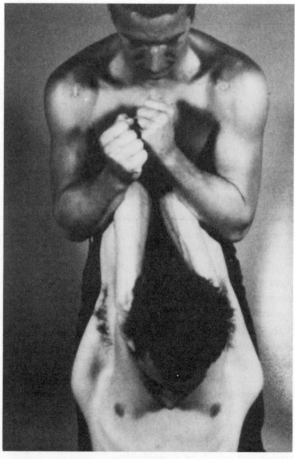

Figure 12.1.   Comparing and competing different degrees in natural flexibility. Each swimmer was able to perform at peak efficiency. If the individual in *a* tried to equal the limits of flexibility in *b*, he may have overstretched musculotendinous units beyond effective ranges. (a) The NCAA division II gold medal winner in the 100-yard freestyle in the year the picture was taken. (b) The NCAA division II gold medal winner in the 200-yard butterfly (teammate). (Photo courtesy of J.V. Ciullo, M.D.)

Relaxation

Relaxation is probably the most important factor, other than stretching itself, in developing flexibility. Relaxation is the opposite of tension. Tension originates in contracted muscles, which result in inflexibility, an insufficient oxygen supply, and fatigue. The ability to relax is important because it decreases tension and its negative consequences, thus allowing one to function more effectively and efficiently. If you want to learn to relax, learn to listen to your body. Stretch slowly and exhale deeply at the moment of maximum stretch. Do not hold your breath. Concentrate on, and be totally aware of, the task at hand to ensure the deepest relaxation.

Warm-up and Cool-Down (Warm-Down)

Warm-up and cool-down exercises are designed to improve performance and reduce the chances of injury. The most important advantages of both active and passive warm-up are:

1. It increases the muscle's temperature.
2. It reduces the muscle's viscosity.
3. It decreases muscular tension.
4. It makes tissues more extensible.

Isolate the Muscle

For stretching to be most beneficial, the proper muscle group must receive the activity. For example, when stretching the hamstrings, make sure that the hip is not rotated. A rotated hip puts more stress on the adductors, or the groin.

Application of the S.A.I.D. Principle

As proposed by Wallis and Logan (1964), strength, endurance, and flexibility should be based on the principle of *specific adaptation to imposed demands*. That is, one should stretch at a velocity not less than 75% of the maximum velocity through the exact plane of motion, range of motion, and at the precise joint angles used while performing skills in their specific activity, for example, high leg kicks as in punting a football. For those movements requiring rapid velocity, a slow stretch should precede the application of the S.A.I.D. principle.

Application of the Overstretching Principle

The physiological principle on which strength development depends is the *overload principle*. The *overstretching principle* is the physiological principle on which flexibility development depends. The difference is that the latter uses stretch in place of resistance. Simply put, such overstretching is a function of the intensity, duration, frequency, and nature of the stretch. Most programs recommend stretching for 6 to 12 seconds in duration. However, 10 to 30 seconds is also commonly recommended. According to Bates (1971), 60 seconds of maintained stretch is optimal in increasing and retaining flexibility. Regarding the frequency or number of repetitions, there also appears to be some differences of opinion. Most programs recommend between 5 to 15 repetitions. However, the best thing to do is experiment. Find out for yourself what is best for you. As a general rule, you should stretch at least once a day for maintenance. Such daily workouts are feasible if interest and motivation can be maintained (Rasch & Burke, 1978). However, empirical evidence suggests that stretching at least twice a day is preferable. The best times appear to be in the morning after awakening (to eliminate morning stiffness and energize oneself) and in the afternoon or early evening after the day's work. However, the best time to stretch is when you feel as if you want to.

The intensity of the stretch should also be up to you. Although stretching will produce some discomfort (especially for beginners), it should not be so great a discomfort as to cause pain. As a general rule, if your muscle begins to quiver and vibrate, if pain persists, or if range decreases, you have overstretched, and either the force or the duration of the stretch should be decreased. Discomfort and pain are subjective matters, so there is no real answer about where to draw the line. The best advice is to use common sense: train, don't strain.

Mechanics

The individual must employ the proper use of mechanics and techniques when stretching. This includes identifying and isolating those muscles and tissues to be stretched and using the appropriate exercise to fulfill that goal. The use of proper mechanics also implies the use of correct technique to reduce risk of injury and impairment of performance. Some examples of incorrect technique are flaring out the rear foot in a hurdler's stretch; executing a turnout from the knees during a plié, and reextension from the flexed position in which the lordosis is regained before the pelvis is derotated. Only through the incorporation of correct mechanics and technique can one achieve optimum results.

Stretch Reflex

Generally speaking stretching should be slow or static. Sudden or painful movements will elicit a stretch reflex causing the muscle to contract. Therefore, ballistic stretching should be avoided, especially during the early stages of a program.

Anticipation and Communication

When stretching with a partner, communicate with each other. It is the responsibility of the person being stretched to inform the partner when the stretch becomes unpleasant or painful. It is the responsibility of the person applying the stretch to anticipate how much overload should be employed. This is a two-way process.

Appropriate Use of Medical Resources

If an injury should occur, determine to the best of your knowledge the extent of the damage. As a general rule, incorporate rest, ice, pressure, and elevation to the injured part of the body—then see a doctor or trainer. The sooner an injury is treated, the earlier rehabilitation can begin and the faster will be the recovery. Again, a good rule of thumb is to use common sense.

Enjoyment

Stretching should be enjoyable and satisfying, and should create a sense of well-being. Enjoyment and pleasure are essentially a matter of satisfying one's motives. However, stretching has the potential to involve varying degrees of pleasantness or unpleasantness. When stretching ceases to be enjoyable, it becomes self-defeating. To paraphrase Iyengar (1979), stretching can be likened to an electric current: Your muscles and connective tissues can be compared to a filament and your body to a light bulb. When the proper flow reaches the bulb, it glows. So, too, can one's body and mind be illuminated.

Summary

Homeostasis is defined as maintenance of a steady state. In order to develop flexibility, one's homeostatic state must be exceeded. As a result of this stress, one enters a new state. This process is called *adaptation*.

The overstretching principle is the physiological principle on which flexibility development depends. It implies that when one stretches regularly, the body will respond with an increased ability to stretch. For stretching to be successful, a movement must actually exceed the momentarily existing range of motion.

Before engaging in a stretching program, one should have some knowledge about anatomy, physiology, and the structure and functions of joints. Flexibility is generally restricted by four conditions: muscle and connective tissue inelasticity, muscle tension, lack of coordination and strength as in the case of active movement, and bone and joint structure.

Review Questions

1. Explain why the public generally accepts the hurt-pain-agony approach to stretching.

2. Explain how the concepts of homeostasis, adaptation, and overstretching relate to the development of flexibility.

3. Explain what factor you feel has the greatest influence on the magnitude of the effects of training.

4. Identify four conditions that limit ROM at a joint.

5. You are coaching a football team. Should you allocate a specific time to stretching, whether this be five seconds or one minute, or encourage each athlete to sustain the stretch until one's individual pain threshold is reached?

6. Make a list of your own ten commandments with reference to stretching.

Answers

1. The public generally accepts the hurt-pain-agony approach to stretching because of a

lack of knowledge and understanding, and because that approach has always been taught.

2. Homeostasis refers to the maintenance of a steady state. Unless one's homeostasis is exceeded, there can be no improvement. Adaptation refers to the new state that is developed after going beyond one's homeostasis. To develop flexibility, one must utilize the overstretching principle. That is, the body will respond to overstretching with an increased ability to stretch.

3. The factor that has the greatest influence on the magnitude of the effects of training is the quality of one's stretching program.

4. ROM is limited by the elasticity of connective tissues, muscle tension, lack of coordination and strength as in the case of active movement, and bone and joint structure.

5. The coach should insist on a set time. However, adequate time should be allowed the individual to stretch both before and after the set time.

6. Share your list with others.

Recommended Readings

Ciullo, J.V., & Zarins, B. (1983). Biomechanics of the musculotendinous unit. In B. Zarins (Ed.), *Clinics in sports medicine* (Vol. 2, pp. 71-85). Philadelphia: W.B. Saunders.

Corbin, C.B. (1984). Flexibility. In J.A. Nicholas & E.B. Hershman (Eds.), *Clinics in sports medicine* (Vol. 3, pp. 101-117). Philadelphia: W.B. Saunders.

Corbin, C.B., & Noble, L. (1980). Flexibility: A major component of physical fitness. *The Journal of Physical Education and Recreation*, **51**(6), 23-24, 57-60.

Frankel, V.H., & Hang, Y.S. (1975). Recent advances in the biomechanics of sport injuries. *Acta Orthopaedica Scandinavica*, **46**(3), 484-497.

Kisner, C., & Colby, L.A. (1985). *Therapeutic exercise: Foundations and techniques*. Philadelphia: F.A. Davis.

Sapega, A.A., Quedenfeld, T.C., Moyer, R.A., & Butler, R.A. (1981). Biophysical factors in range-of-motion exercise. *The Physician and Sportsmedicine*, **9**(12), 57-65.

PART II

Functional Anatomy

CHAPTER 13

The Lower Extremity and Pelvic Girdle

For our purposes, the lower extremity and pelvic girdle shall be considered to consist of the foot, ankle joint, leg, knee joint, thigh, gluteal region, iliac region, and hip joint. This section contains an analysis of this anatomical area's structure, function, limits on range of motion, potential for injury, and preferred methodology of stretching. (Stretching exercises from Part 3 of this book are referred to where appropriate.)

The Foot

The foot is a very complicated structure. It has three major anatomical parts: the hindfoot, consisting of the calcaneus and talus; the midfoot, comprised of the navicular, cuboid, and three cuneiforms; and the forefoot, formed by the metatarsals and phalanges (see Figure 13.1). It contains 26 bones (7 tarsals, 5 metatarsals, and 14 phalanges) and 4 layers of interwoven and overlapping fascia, muscles, tendons, and ligaments. The structure of the foot is similar to the hand, but with differences that adapt it to the functions of weight bearing, shock absorption, and propulsion.

The foot is an elastic, arched structure (Luttgens & Wells, 1982). The plantar vault is an architectural component of that structure that blends all the elements of the foot—joints, ligaments, and muscles—into a unified system. It acts as the shock-absorber essential for the flexibility of the foot. However, the curvature and orientation of the vault depend upon a delicate balance of muscles (Kapandji, 1982). For example, with *pes cavus* or *claw feet*, there is an unusually high arch, which can result from contractures of the plantar aponeurosis or from the use of shoes with soles that are too rigid (Cailliet,

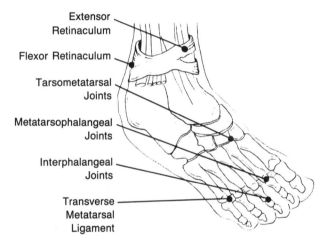

Figure 13.1. The bones and joints of the foot. *Note.* From *Living Anatomy* (p. 139) by J.E. Donnelly, 1982, Champaign, IL: Human Kinetics. Copyright 1982 by J.E. Donnelly. Reprinted by permission.

1977; Kapandji, 1982). Cailliet recommends exercises for this condition designed to stretch the toe extensors and distal toe flexors.

The Significance of a Flexible Foot and Ankle

A rigid system absorbs less energy than a flexible one. Such a·system is less efficient and more prone to breakdown. On the other hand, a supple foot and ankle absorb energy efficiently, resulting in less chance for injury. For those involved in ballet, flexibility is a must. As explained by Hamilton (1978d):

Flexibility is needed in the instep or midfoot so that the foot in the pointe position becomes the projection of the axis of the tibia (shinbone). This requires a total of ninety degrees of plantar flexion (combining motion at the ankle and instep), and actually, a few degrees more if the downward movement is going to compensate for the recurvatum most dancers have at the knee. If this motion is not present, the dancer will not be "all the way up" on pointe or demi-pointe. There is a tremendous difference between being all the way up and almost all the way up in terms of the extra energy required to maintain the pointe position. The result is chronic overstrain of the achilles and other tendons. (p. 85)

It seems appropriate here to address the question, "At what age should young girls begin working on full pointe?" Hamilton (1978a; 1978d), the official doctor of the New York City Ballet, subscribes to George Balanchine's view that students should not work on pointe until they have the strength and training to do something when they get up there. This is usually about the age of twelve.

The Significance of Exercise

Connective tissues and muscles maintain their strength and elasticity only when they are used. One reason for the great increase in foot problems is the lack of exercise. Too many people today, young and old, neglect walking, which is the best activity for maintaining the elements that help support the foot (Thompson, 1981).

Limits on Range of Motion

The ranges of motion that take place within the foot depend on a variety of things: bony structure, joint articulation, fascia, ligaments, musculature, and tendon support. Like other parts of the body, the foot can become more flexible if its tissues are stretched. But often this part of the body is neglected, for working on flexibility requires diligence and hard practice.

Flexion of the Interphalangeal and Metatarsophalangeal Joints of the Toes.
Flexion of the interphalangeal and metatarsophalangeal joints involves bending or drawing the toes toward the sole of the foot. Flexion at these joints ranges from 0 to 90 degrees and 0 to 35 degrees respectively. Flexion is produced by both the intrinsic and extrinsic phalangeal flexors—that is, by muscles that have their origin and insertion on the bones within the foot, and by muscles that have their origin outside of the foot. Factors limiting range of motion in the

foot are: contractile insufficiency, tension of the extensor muscle tendons of the toes, and contact of the soft parts of the phalanges.

Extension of the Interphalangeal and Metatarsophalangeal Joints of the Toes.
Extension of the interphalangeal and metatarsophalangeal joints involves drawing the phalanges away from the sole of the foot. Extension of the phalanges ranges from 0 to 80 degrees. This movement is produced primarily by the extrinsic extensors of the foot. Factors limiting range of motion here are contractile insufficiency and tension of the plantar and collateral ligaments of the toe joints. Subotnick (1977) points out that extension may also be limited by tight plantar fascia or inflammation of the plantar fascia (i.e., plantar fasciitis). The latter may cause severe pain when running on the balls of the feet.

The Ankle or Talocrural Joint

The ankle or talocrural joint is an example of a hinge joint. It is formed by the tibia, fibula, and talus. The relationship of these three bones is maintained by a fibrous capsule, ligaments, and musculotendinous structures. The medial or deltoid ligament has four components: the posterior tibiotalar, the tibiocalcanean, the tibionavicular, and the anterior tibiotalar. The *lateral collateral ligament* is comprised of three bands: the anterior talofibular, the posterior talofibular, and the calcaneofibular (see Figure 13.2). Because the bony stability is greater laterally than medially and the deltoid ligament is stronger than the lateral collateral ligaments, the joint is predisposed towards inversion. This is of particular importance because the vast majority of all ankle ligament injuries involve the lateral side with the common inversion sprain.

The Effects of Excessive Stress

The bone structure of an ankle and foot can be modified by excessive stress. For instance, it has been reported that dancers who begin training before age 12 will exhibit architectural changes in the tarsal bones that will allow for increased mobility and plantar flexion of the forefoot (Ende & Wickstrom, 1982; Nikolic & Zimmermann, 1968). However, excessive stress can also result in decreased range of motion. Examples are the formation of spurs on the anterior and posterior lips of the talus (Brodelius, 1961; Ende & Wickstrom, 1982; Hamilton, 1978c, 1978d; Howse, 1972),

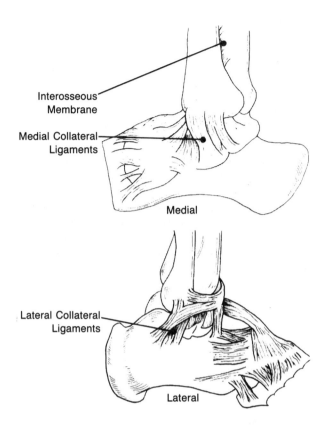

Figure 13.2. Medial and lateral views of the ligaments of the ankle. *Note.* From *Living Anatomy* (p. 137) by J.E. Donnelly, 1982, Champaign, IL: Human Kinetics. Copyright 1982 by J.E. Donnelly. Reprinted by permission.

which can result in asymmetrical pliés for dancers (Ende & Wickstrom, 1982; Schneider, King, Bronson, & Miller, 1974). Another problem with excessive stress is impingement of osteophytes or small fractures on the tibia at the dorsal neck of the anterior crown of the talus (Ryan, 1976). Ankle motion can also be limited by the presence of an extra bone behind the ankle called *os trigonum* (Brodelius, 1961; Ende & Wickstrom, 1982; Hamilton, 1978b; Howse, 1972).

Limits on Range of Motion

The ranges of motion which take place within the ankle depend on a number of things: bony structure, joint articulation, fascia, ligaments, musculature, and tendon support. Here, too, the tissues of the joint are capable of being stretched and its flexibility enhanced, as seen most often in ballet dancers.

Eversion. Eversion of the ankle involves turning the sole of the foot so that it tends to face laterally (see Figure 13.3a & c). This movement is produced primarily by the peroneus longus and peroneus

brevis. Eversion ranges from 0 to 20 degrees. The factors limiting this motion are contractile insufficiency, tension of the deltoid/medial tarsal ligaments, tension of the tibialis anterior and tibialis posterior muscles, and contact of the tarsal bones laterally.

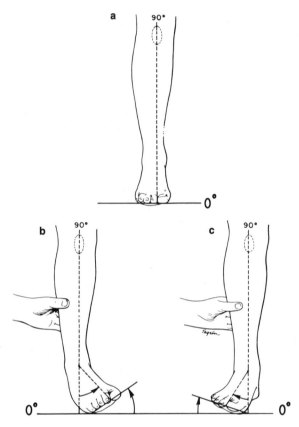

Figure 13.3. Inversion and eversion of the ankle. (a) Zero starting position. (b) Inversion. (c) Eversion. *Note.* From *Manual of Orthopaedic Surgery* (p. 61), 1985, Park Ridge, IL: American Orthopaedic Association. Copyright 1972 by The American Orthopaedic Association. Reprinted by permission.

Inversion. Inversion of the ankle involves turning the sole of the foot so that it tends to face medially (see Figure 13.3b). The movement is produced primarily by the tibialis anterior and tibialis posterior, and assisted by the flexor digitorum longus, flexor hallucis longus, and medial head of the gastrocnemius. Inversion of the ankle ranges from 0 to 45 degrees. The factors limiting the range of motion are contractile insufficiency; tension of the interosseous talocalcanean ligament; the other tarsal interosseous ligaments; the calcaneofibular ligament; tension of the peroneus longus and peroneus brevis; and contact of the tarsal bones medially.

Plantar Flexion.   Plantar flexion of the ankle involves drawing the foot away from the tibia (i.e., extension of the foot). This movement is produced primarily by the gastrocnemius and soleus, and assisted by the tibialis posterior, peroneus longus, peroneus brevis, flexor hallucis longus, flexor digitorum longus, and plantaris. Ankle plantar flexion ranges from 0 to 50 degrees. Factors limiting range of motion are contractile insufficiency; tension of the anterior talofibular ligament; tension of the anterior tibiotalar ligament; tension of the dorsiflexor muscles; and contact of the posterior portion of the talus with the tibia.

Ankle Dorsiflexion.   Dorsiflexion of the ankle involves drawing the foot upward and toward the tibia (i.e., flexion of the foot) (see Figure 13.4). Ankle dorsiflexion is produced primarily by the tibialis anterior, and assisted by the extensor digitorum longus, extensor hallucis longus, and peroneus tertius. Dorsiflexion ranges from 0 to 20 degrees. Factors limiting range of motion are contractile insufficiency; tension of the peroneus longus and peroneus brevis muscles; tension of the calcareal tendon; tension of the deltoid ligament; tension of the calcaneofibular ligament; and contact of the talus with the anterior margin of the tibial surface.

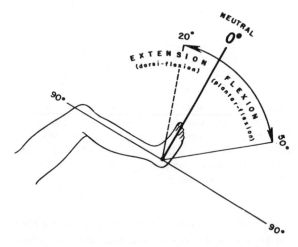

Figure 13.4.   Flexion and extension of the ankle. *Note.* From *Manual of Orthopaedic Surgery* (p. 68), 1985, Park Ridge, IL: American Orthopaedic Association. Copyright 1972 by The American Orthopaedic Association. Reprinted by permission.

Injury Prevention

The ankle and foot are susceptible to numerous injuries. Among the more common are fascial and ligamentous strains and sprains, tendinitis, and stress fractures. Preventive action includes proper

conditioning, adequate warm-up, utilization of proper technique, avoiding hard surfaces, resting when fatigued, and avoiding overuse.

The Lower Leg

The crus, or leg, is the segment of the lower limb between the knee and ankle. It is analogous to the smaller forearm segment of the upper limb. The lower leg is made up of two bones: the tibia, or shinbone, and its smaller companion, the fibula (see Figure 13.5). The two bones are connected together by the interosseous membrane. Surrounding the tibia and fibula are a number of muscles that are susceptible to injury if not adequately stretched before activation.

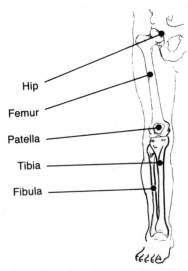

Figure 13.5.   The bones of the upper and lower limb, anterior view. *Note.* From *Living Anatomy* (p. 137) by J.E. Donnelly, 1982, Champaign, IL: Human Kinetics. Copyright 1982 by J.E. Donnelly. Reprinted by permission.

The Posterior Muscles

The calf is comprised of the muscles in the lower posterior (back) portion of the leg. The calf has three superficial crucial muscles—the gastrocnemius, soleus, and plantaris—and four deep crucial muscles—the popliteus, flexor hallucis longus, flexor digitorum longus, and tibialis posterior. The primary function of the superficial muscles is plantar flexion (extension) of the ankle and flexion of the knee; the primary function of the deep muscles is flexion of the toes and inversion of the foot.

The gastrocnemius is the most superficial muscle, is comprised of two heads, and forms the greater part of the calf. The soleus is a broad, flat muscle situated immediately deep or anterior to the gastrocnemius. Together, they form a muscular mass called the triceps surae. The triceps surae contributes nine-tenths to the total flexion force of the posterior muscles. The tendons of the gastrocnemius and soleus form the tendo calcaneus.

The tendo calcaneus, or Achilles tendon, is the largest and strongest tendon in the body. It is attached to the posterior surface of the calcaneus. The strength of the tendon approximates 18,000 pounds per square inch. Despite the tendon's tremendous strength, it is not invulnerable to injury. The vulnerability of the Achilles tendon will be discussed in a later section.

Injuries to the Posterior Muscles and Tendo Calcaneus.

Pulls or strains of the calf are not uncommon. They are caused by a number of things: cold muscles, inadequate warm-up, overuse, fatigue, improper technique, working on a hard surface, or stepping unexpectedly in a hole. A pull of the calf has been dubiously named *tennis leg*—dubiously for it is often observed in sports and activities other than tennis. This injury may be associated with rupture of the plantaris muscle (or, more commonly, the gastrocnemius). The plantaris is a small vestigial muscle located between the gastrocnemius and the soleus. The plantaris possesses very little belly and is mostly tendon. The mechanism of the injury is thought to be a sudden dorsiflexion of the foot while it is supinated and in plantar flexion with the knee joint in extension (Ryan, 1972). Another explanation is that the plantaris is mostly tendinous, unlike the two larger muscles that surround it, and so lacks the ability to respond immediately as opposed to its surrounding muscles. Hence, due to faulty reciprocal innervation, it is often slow to contract and relax and consequently is easily pulled or ruptured (Dollan & Holliday, 1974).

The most common type of injury to the Achilles tendon is tendinitis, a condition associated with tenderness and swelling. Treatment of tendinitis includes rest, ice, mild anti-inflammatory medicines, and appropriate medical assistance. However, the most catastrophic injury to a tendon is rupture. Rupture can be likened to the giving way of an old, frayed rope, because the fibers of a tendon are not straight, but coiled like rope. Treatment consists of either prolonged immobilization in a cast, or surgical repair. Obviously, a preventive approach that includes enhancing both the tendon's flexibility and strength is the most practical and prudent course of action to follow.

Stretching the Posterior Crural Muscles and Tendo Calcaneus.

The method used to stretch the lower leg's posterior muscles and tendons is virtually identical to the mechanism that often initiates injury. To stretch these muscles, the feet are slowly dorsiflexed while they are supinated and in plantar flexion with the knee joint in extension. Injury is due to a rapid, or ballistic, dorsiflexion; prevention of injury is aided by slow stretching, showing once again that static stretching is the safer technique. Proper stretching of these muscles can be achieved in a modified hurdler's stretch position when one pulls up on the toes toward the body. If the toes cannot be reached, a towel may be used. Another commonly employed stretch is to stand about three feet from a wall and lean forward while keeping the heels down. More advanced (and controversial) stretches include the ballet demi pliés (see Exercises #19-40).

The Anterior and Lateral Crural Muscles

The anterior muscles are found toward the front of the leg. This group consists of four muscles: the tibialis anterior is situated just outside the tibia, and is the major dorsiflexor of the ankle joint and invertor of the foot. The extensor hallucis longus, the extensor digitorum longus, and the peroneus teritus assist in dorsiflexion with the former two also extending the toes.

There is another set of crural muscles, called the lateral crural muscles, which are situated on the lateral side of the leg. The group consists of the peroneus longus muscle and the peroneus brevis muscle. Both assist in eversion of the feet, while the former can also plantar-flex the feet.

Injuries.

"Shinsplints" are one of the most common injuries to the anterior and lateral regions of the leg. This catch-all syndrome is thought to be a microscopic tearing of the attachments of the muscles from the tibia, resulting in tenderness and/or a dull pain. The etiology of shinsplints has been vaguely attributed to a number of causes, including practicing on hard surfaces, improper warm-up, poor technique, fallen arches, improper body balance from low back strain, inherited tendency, lack of flexibility, fatigue, and overuse. Shinsplints can be treated with ice, warm soaks, whirlpool, gentle massage, stretching, taping, reduced activity, or rest.

Stretching.

The anterior crural muscles can be stretched by slowly plantar-flexing and/or inverting the ankle. A safe method is to apply a manual stretch by extending the ankle with one leg crossed over the other while in a sitting position (see Exercise #7). Another easily employed method is to stand and lean against a wall with one foot turned under. Then one's weight is shifted onto the top of the foot to develop the stretch (see Exercise #6). A method often cited in yoga texts is the sitting on the shins with the toes facing backwards. In time, more weight is gradually shifted backward onto the heels (see Exercises #8 & 9). However, it should be pointed out that this method may present a potential risk for those with bad knees.

The easiest and safest method to stretch the lateral crural muscles is to apply a manual stretch by slowly inverting the ankle with one leg crossed over the other while in a sitting position (see Exercise #14). A second method is to assume a modified hurdler's stretch position, reach down and grasp the outer portion of your foot (or use a towel if it cannot be reached), and slowly turn the outside of the foot medially (see Exercise #15). Another effective stretch can also be applied by standing about one foot from a pillar with the feet hip width and toed-in. Then, slowly flex at the waist and shift the hips backwards to form a 45-degree angle with the legs (see Exercise #18).

The Genual or Knee Joint

The genual, or knee joint, is the largest joint in the body. It is formed by the articulation of three bones: the femur, tibia, and fibula (see Figure 13.5). The knee is an example of a modified hinge joint. Since the bony arrangement is architecturally weak, compensation must be provided by firm support of ligaments (nine in total) and muscle.

Limits on Range of Motion

Medial and lateral rotations of the tibia are possible only to a slight degree. The knee moves almost exclusively in flexion and extension, which are the motions that will be analyzed here.

Flexion. Flexion of the knee involves drawing the heel up to the back of the thigh (see Figure 13.6). Flexion can be carried to about 120 degrees with the hip joint extended, to about 135 degrees when the hip joint is flexed, and to about 160 degrees when a passive element, such as sitting on the heels, is introduced. During active shortening, flexion of the unweighted knee is performed by two sets of biarticular muscles: the hamstrings (hip and knee), and the gastrocnemius (knee and ankle). Range of motion is limited by contractile

insufficiency; tension of the quadriceps extensor and its tendon; tension in the anterior parts of the capsule; tension of the posterior cruciate ligament; tension of both cruciate ligaments in extreme passive flexion; and contact of the posterior portion of the leg with the posterior position of the thigh and buttocks.

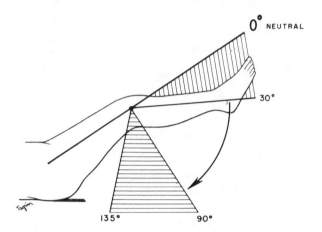

Figure 13.6. Flexion of the knee. *Note.* From *Manual of Orthopaedic Surgery* (p. 68), 1985, Park Ridge, IL: American Orthopaedic Association. Copyright 1972 by The American Orthopaedic Association. Reprinted by permission.

Extension. Extension of the knee is the return movement from flexion. Extension beyond 0 degrees is called *hyperextension, recurvatum,* or *swayback* knee (see Figure 13.7), and is caused by ligamentous instability or bony deformity. If hyperextension is present, stretching exercises that further extend the knee should be avoided. Specifically, one must be careful not to lock or press back the knee joint. Instead, bend the knee slightly, and bring it back to a straight, but strong, position. Then raise the kneecaps up toward the thigh (Follan, 1981).

Extension of the knee is produced by the powerful quadriceps. Factors limiting range of motion are contractile insufficiency; tension in the hamstring and gastrocnemius muscles; and tension of both cruciate ligaments, the tibial and fibular collateral ligaments, the posterior aspect of the capsule, and the oblique posterior ligament. The locking of the knee in flexion may also restrict extension, and may be due to a mechanical internal derangement such as a loose body or torn meniscus. Remember, the knee is a sliding or gliding mechanism. Any foreign object that is interposed between two surfaces will block motion in the same fashion that a wedge beneath a door will hold it fast.

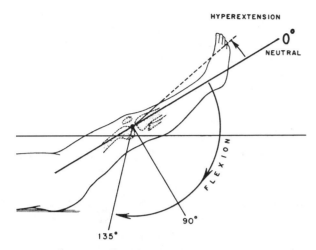

Figure 13.7. Extension and hyperextension of the knee. *Note.* From *Manual of Orthopaedic Surgery* (p. 79), 1985, Park Ridge, IL: American Orthopaedic Association. Copyright 1972 by The American Orthopaedic Association. Reprinted by permission.

The Mechanical and Structural Disadvantages of the Knee

One of the potentially detrimental aspects of the knee joint is that it is partially controlled by two-joint muscles. The hamstrings, which function to flex the knee as well as extend the hip, are an example, as well as the rectus femoris, which extends the knee and flexes the hip (Fujiwara & Basmajian, 1975; Kelley, 1971). Trouble develops when both muscle groups are simultaneously moved to their extremes. Consequently, the tension on the muscles and/or tendons may become so great as to cause an injury. Kelley clearly illustrates how this can happen during the act of sprinting: The tension on the rectus femoris must be considerable when the trailing leg is in knee flexion and hip extension. The hamstrings must suffer the same sort of stress when a hurdler's leading leg undergoes simultaneous hip flexion and nearly complete knee extension, when a cheerleader or dancer performs high leg kicks, or when a high jumper uses the straddle technique.

The Upper Leg

The thigh is the segment of the upper limb between the hip and knee. This segment contains a single bone, the femur (see Figure 13.8). The femur is the longest and strongest bone in the body, and is surrounded by a number of muscles called the femoral muscles (see Figure 13.9).

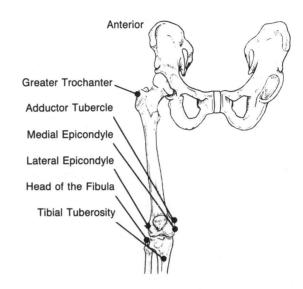

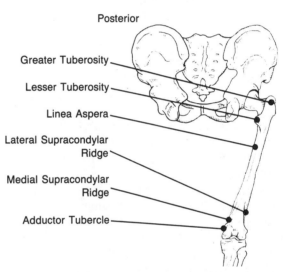

Figure 13.8. The femur and hip joint, anterior and posterior views. *Note.* From *Living Anatomy* (p. 114) by J.E. Donnelly, 1982, Champaign, IL: Human Kinetics. Copyright 1982 by J.E. Donnelly. Reprinted by permission.

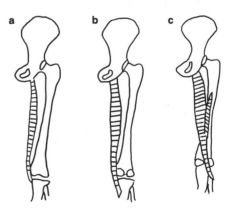

Figure 13.9. The hamstrings. (a) The semitendinosus. (b) The semimembranosus. (c) The biceps femoris.

The Posterior Femoral Muscles

The posterior (or rear) portion of the thigh is made up of three muscles. In layman's terminology, these muscles are known as the *hamstrings*. This word evolved from the Anglo-Saxon *hamm*, meaning *back of thigh*. In medical terminology, the muscles have very long names derived from their physical composition.

The biceps femoris is found posterior and laterally in the thigh, and is accordingly named because it has two heads. The semitendinosus is located posterior and medially in the thigh, and is so-named because the tendon is of remarkable length. Literally, the name implies that the muscle is half tendon. Finally, there is the semimembranosus, which lies on the posteriomedial aspect of the thigh. The muscle is so-called because of the flattened membraneous form of its upper attachment.

The major responsibilities of the hamstrings are to produce both flexion of the knee joint and extension of the hip joint. In flexion at the hip and in leaning forward, they are active as supporters against gravity. When the knee is semiflexed, the biceps femoris can act as a lateral rotator, and the other hamstrings as medial rotators of the leg. When the hip joint is extended, the biceps also laterally rotate the thigh while the other hamstrings act as medial rotators. The hamstrings-to-quadriceps torque ratio varies in selected populations. Parker, Ruhling, Holt, Bauman, and Drayna (1983) found that high school football players had a ratio between 47% and 65%. In contrast, Davies, Kirkendall, Leigh, Lui, Reinbold, and Wilson (1981) reported ratios between 51% and 64.9% for professional football players. However, Gilliam, Villanacci, Freedson, and Sady (1979) calculated ratios in the 40% to 70% range for children between the ages of 7 and 13 years.

Causes and Mechanisms of Injury. The hamstring strain, commonly known as a pulled hamstring, is caused by a violent stretch or rapid contraction of the hamstring muscle group causing rupture within the musculotendinous unit (American Medical Association Subcommittee on Classification of Sports Injuries, 1966). The injury is time-consuming, easily aggravated, psychologically devastating, and almost literally a "pain in the butt." A pulled hamstring may occur in the muscle's belly or near the ends in the tendon areas. Therefore, the pull may occur just below the hip or posteriorly at midthigh level.

For years, numerous people have speculated about the predisposing factors that might cause the ham-

string muscle group to become strained. Originally, research suggested that a strength-ratio imbalance between the hamstrings and quadriceps was such a factor (Burkett, 1970). Currently, however, researchers are inclined to favor the idea that a decrease in the 50% to 60% hamstring-to-quadricep muscle strength ratio predisposes such injuries (Klafs & Arnheim, 1977; Klein & Allman, 1969; Liemohn, 1978; Sutton, 1984). An explanation of this theory by Burkett (1975) is based on the fact that during parts of some movements, such as running, both the hamstrings and quadriceps contract at the same time. Thus opposing forces are in action. If one of these forces is greater than the other and resistance is maintained, something must give, and it is usually the hamstring muscles which are weaker than the quadriceps.

Research by Burkett (1971) has indicated that a strength-ratio imbalance between the right and left hamstrings may also initiate an injury. Burkett's study found that a strength difference of 10% or more would likely result in strain to the weaker hamstring. Resistance training could help to maintain these critical strength-ratio balances. However, theories vary regarding exact optimum ratios.

Another theory that explains the pulled hamstring is based on the neuro-mechanism. According to Burkett (1975), the cause of the injury could be due to the dual innervation of the biceps femoris and its asynchronous stimulation:

1. the stimulation to the short head is more intense than to the long head, causing an imbalance in the contraction phase,
2. the intensity of the stimulation doesn't change but the timing of the stimulation to the two different heads is asynchronous,
3. both 1 and 2, and
4. the change from prime mover stabilizer causes a lag in stimulation.

However, probably one of the most frequently cited causes of the problem is lack of flexibility. All things being equal, the more flexible a person, the less the chance of injury. Conversely, the more inflexible a person, the greater the likelihood of a pull. One explanation by Klein and Roberts (1976) is that when the hip flexors are tight and the pelvis tipped forward, the hamstrings are actually in a state of overstretch, because the origin of the attachment on the pelvis is lifted upward and the distance between the origin and insertion of the muscle is lengthened. Consequently, this action may account for early hamstring fatigue, one of the fundamental causes of hamstring injury.

Another explanation is that during exercise muscles swell and shorten. If the muscles are not flexible, they will be more susceptible to strain during the next exercise period. Consequently, there is increased risk of injury.

Among other possible causes of pulled hamstrings are: (a) overuse, (b) poor training methods and techniques, (c) lack of endurance, (d) fatigue, (e) structural abnormalities (e.g., lumbar lordosis, leg length discrepancy, or flat feet, (f) poor posture, (g) dehydration, (h) mineral deficiency (e.g., magnesium), and (i) trauma (Corbin & Noble, 1980; O'Neil, 1976; Taunton, 1982).

A recent review of the literature by Sutton (1984) clearly substantiates the notion that there is probably no single factor that predisposes one to hamstring strain. Furthermore, due to the number of confounding variables, an accurate prediction of those individuals who will suffer from hamstring strain is not yet possible with tests currently used. Therefore, more research is still needed. Nonetheless, common sense suggests the incorporation of lengthening and strengthening programs, along with the manipulation of those variables that are thought to predispose one to hamstring strains. An ounce of prevention is worth a pound of cure.

Stretching. Stretching the hamstrings occurs with flexion of the hip (i.e., decreasing the angle between the thigh and chest). This is usually accomplished either by extending the knees from a standing position with the hands on the floor (see Exercises #48 & 51), or by lowering the chest towards the floor while sitting or standing with one or both legs extended (see Exercises #41, 43, 44, 46, 47, & 50-58). Because there is a significant interrelationship between the hamstrings, pelvis, and lower back, you can also stretch your lower back muscles in the manner described. This will be discussed later in more detail.

Probably the most common method used to stretch the hamstrings is the hurdler's stretch (see Figure 13.10). When performing a regular hurdler's stretch, extend the leg to be stretched forward and flex the opposite leg so that the heel is next to the buttocks and hip. Remember, though, that this technique has several disadvantages. For those who have bad knees, flexion of the knee joint in this position may be painful and dangerous (Rapoport, 1984). This problem is further compounded if the rear foot is allowed to flare out to the side, because this may result in overstretching of the medial collateral ligaments (Anderson, 1980). Another disadvantage is that for most people who have tight hip flexors, the position

results in a slight sideward tilting of the pelvis and an improper stretch. When the position is correct, the body's weight is evenly distributed on both tuberosities of the ischium, and both crests of the iliac are parallel. This sideward tilting of the pelvis can be corrected by placing folded blankets and mats under the lower tuberosity until they become level. Another substantial problem with this technique is the increased strain imposed on the lower back.

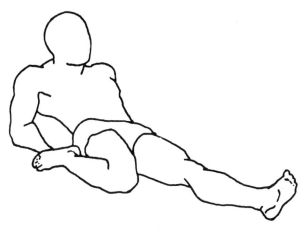

Figure 13.10. The hurdler's stretch. Note the rear foot is flared out to the side, thus placing stress on the medial aspect of the knee.

To guard against excessive stress on the lower back, two possible courses of action are plausible. First, the stretch can be initiated sitting on a bench or table approximately crotch-level (Barney, Hirst, & Jenson, 1972; Myers, 1983). With this technique, the lower leg hangs freely over the edge while the opposing leg is extended on the supporting surface. Then lower the trunk towards the thighs while keeping the upper back extended (see Exercise #43). Another method advocated by numerous experts (Anderson, 1980; Beaulieu, 1981; Cailliet, 1981) is to sit upright on the floor, flex the nonstretched leg so that the knee and thigh are brought close to the chest and the foot is placed flat on the floor. During the forward stretch, the flexed leg is rotated outward and the knee is allowed to abduct. Thus one is free to reach for the toes. In yoga, the *trianga mukhaikapada pashimottanasana* corresponds to the regular hurdler's stretch and the *marichyasana* to the modified version. If the flexed leg is fully abducted so that the outer side of the thigh and calf rests on the floor and the heel is placed against the inner side of the opposite thigh, this is called *janu sirsasana* (Iyengar, 1979) (see Exercise #41).

The Medial Femoral Muscles

The medial (toward the midline, or inside) portion of the thigh is comprised of five muscles. This region is commonly known as the groin. The word *groin* is actually the name applied to the region which includes the upper part of the front of the thigh and the lower part of the abdomen. In medical terminology, the muscles of the medial femoral group are called the adductor muscles. As with other muscles, the names are derived from their physical composition and/or function.

The muscles in this region are the adductor brevis, adductor longus, adductor magnus, gracilis, and pectineus. The primary functions of these muscles are to adduct, flex, and rotate the thigh medially. Furthermore, they serve to restrict abduction along with the ligaments of the hips (see Figure 13.11).

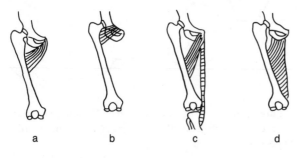

Figure 13.11.   The adductors (groin). (a) The adductor brevis. (b) The pectineus. (c) The adductor magnus. (d) The adductor longus.

Causes and Mechanisms of Injury.   Like the hamstrings, the groin is prone to strain. However, unlike the hamstrings, these injuries are more difficult to manage because they are located in an area that is awkward both to treat and support. The cause of the groin strain is virtually the same as that of the pulled hamstring. With diligent and disciplined conditioning, the risk of groin strain can be reduced.

Stretching.   Stretching the adductors is possible by abduction of the hip, that is, straddling the legs. This can be done while standing, sitting, kneeling, or lying, and the knees may be extended or flexed during the stretch (see Exercises #63-90).

A method that deserves special attention is the practicing of a straddle or Japanese split from a standing position. Here, one flexes at the hips and slowly straddles the legs as widely as possible. However, Biesterfeldt (1974) points out that this technique presents potential risks. Japanese splits apply direct sideward force on the knees. For those who are not fully mature, such forces can, if con-

tinued over some time, result in permanent deformity, such as loose and knocked knees. Obviously, the use of a partner applying pressure on the outside of the knees while standing from behind must be totally avoided.

The Anterior Femoral Muscles

The anterior (or front) portion of the thigh is made up of the four quadricep muscles, the sartorius muscle, the tensor fascia lata, the gluteal aponeurosis, and the iliotibial band. The quadriceps are commonly known as the *quads*. Each of the quads is named according to its respective position. Thus the rectus femoris is found on top of the femur; the vastus lateralis is located on the outside of the femur; the vastus medialis is positioned on the medial or inside of the thigh; and the vastus intermedialis is situated between the femur and rectus femoris (see Figure 13.12). The sartorius is named after the custom of tailors to sit cross-legged. All the quads function to extend the knee, while the rectus also produces flexion of the hip. In contrast, the sartorius flexes both the hip and the knee and rotates the lower limb laterally when the foot is off the ground. Lastly, the tensor fasciae lata assists in flexion and abduction of the hip joint and inward rotation of the thigh.

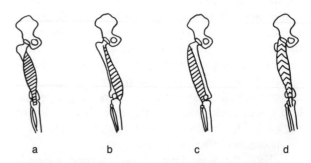

Figure 13.12.   The quadriceps. (a) The vastus intermedialis. (b) The vastus medialis. (c) The vastus lateralis. (d) The rectus femoris.

Causes and Mechanisms of Injury.   Injuries to the thigh are not uncommon. Stiffness, soreness, and tenderness are associated with a number of possible causes, including insufficient warm-up and stretching, overtraining, and fatigue. Here, too, a preventive approach is the most practical and prudent course of action to follow.

Stretching.   There are three principal kinds of stretching exercises for the quads: (a) bringing the heel(s) to the buttocks without hip extension;

(b) bringing the heel(s) to the buttocks with hip extension; and (c) hip extension with the legs relatively straight (see Exercises #91-110). The former methods will apply tension to all the quads while the latter method concentrates mainly on the rectus femoris and other hip flexors. For those with bad knees only the latter method should be used.

The Iliac Region

The iliac region is so named because of its direct anatomic relationship with the ilium. This region is made up of three muscles: The psoas major arises from the anterior surface and lower borders of the transverse processes of all the lumbar vertebrae and is attached to the lesser trochanter of the femur. It serves as a flexor of the hip. In front of the psoas major within the abdomen is the psoas minor, which is a weak flexor of the hip. The iliacus originates at the iliac fossa and inserts into the lateral side of the tendon of the psoas major. This muscle assists in forward tilt of the pelvis, flexion of the hip joint, and outward rotation of the thigh.

The muscles of the iliac region are also susceptible to strain. A test designed to reflect a strain in the deep iliopsoas muscle requires one to sit on the edge of a table with both legs hanging over the end, then attempt to lift the affected thigh upward against a resistance. A strain of the iliopsoas would be indicated by a leg pain in the groin area. This injury can significantly impair movement. Without the full usage of the iliopsoas, one is unable to maintain an upright posture easily or to move the thigh effectively.

The Gluteal Region

The gluteal region is often referred to as the buttocks. This region consists of three glutei, and six smaller, more deeply situated muscles. The gluteus maximus is the largest and most superficial muscle in the region. It is responsible for extension of the hip joint and assists in outward rotation of the thigh. The gluteus minimus is the smallest and deepest of the three gluteal muscles. The gluteus medius is the intermediate muscle in both size and location. Both of these muscles abduct the hip joint and assist with inward rotation of the thigh. The six remaining muscles—the piriformis, obturator externus, obturator internus, quadratus femoris, gemellus inferior, and gemellus superior—function to produce outward rotation of the thigh.

Causes and Mechanisms of Injury

Injuries to the gluteal region are not uncommon. Like other muscle groups, soreness and strains can occur in this region for a host of reasons, the most common of which are overtraining and the use of poor technique. As with groin injuries, this area is awkward both to treat and to support.

Stretching

Stretching the muscles of the gluteal region is difficult, and is usually accomplished by flexing the hip joint with the knees pulled toward the chest. Another method is to pull your ankle or knee to the opposite shoulder (see Exercises #120 & 128).

The Coxal or Hip Joint

The coxal, or hip joint, is perhaps the most striking example in the body of a ball and socket joint. It consists of the globular femoral head, which articulates with the deep, cup-shaped fossa of the acetabulum. It is because of the ball and socket arrangement that the hip is endowed with the ability to cover a wide range of motions.

Factors Affecting Stability and Ranges of Motion

Although the joint possesses considerable mobility, its chief function is to provide stability. There are many factors that contribute to the stability of the hip joint and determine its ultimate ranges of motion. These factors will be discussed below.

The Acetabulum. The acetabulum is a somewhat hemispherical cavity that articulates with the femoral head. It is formed from the union of the ilium, ischium, and pubic bones. When viewed from the anterior, it faces forward, downward, and laterally—a position that enhances stability.

Another factor that assists in creating stability is the acetabular labrum, which is a fibrocartilagenous rim attached to the margin of the acetabulum, thus increasing the depth of the joint and acting like a collar for the femoral head. It improves the fit between the two joining surfaces of the joint and tends to keep the head firmly in place.

The Shape of the Pelvis. The shape of the acetabulum is in part determined by the shape of the pelvis. However, the shape of the pelvis is to a major extent determined by one's sex. The female pelvis differs from that of the male in those particulars which render it better adapted to pregnancy and childbearing. A woman's pelvis is more shallow and shorter, the bones lighter and smoother, the coccyx more movable, and the subpubic arch angle more acute (i.e., greater than a right angle). It is also wider and almost cylindrical. As a result, the heads of the bones are more widely separate in women. Because the thighs grow toward the center line of the body as they approach the knees, this outward flare at the hips has a tendency to bring the knees of a woman somewhat closer together than a man's (see Figure 13.13). The broader hips give the female a much greater potential for range of motion, and thus the ability to do splits and high extensions more easily (Hamilton, 1978b).

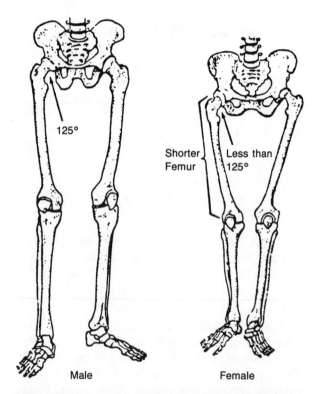

Figure 13.13. A comparison of the male and female outward flaring of the hips. The femoral angle is less than 125° in some women, giving a greater tendency to knock-knees. *Note.* From *Biology of Women* (p. 24) by E. Sloane, 1980, New York: John Wiley and Sons. Copyright 1980 by John Wiley & Sons, Inc. Reprinted by permission.

The Angle of Inclination and Declination. The head of the femur forms two distinct angles with the shaft of the femur, the angle of inclination and the angle of declination. The angle of inclination is the measure of the neck-shaft angle in the frontal plane. At birth, newborns have angles of almost 150 degrees. However, this decreases with age. By

adulthood, the average angle is about 125 degrees (see Figure 13.14).

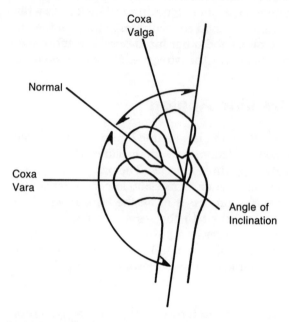

Figure 13.14. The angle of inclination. This angle is formed by a line drawn through the femoral shaft center and one bisecting the head and neck. Coxa Vara is angulation less than normal and Coxa Valga is angulation beyond the normal.

When the angle of inclination is larger than 125 degrees in an adult the resulting deformity is known as coxa valga. In extreme cases, it may reach a straight angle of 180 degrees. With coxa valga, there are no skeletal checks to restrict ranges of motion, thus promoting dislocation (Kapandji, 1982; Steindler, 1977).

If the angle of inclination is less than 125 degrees, the deformity is termed coxa vara. This results in a flaring or widening of the hips. With coxa vara, there is a restriction of the ability to abduct due to impingement of the greater trochanter against the ilium. Furthermore, inward rotation of the femur becomes limited (Steindler, 1977).

The angle of declination is the measure of the degree of forward angulation of the femur's head in relation to its shaft. In other words, it is the angle between the axis of the femoral neck and the frontal plane. This angle is normally rather high at birth (40 degrees). However, with age, it decreases to about 12 to 15 degrees. The term for this angulation is the anteversion angle. A decrease of this angle is called retroversion (see Figure 13.15).

An angle of anteversion produces an increased internal torsion or rotation of the femur and leg, resulting in an in-toeing or a pigeon-toed gait. In contrast, retroversion produces an external torsion or rotation of the femur and leg, resulting in an outward-toeing or duck-toed gait. In ballet, this is referred to as a *turnout*. The turnout is important because it allows one to increase range of motion. This technique will be explained later. However, we can briefly state here that the conditions ideal for ballet (and certain sports) are a long neck with a low-shaft angle for maximum range of motion, and retroversion for good, natural turnout. Unfortunately, this combination is extremely rare (Hamilton, 1978a).

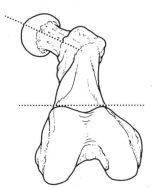

Figure 13.15. The angle of declination. Anteversion is angulation beyond "normal." In contrast, retroversion is angulation below "normal."

The Articular Capsule and Ligaments. Although it is primarily the bony design that determines the degree of motion of the hip, other factors do play a role. Probably the most important limiting factor is the articular capsule and the powerful ligamentous support apparatus. The heavy fibrous articular capsule, like a sleeve, encloses the hip joint and the greater part of the femoral neck. Integrated into the capsule are the ligaments. At the hip, the principal ligaments are the iliofemoral, ishiofemoral, pubofemoral, and ligamentum teres. Their mechanism of checking joint motion will be discussed later.

Muscular Reinforcement and Coordination. The stability of the joint is further enhanced by those muscles that run roughly parallel to the femoral neck. They help keep the femoral head in contact with the acetabulum. These muscles are the piriformis, obturator externus, gluteus medius, and gluteus minimus.

Another factor to take into consideration is the role that the muscles play in creating motion during active stretching. For example, in abduction (the moving apart of the legs), the limiting factor may be the lack of strength and/or coordination of the agonists to create the movement. In this instance, that would be the abductor muscles.

Finally, it must be remembered that resistance of the antagonistic or opposing muscle group and its respective connective tissue sheaths are also a major limiting factor in one's range of motion. Thus, during abduction, the major inhibitors are the adductor muscles and their respective tissue sheaths.

Limits on Range of Motion

Altogether, there are six major movements of the hip excluding circumduction. These are flexion, extension, abduction, adduction, medial rotation, and lateral rotation. Following is an analysis of these movements.

Flexion. Hip flexion is defined as a decrease in the angle between the thigh and abdomen. Flexion of the hip with the knee flexed ranges from 0 to 120 degrees (see Figure 13.16). With the knee extended, range is usually limited to about 90 degrees (see Figure 13.17). Tests for measuring hamstring

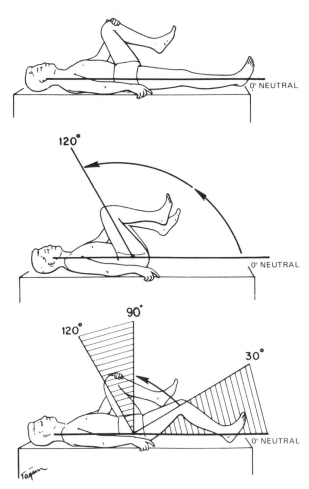

Figure 13.16. Hip flexion. *Note.* From *Manual of Orthopaedic Surgery* (p. 102), 1985, Park Ridge, IL: American Orthopaedic Association. Copyright 1972 by The American Orthopaedic Association. Reprinted by permission.

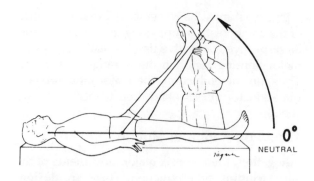

Figure 13.17. The straight leg raising test. *Note.* From *Manual of Orthopaedic Surgery* (p. 130), 1985, Park Ridge, IL: American Orthopaedic Association. Copyright 1972 by The American Orthopaedic Association. Reprinted by permission.

muscle tightness include the passive toe-touch test, the passive unilateral straight-leg-raising (SLR) test, and the active unilateral SLR test (see Figure 13.18). The SLR test is also important because it can be used as a neurological test. These would include lumbar nerve root compression, sciatic normality, and disk protrusion (Bohannon, Gajdosik, & LeVeau, 1985; Gajdosik & Lusin, 1983; Urban, 1981).

There are a number of instruments that can be used to assess the SLR test (Hsieh, Walker, & Gillis, 1983). However, recent studies have found that various factors may influence the results of the test. For example, Bohannon et al. (1985) found pelvic rotation to begin within 9 degrees at the beginning of the passive SLR test, and that the

The straight leg raising test for hamstring length is actually a combination of hip flexion and flexion of the lumbar spine. Having the low back flat on the table is a prerequisite to accurate testing.

Normal length of right hamstring, low back, and left hip flexor muscles.

With the low back flat on the table, and the left leg held down to stabilize the pelvis and prevent excessive flexion of the lumbar spine, the right leg with the knee straight can be raised passively to an angle of 80° to 85° hip flexion. This range of motion indicates normal hamstring length.

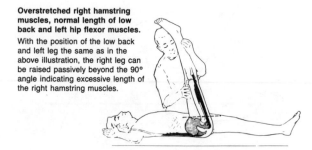

Normal length of right hamstring muscles, short low back and left hip flexor muscles.

Although the right hamstring muscles are normal in length, straight leg raising is restricted because the shortness of the left hip flexor and low back muscles hold the lumbar spine in hyper-extension maintaining the pelvis in anterior tilt when the left leg is held down on the table. To avoid the misdiagnosis of short hamstrings in this case, the left thigh should be allowed to flex sufficiently to flatten the low back, and be stabilized in that position while raising the right leg. Restriction of, or excessive lumbar spine flexion affects the test for hamstring length.

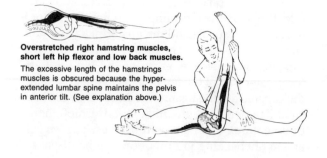

Overstretched right hamstring muscles, normal length of low back and left hip flexor muscles.

With the position of the low back and left leg the same as in the above illustration, the right leg can be raised passively beyond the 90° angle indicating excessive length of the right hamstring muscles.

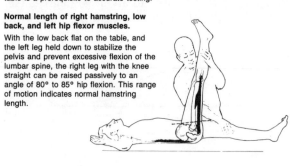

Overstretched right hamstring muscles, short left hip flexor and low back muscles.

The excessive length of the hamstrings muscles is obscured because the hyper-extended lumbar spine maintains the pelvis in anterior tilt. (See explanation above.)

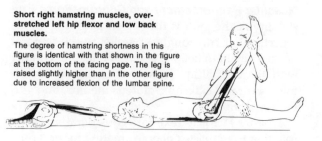

Short right hamstring muscles, normal length of low back and left hip flexor muscles.

With the position of the low back and left leg the same as in the above illustrations, the right leg can be raised passively only to an angle of approximately 50°, indicating a marked shortness of the hamstring muscles.

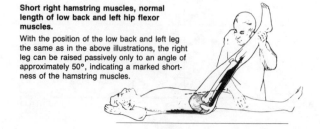

Short right hamstring muscles, over-stretched left hip flexor and low back muscles.

The degree of hamstring shortness in this figure is identical with that shown in the figure at the bottom of the facing page. The leg is raised slightly higher than in the other figure due to increased flexion of the lumbar spine.

Figure 13.18. Tests for length of hamstring muscles. *Note.* From *Muscles Testing and Function* (2nd ed., p. 166) by H.O. Kendall, F.P. Kendall, and G.E. Wadsworth, 1971, Baltimore: Williams and Wilkins. Copyright 1971 by The Williams and Wilkins Company. Reprinted by permission.

angle of pelvic rotation increased in conjunction with the angle of the straight-leg-raising. Yet in a study of the active SLR test (Mayhew, Norton, & Sahrmann, 1983), the findings indicated that the degree of participation of the contralateral hamstrings and abdominal muscles may contribute to potential variations. In addition to the above, the pull of the gastrocnemius may influence the degree of movement. Hence, to minimize the pull, the ankle should be allowed to plantar-flex slightly.

Flexion of the hip is produced primarily by the psoas major and iliacus, and assisted by the rectus femoris, sartorius, tensor fasciae latae, pectineus, adductor brevis, adductor longus, and adductor magnus. Range of motion is checked by contractile insufficiency, contacting the thigh with the abdomen, and tension of the hamstring muscles. During flexion, all ligaments are relaxed. Thus they provide no resistance.

Extension. Hip extension involves the return from flexion to the anatomical, or neutral, position. Extension beyond the anatomical position is called hyperextension, as shown in Figure 13.19. Active range of motion is 10 degrees with the knee flexed

and 20 degrees with the knee extended. In contrast, passive hyperextension attains a range of 20 degrees when one lunges forward, and reaches 30 degrees when the lower limb is forcibly pulled back (Kapandji, 1982). To achieve a true test for the hip flexor muscles (that helps limit hyperextension), it is necessary to lie with your back flat on a table with one leg flexed at the hip and one leg (the leg with the hip to be tested) hanging over the edge. If the thigh fails to touch the table while the back is held flat, then tightness of the hip flexors is indicated (Kendall, Kendall, & Wadsworth, 1971).

Extension of the hip is produced primarily by the gluteus maximus, semitendinosus, semimembranosus, and biceps femoris. Range of motion is limited by contractile insufficiency; tension of the hip flexor muscles; locking of the spine to prevent anterior tilting of the pelvis via exaggeration of the lumbar lordosis; and tension by all the ligaments. These things make it difficult to execute a split with the hips squared and the rear hip turned in.

Abduction.   Abduction of the hip may be defined as the movement of the lower limb laterally away from the axis of the body (see Figure 13.20). It is

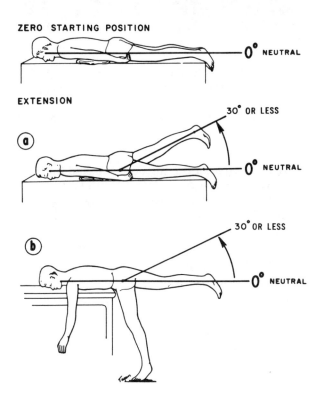

Figure 13.19. The hip (extension). *Note.* From *Joint Motion Method of Measurement and Recording* (p. 59), 1965, Edinburgh: Churchill Livingstone. Copyright 1965 by The American Academy of Orthopaedic Surgeons. Reprinted by permission.

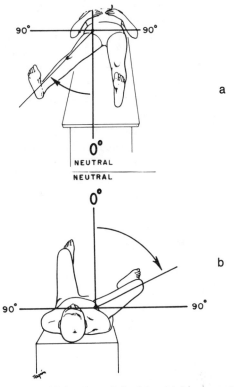

Figure 13.20. Abduction of the hip. (a) In extension. (b) In flexion. *Note.* From *Manual of Orthopaedic Surgery* (p. 104), 1985, Park Ridge, IL: American Orthopaedic Association. Copyright 1972 by The American Orthopaedic Association. Reprinted by permission.

produced primarily by the gluteus medius and gluteus minimus, and assisted by the tensor fasciae lata and the sartorius. In one hip, abduction ranges from 0 to 45 degrees. However, in practice abduction at one joint is automatically followed by a similar degree of abduction at the other. This becomes obvious after 30 degrees of abduction, when a tilting of the pelvis can be clearly seen. Thus abduction is the result of a 15-degree abduction in each limb. In further describing this motion, Kapandji (1982) points out that as abduction continues, the vertebral column as a whole compensates for pelvic tilt by bending laterally towards the supporting side. Thus, here too, the vertebral column is involved in movements of the hip.

Abduction of the hip is limited by several elements: contractile insufficiency, tension of the hip adductor muscles, tension of the pubofemoral and iliofemoral ligaments, and impact of the femoral neck on the acetabular rim. It should also be mentioned that the vertebral column and pelvis can serve as restraining factors, because the vertebral column is involved in movements of the hip, and any restrictions on the column could in turn restrict compensatory actions for excessive pelvic tilting.

How, then, can one maximize one's range of abduction? Are there any secrets? The answer is yes! For example, let's examine the straddle split as shown in Figure 13.21. This skill can be performed passively on the floor, or actively in the air. In either case, when executed to the ultimate position (180 degrees), pure abduction does not take place. Rather, the pelvis is tilted anteriorly (i.e., forward) while the vertebral column is hyperextended. Thus the hip is put into a position of abduction and flexion. This is because, after a certain point, movement is transferred to the pelvis, and thereafter through the spine. The purpose in particular here is to reduce and minimize the checking/restraining action of the iliofemoral ligament because during hip flexion, as you will recall, all ligaments are relaxed.

Another technique used to enhance one's range of abduction is the use of the turnout. The rationale of a turnout is twofold. First, the turnout incorporates a lateral rotation of the hip joint, which results in a relaxing of the ischiofemoral ligament. (However, all the anterior ligaments of the hip become taut, especially those bandings running horizontally, that is, the iliotrochanter band and pubofemoral ligament.) The second rationale for the turnout is more significant. Following is a concise explanation by Chujoy and Manchester (1967):

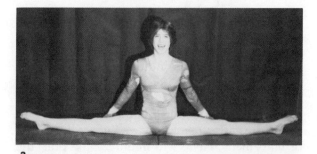

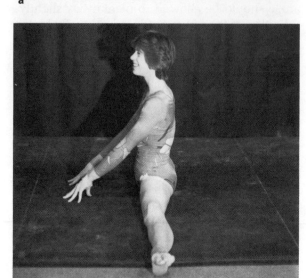

Figure 13.21.   The straddle split. (a) Front view. (b) Side view. *Note.* From *Coaching Women's Gymnastics* (p. 80) by B. Sands, 1984, Champaign, IL: Human Kinetics. Copyright 1984 by B. Sands. Reprinted by permission.

The principle of the turn-out is based on the anatomical structure of the hip joints. In normal positions the movements of the legs are limited by the structure of the joint between the pelvis and the hips. As the leg is drawn to the side the hip-neck meets the brim of the acetabulum and further movement is impossible. But, if the leg is turned out, the big (greater) trochanter recedes and the brim of the acetabulum meets the flat side-surface of the hip-neck. This allows the dancer to extend the leg so that it forms an angle of ninety degrees or more with the other leg. The turn-out is not an aesthetic conception but an anatomical and technical necessity for the ballet dancer. It is the turn-out that makes the difference between a limited number of steps on one plane and the possibility of control of all dance movements in space. (p. 923)

Regrettably, turnout is often forced by those who cannot make the totally external position. Consequently, this places increased external torsion on the knees and can produce medial knee strain and patellar subluxation. The effect is similar to a football player firmly planting his cleated shoe in the ground and then rotating his leg (Miller, Schneider, Bronson, & McClain, 1975). The most common method of forcing the turnout in ballet is called *screwing the knee*. This is accomplished by assuming a demi plié (half-knee bend) position, allowing a 180-degree position of the feet, then straightening the knees without moving the feet (Ende & Wickstrom, 1982; Ryan, 1976; Teitz, 1982) (see Exercises #30-34).

Since the turnout at the hip is mostly determined by the bony design and to a lesser degree by the surrounding hip joint capsule and connective tissue, we must ask the question, "To what extent can this be affected by training?" According to Hamilton (1978a), the consensus of medical literature indicates that spontaneous changes in anteversion occur most rapidly from birth to age 8, and that the process is close to completion by age 10. However, it is not completely finished until about age 16. Later attempts to correct anteversion seem to have little effect. Rather, a compensatory external rotation deformity is created in the tibia below the knee.

Adduction. Adduction of the hip may be defined as the movement of the lower limb toward the midline of the body. This movement is produced primarily by the adductor longus, adductor brevis, and adductor magnus, and assisted by the pectineus and gracilis. Range of motion is limited by contractile insufficiency and contact with the opposite leg. When the thigh is flexed, the range increases from 0 to 60 degrees. Here motion is further restricted by tension of the abductory muscles, tension of the iliofemoral ligament, and tension of the ligament of the femur's head.

Medial Rotation. Medial rotation of the hip is defined as internal or inward rotation of the femur (see Figure 13.22). This movement is produced by the tensor fasciae lata, gluteus minimus, and gluteus medius. With the knee joint flexed, it ranges from 0 to 45 degrees, and somewhat less with the leg extended. Medial rotation is limited by contractile insufficiency, tension of the hip lateral rotators, and tension of the ischiofemoral ligament with the hip flexed, and the iliofemoral ligament when extended.

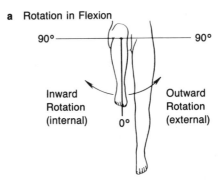

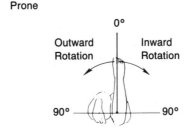

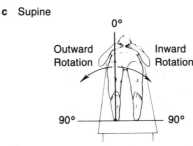

Figure 13.22. Medial (inward) and lateral (outward) hip rotation. (a) In flexion. (b) In extension—prone. (c) In extension—supine. *Note.* From *Manual of Orthopaedic Surgery* (pp. 103-104), 1985, Park Ridge, IL: American Orthopaedic Association. Copyright 1972 by The American Orthopaedic Association. Reprinted by permission.

Mann, Baxter, and Lutter (1981) contend that stretching of the hip by medial rotation is important because it can often eliminate knee pain associated with running. For instance, limited hip, pelvic, or back rotation can place more torque on the knee, leg, and ankle during running, especially during the foot-plant phases of running. Furthermore, if there is an external rotational deformity of the hip, more torque is placed on the knee as the speed is increased and the lower extremity attempts to rotate internally. Hence the importance of stretching the medial rotators.

Lateral Rotation. Lateral rotation of the hip is defined as external or outward rotation of the femur (see Figure 13.22). Lateral rotation is produced by the obturator muscles, gemelli and quadratus femoris, and assisted by the piriformis, gluteus maximus, and sartorius. Range of motion is from 0 to 45 degrees with the knee joint flexed. The movement is limited by contractile insufficiency, tension of the hip medial rotators, and tension of the iliofemoral ligament. Lateral rotation is seen in many yoga postures such as the easy posture, perfect posture, and lotus posture (see Exercise #132).

Review Questions

1. You are an instructor of young dancers. Explain how you will determine when it is appropriate for one to start on pointe work.

2. Design a program to reduce the potential incidence of inversion sprains. Cite specific exercises and additional measures that you will initiate.

3. Design a series of exercises to stretch and strengthen the Achilles tendon.

4. What is the appropriate course of action to follow if an athlete reports to you a locking of the knee that occurs many times throughout the day? What are some potential causes?

5. Describe a series of tests to measure hamstring flexibility.

6. Explain the statement, "There is probably no single factor that predisposes one to hamstring strain."

7. Explain why the hurdler's stretch is no longer recommended as part of a stretching program. What would be an appropriate substitute?

8. Explain how stretching the quadriceps might be potentially dangerous for those with bad knees.

9. Draw a diagram and label the hamstrings, quadriceps, and groin muscles.

10. Explain why females have a greater predisposition for ROM in the pelvic region.

11. Explain why the straight-leg-raising test (either active or passive) is apt to be inaccurate.

12. Explain the anatomical advantages associated with a turnout in order to enhance one's range of abduction.

13. Explain the dangers associated with an improper turnout.

14. Draw a diagram of the pelvis and label its major parts.

Answers

1. Pointe work should begin when one has the strength and skill to do something in the desired position. For most, this will be at about age 12.

2. To reduce the potential incidence of inversion sprains, one must enhance the strength, endurance, and skill level. With regard to the first, one should use hand resistance exercises in all directions about the ankle joint. Perform one or two sets of 10 to 15 contractions. Additional measures would include the use of proper equipment, footwear, and ankle taping.

3. See Exercises #19 to 40 to enhance flexibility. You can strengthen the Achilles tendon by doing toe rises while holding a barbell (see Exercise #233).

4. One should immediately seek professional help. Potential causes of a locking of the knee include a torn meniscus and bone chips.

5. Hamstring flexibility can be tested with the passive straight-leg-raising test from either a standing or supine position.

6. Because there are a number of confounding variables, there is probably no single factor that predisposes one to hamstring strain.

7. The hurdler's stretch is no longer recommended because it may cause overstretching of the medial collateral ligaments. This risk can be reduced either by stretching on a table with one leg hanging over the edge or by assuming the hurdler's stretch position with the nonstretched leg flexed and abducted onto the floor.

8. Those with bad knees have a greater predisposition to injury because those exercises that bring the heels to the buttocks may place considerable force on the muscles and ligaments being stretched.

9. See Figures 13.9, 13.11, and 13.12.

10. Females have a greater predisposition for ROM in the pelvic region because the pelvis is more shallow and wider than that of males.

11. The straight-leg-raising test is apt to be inaccurate because of the measuring instrument, errors in measurement, competency of the evaluator, and the motivation of the person being tested.

12. A turnout is important because it allows one to increase range of motion. This is accomplished by the relaxing of the ischiofemoral ligament and by making the big (greater) trochanter recede. Thus the brim of the acetabulum meets the flat side-surface of the hip-neck.

13. An improper turnout can produce medial knee strain and patellar subluxation.

14. See Figure 8.1a, 8.1b, and 13.13.

Recommended Readings

Agre, J.C. (1985). Hamstring injuries proposed aetiological factors, prevention, and treatment. *Sports Medicine, 2*(1), 21-33.

Arnheim, D.D. (1980). *Dance injuries. Their prevention and care* (2nd ed.). St. Louis: C.V. Mosby.

Distefano, V.J. (1981). Anatomy and biomechanics of the ankle and foot. *Athletic Training, 16*(1), 43-47.

Gelabert, R. (1977, Feb). Turning out. *Dance Magazine*, pp. 86-87.

Gelabert, R. (1980). Preventing dancers' injuries. *The Physician and Sportsmedicine, 8*(4), 69-76.

Grace, T.G. (1985). Muscle imbalance and extremity injury: A perplexing relationship. *Sports Medicine, 2*(2), 77-82.

Hamilton, W. (1982, Oct). The best body for ballet. *Dance Magazine*, pp. 82-83.

Henricson, A., Larsson, A., Olsson, E., & Westlin, N. (1983). The effect of stretching on the range of motion of the ankle joint in badminton players. *The Journal of Orthopaedic and Sports Physical Therapy, 5*(2), 74-77.

Jacobs, M., & Young, R. (1978). Snapping hip phenomenon among dancers. *The American Corrective Therapy Journal, 32*(3), 92-98.

Mack, R.P. (1975). Ankle injuries in athletics. *Athletic Training, 10*(2), 94-95.

Mayhew, T.P., Norton, B.J., & Sahrmann, S.A. (1983). Electromyographic study of the relationship between hamstring and abdominal muscles during unilateral straight leg raise. *Physical Therapy, 63*(11), 1769-1773.

Millar, A.P. (1975). An early stretching routine in hamstring strains. *The Australian Journal of Sports Medicine, 7*(5), 107-109.

Möller, M.H.L., Öberg, B.E., & Gillquist, J. (1985). Stretching exercise and soccer: Effect of stretching on range of motion in the lower extremity in connection with soccer training. *The International Journal of Sports Medicine, 6*, 50-52.

Myers, M. (1982, June). Is the grand plié obsolete? *Dance Magazine*, pp. 78-80.

Pruett, D.M., & Rohan, J. (1984). Limitation of movement due to hip joint ligaments and implications for teaching exercise and dance. *The Florida Journal of Health, Physical Education, Recreation and Dance, 22*(2), 5-6.

Roberts, W. (1963). The locking mechanism of the hip joint. *Anatomical Record, 147*(3), 321-324.

Sammarco, G.J. (1975). Biomechanics of the foot and ankle—injuries of the foot. *Athletic Training 10*(2), 96-98.

Singleton, M.C., & LeVeau, B.F. (1975). The hip joint: Structure, stability, and stress. *Physical Therapy, 55*(9), 957-973.

Smart, G.W., Taunton, J.E., & Clement, D.B. (1980). Achilles tendon disorders in runners—a review. *Medicine and Science in Sports and Exercise, 12*(4), 231-243.

Teitz, C.C., Harrington, R.M., & Wiley, H. (1985). Pressures on the foot in pointe shoes. *Foot & Ankle, 5*(5), 216-221.

Urban, L.M. (1981). The straight-leg raise test—a review. *The Orthopaedic and Sports Physical Therapy Journal, 2*(3), 117-133.

Williams, P.L., & Warwick, R. (1980). *Gray's anatomy* (36th British ed.). Philadelphia: W.B. Saunders.

CHAPTER 14

The Vertebral Column

The vertebral column is a truly unique and amazing structure. In the layperson's terminology it is called the backbone, a term which has obvious validity with respect to its position in the body, but which offers little help in structural and movement matters. In fact, the vertebral column is not a single bone. Rather, it is a stack of thirty-three bones that are flexibly connected one above the other (Kelley, 1971).

Gross Anatomy

The vertebral column is made up of a series of separate bones, the vertebrae, linked together by a larger number of cartilage disks and ligaments. Altogether, the column consists of thirty-three vertebrae, which are generally arranged into five divisions:

- the seven cervical vertebrae (neck),
- the twelve thoracic vertebrae (rib cage),
- the five lumbar vertebrae (lower back),
- the five sacral vertebrae (base of the spine),
- the four coccygeal vertebrae (coccyx).

In the adult, the sacrum is a single bone that results from the fusion of five sacral vertebrae. Similarly, the coccyx is a single bone that results from the fusion of the four coccygeal vertebrae. Therefore, between the last nine vertebrae, there is a substantial amount of stability, and virtually no mobility (see Figure 14.1).

An important feature of the vertebral column is the presence of four distinct curves. At birth, an infant's spine has only one long curve. This curve extends over its entire length and is convexed posteriorly (C-shaped). However, once the infant starts to raise its head, the cervical curve begins to develop. This is referred to as cervical lordosis. Later, when the child begins to stand and walk, the lumbar curve develops in the lower back (see Figure 14.2b).

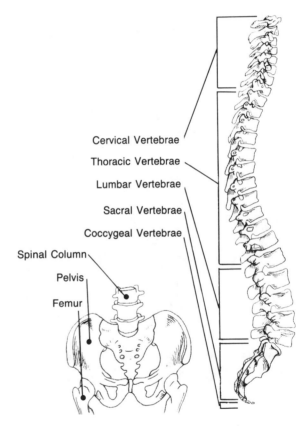

Figure 14.1. Lateral view of the spine, anterior view of the spine and pelvis. *Note.* From *Living Anatomy* (p. 81) by J.E. Donnelly, 1982, Champaign, IL: Human Kinetics. Copyright 1982 by J.E. Donnelly. Reprinted by permission.

Abnormal vertebral curves may be present in some persons (see Figure 14.2). Deformities in flexion are called kyphosis. Kyphosis is the result of a forward bend in the thoracic region, and is seen in those who have a "hunchback." Another deformity is the "sway-back" appearance called lordosis. Lordosis is the result of an excessive extension most commonly seen only in the lumbar area. It is accompanied by a forward protrusion of the abdomen, and a backward protrusion of the buttocks. Deformities producing a lateral deviation are called *scoliosis*. Scoliosis is almost always primarily in the thoracic region.

This structure can be better appreciated and understood by considering a number of analogies. The vertebral column can be thought of as a massive transmitting and receiving tower supported by guy wires. The tower is made up of the bony vertebral column, the disks, and the ligaments. The guy wires are the muscles that support the system and hold it erect. The base of the system is the sacrum and pelvis, and the head is both receiver and transmitter. Yet another way to visualize the column is to imagine it as a flexible boom, like the mast of a sailboat. Hence, it is essentially the fulcrum of a lever.

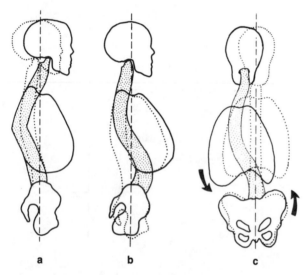

Figure 14.2. Abnormal curvature of the vertebral column. (a) Kyphosis. (b) Lordosis. (c) Scoliosis.

Function

The vertebral column has a number of different functions. Probably the most important function is that it serves to protect the spinal cord. It also provides a firm support for the trunk and appendages. Thus it serves as a sustaining rod for the maintenance of the upright position of the body. Because the column is the fulcrum of a lever system, it produces a considerable mechanical advantage in terms of loading. The vertebral column also provides for muscular attachments, serves as an anchor for the rib cage, acts as a shock absorber, and provides a combination of strength and flexibility that affords maximal protection and stability with minimal restriction of mobility.

The Vertebrae

The typical vertebra is made up of two major parts. These are the forward vertebral body (found anteriorly) and the backward vertebral arch (located posteriorly). However, if a vertebra is dismantled, it is found actually to consist of several fused parts. For a clearer understanding, we can compare a single vertebra with the structure of a house (Hoppenfeld, 1967).

The basic foundation of the house is the body. The body is the largest part of the vertebra. It is located anteriorly, is cylindrical in shape, and is wider than it is tall. It is the weight-bearing part of the vertebra. Next is the vertebral arch. This is composed of seven smaller structures. Two of these are the pedicles, which form the supporting sides or walls. Obviously they, too, are built to withstand great forces placed upon them. Then there are the two laminae, which form the roof of the house. Extending laterally from each pedicle-laminae are the transverse processes. These may be thought of as the eaves or wings of the house. Lastly there is the spinous process that makes up the chimney of the roof. The spinous process is the most posterior part of the vertebra. Therefore, this part is seen when one bends forward (see Figure 14.3).

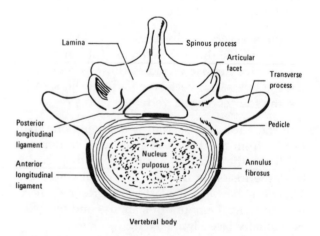

Figure 14.3. The vertebral segment. As viewed from above, the vertebral segment is divided into the anterior and posterior segments. The anterior portion is the vertebral body and the disk structures. The posterior portion consists of the lamina, pedicles, and facets. In this segment the posterior longitudinal ligament is incomplete, placing it at the lower lumbar (L_5) level. *Note.* From *Low Back Pain Syndrome* (3rd ed., p.7) by R. Cailliet, 1981, Philadelphia: F.A. Davis. Copyright 1981 by F.A. Davis Company. Reprinted by permission.

The Disks

Between the vertebral bodies and uniting them are 23 intervertebral disks. Altogether, the disks make up approximately one-quarter of the total length of the vertebral column. They function chiefly as hydraulic shock absorbers that permit compression and distortion. Therefore, they allow motion between the vertebrae (extension, flexion, rotation, or combinations of these motions).

Another factor that is extremely important is the thickness of the disk. The amount of movement that can occur in any part of the vertebral column depends in large part upon the ratio between the height of the intervertebral disks and the height of the bony part of the column. Kapandji (1982) concisely describes the significance of the disks. As is apparent, disk thickness varies with disk position in the vertebral column. The regions from thickest to thinnest are the lumbar (9 mm), thoracic (5 mm), and cervical (3 mm). However, more important than the absolute thickness is the ratio of the disk thickness to the height of the vertebral body. In fact, Kapandji states that this ratio accounts for the mobility of the particular segment of the vertebral column because the greater the ratio the greater the mobility. Thus the cervical region is most mobile since its disk to body ratio is 2/5, or 40%. In contrast, the lumbar region is slightly less mobile with a ratio of 1/3, or 33%. Lastly, there is the thoracic region. This region is the least mobile with a ratio of 1/5, or 20%. Hence, the disks play a major role in ultimately determining potential range of movement in the back.

The disk consists of two parts: the nucleus pulposus and the annulus fibrosus. The liquid and elastic properties of the nucleus pulposus and annulus fibrosus, acting in combination, enable the disk to withstand great loads.

The Nucleus Pulposus

The nucleus pulposus is composed of an incompressible gel-like material that is encased in an elastic container. A protein-polysaccharide makes up its chemical composition. The nucleus is strongly hydropholic; that is, it has a strong affinity to or attraction for water. In fact, it can bind nine times its volume of water (the inhibition pressure of the nucleus has been found to reach 250 mmHg). According to Püschel (1930), at birth the water content of the nucleus is 88%. Consequently, it cannot be compressed. Furthermore, since it exists for all practical purposes as a closed container, it must conform to Pascal's law: "Any external force exerted on a unit of a confined liquid is transmitted

undiminished to every unit of the interior of the containing vessel" (Cailliet, 1981a). In other words, a pressure applied to a liquid is transmitted unchanged to all parts of the liquid, and to the walls of the vessel that contain it. Thus the nucleus acts as a hydraulic shock absorber.

However, as the nucleus ages, it loses its water-binding capacity. Consequently, by the age of 70, the water content diminishes to just 66%. The causes and implications of this dehydration are extremely significant. First, the dehydration appears to be a natural process of aging. That is, it appears to be a by-product of attrition due to continual stress and wear and tear. This can be explained by a decrease in the content of the protein-polysaccharide as well as by the gradual replacement of the gelatinous material of the nucleus by fibrocartilage. Hence, there is a decrease in the fluid content. Lastly, after the second decade, the disk's vascular supply disappears. By the third decade, the disk, now avascular, receives its nutrition by diffusion of lymph through the vertebral end plates. This can explain the loss of both flexibility and height in the aged, as well as the impaired ability of the aged to regain elasticity in an injured disk (Cailliet, 1981a).

What, then, is the function of the nucleus pulposus? As stated earlier, its chief function is that of a hydraulic shock absorber. Specifically, it serves to receive primarily vertical forces from vertebral bodies, and to redistribute them radically in a horizontal plane. Then the annulus fibrosus resists the created tension. To better understand this action, imagine the nucleus as a movable swivel (see Figure 14.4). A summary of these actions is presented in Table 14.1.

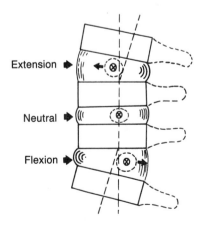

Figure 14.4. The fulcrum of movement in flexion and extension of the lumbar spine. *Note.* From *A Practical Guide to Management of the Painful Neck and Back* (p. 37) by J.W. Fisk and B.S. Rose, 1977, Springfield, IL: Charles C Thomas. Copyright 1977 by Charles C Thomas Publisher. Reprinted by permission.

Table 14.1   Functions of the Nucleus Pulposus

Action	Flexion	Extension	Lateral Flexion
The upper vertebrae will tilt:	Anteriorly	Posteriorly	Toward the side of flexion
THEREFORE, The disk will flatten:	Anteriorly	Posteriorly	Toward the side of flexion
THEREFORE, The disk will enlarge:	Posteriorly	Anteriorly	Toward the side opposite of flexion
THEREFORE, The nucleus will be driven:	Posteriorly	Anteriorly	Toward the side opposite of flexion

The Annulus Fibrosus

The annulus fibrosus consists of approximately 20 concentric fibers. These elastic fibers are woven so that one layer runs at an angle to the preceding layer. Therefore, they seem to cross each other obliquely. This special pattern allows a controlled motion to take place. For example, when a shearing force is applied (i.e., a force that tends to cause one layer of an object to slide over another layer), the oblique fibers in one direction will tighten, while the opposing oblique fibers relax (see Figure 14.5).

As stated earlier, the annulus fibrosus must receive the ultimate effects of most forces trans-mitted from one vertebral body to another. This may seem strange because the major loading of the disk is in the form of vertical compression and the annulus fibrosus is best constructed to resist shear. However, the nucleus pulposus transforms the vertical thrust into a radical or shear force. Then the shear force is restricted by the elastic and tensile strength of the fibers.

Similar to the nucleus pulposus, the annulus fibrosus loses a great deal of its elasticity and resiliency with age. In young and undamaged disks, the fibroelastic tissue of the annulus fibrosus is predominantly elastic. However, in the process of aging, or as a residual of injury, there is a relative increase in the percentage of fibrous elements. As this increase occurs, the disk loses its elasticity, and its recoil hydraulic mechanism decreases. In the older annulus fibrosus there is a replacement of the highly elastin collagen fibrils by large fibrotic bands of collagen tissue devoid of mucoid material. The disk is therefore less elastic (Bick, 1961; Cailliet, 1981a; Panagiotacopulos, Knauss, & Bloch, 1979; Walker, 1981).

Furthermore, as the disk becomes more and more inelastic, it becomes more and more susceptible to injury and trauma. Then each episode of trauma sets the stage for extrusion of the nucleus pulposus into the tears of the annulus fibrosus. Thus even a minor stress might tip the scales or be the straw that breaks the camel's back (Cailliet, 1981a). Then the vicious cycle is repeated again.

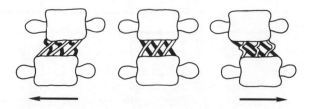

Figure 14.5.   Controlled motion. The elastic fibers of the annulus fibrosus are in part responsible for the controlled motion that takes place in the vertebral column. When a horizontal force is applied to the vertebrae, the oblique fibers in one direction will tighten, while those in the other relax. With a force in the opposite direction, the opposite set of oblique fibers tightens, and the remaining obliquely directed fibers relax.

Furthermore, due to the reduced vascular supply to the disk, the ability of an injured disk to regain its elasticity is bound to be stronger in the young. No wonder that herniation, rupture, or bulging of the disk are found more often in the aged than in the young (Bick, 1961; Cailliet, 1981a; Panagiotacopulos, Knauss, & Bloch, 1979).

The Vertebral Ligaments

Ligamentous structures and other connective tissues also contribute to the stability of the spine (see Figure 14.6). Their function is to limit or modify movement occurring at a joint. For stability to be maximal, ligaments must be short, thick, and strong. However, for maximal range of motion, ligaments need to be long. Ideally, the structures should be suited for an optimum degree of mobility as well as for an optimum stability. Hence long, thick, and strong ligaments would be preferred. However, this is seldom the case.

How effectively a ligament checks excessive movement does not depend only upon its length and size, but also upon its distance from the axis

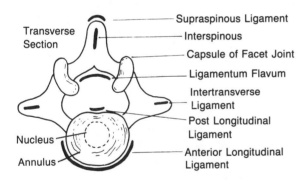

Transverse Section
— Supraspinous Ligament
— Interspinous
— Capsule of Facet Joint
— Ligamentum Flavum
— Intertransverse Ligament
— Post Longitudinal Ligament
Nucleus
Annulus
— Anterior Longitudinal Ligament

Lateral Section

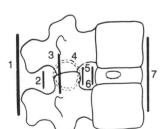

1. Supraspinous
2. Interspinous
3. Intertraverse
4. Facet Joint Capsule
5. Ligamentum Flavum
6. Posterior Longitudinal
7. Anterior Longitudinal

Figure 14.6. Restraining ligaments of the spine. *Note.* From *A Practical Guide to Management of the Painful Neck and Back* (p. 36) by J.W. Fisk and B.S. Rose, 1977, Springfield, IL: Charles C Thomas. Copyright 1977 by Charles C Thomas Publisher. Reprinted by permission.

of motion. That is, the greatest strain will fall on those ligaments and structures farthest away from the axis or fulcrum of movement. Conversely, those closest to the center of rotation will produce the smallest contribution to checking excessive movement.

Flexion and Extension

Because the greatest load falls on those ligaments farthest away from the fulcrum of movement, the structures limiting flexion, working from the nucleus pulposus outwards, would be: (a) the posterior annulus fibrosus, (b) the posterior longitudinal ligament, (c) the ligamentum flavum, (d) the facet joint capsule, (e) the intertransverse ligaments, (f) the interspinous ligaments, and (g) the supraspinous ligaments. Other structures that might assist in limiting and/or restricting flexion are the erector spinae muscles of the lower back and the lower lumbodorsal fascia. The latter is a dense, fascial sheath of connective tissue that encompasses the erector spinae muscles (Farfan, 1973; Fisk & Rose, 1977). Insofar as extension is concerned, this type of movement would be limited by the anterior annulus fibrosus and the anterior longitudinal ligaments.

Lateral Flexion

Lateral flexion is limited by all ligamentous structures to the midline. Again, the greatest load will fall on those structures farthest away from the fulcrum of movement. Accordingly, the three layers of lumbodorsal fascia and the facet capsular ligaments are of major importance, and the intertransverse and anterior longitudinal ligaments are of less importance.

Limits on Range of Motion of the Thoracic-Lumbar Region

The range of movement between any two successive vertebrae is slight. However, the sum total of these movements is of considerable magnitude when the vertebral column is considered as a whole. Furthermore, various ranges of motion have been ascribed to the regions of the vertebral column depending upon numerous factors. Following is an analysis of the thoracic and lumbar regions of the trunk in relation to flexion, extension, and lateral flexion.

Trunk Flexion

Flexion of the trunk is defined as bending or drawing the chest towards the thighs as shown in Figure 14.7. This movement is produced primarily by the rectus abdominis, and assisted by the external and internal abdominal oblique muscles. Range of motion is limited by contractile insufficiency; tension of the spinal extensor muscles; tension of the posterior annulus fibrosus, the posterior longitudinal ligament, the ligamentum flava, the facet joint capsule, the intertransverse ligaments, the interspinous ligaments, and the supraspinous ligaments; apposition of the lower lips of the vertebral bodies anteriorly with surfaces of subjacent vertebrae; compression of the ventral parts of the intervertebral fibrocartilage; and contact of the ribs with the abdomen. Flexion of the trunk takes place almost exclusively in the lumbar region. This is a consequence of the almost complete absence of an upward inclination of the superior articular surfaces (i.e., the orientation of the articular facets) in the thoracic region.

Trunk Extension

Extension of the trunk is defined as bending dorsally (see Figure 14.8). This movement is associated with an accentuation of the lumbar curvature, and is produced by the erector spinae muscles of the lower back. Range of motion is restricted by contractile insufficiency; tension of the anterior abdominal muscles; tension of the anterior annulus fibrosus and anterior longitudinal ligaments; contact of the spinous processes; and contact of the caudal articular margins with the laminae.

Lateral Trunk Flexion

Lateral flexion of the trunk is defined as a sideward inclination of the torso (see Figure 14.9). This movement is produced by the external and internal

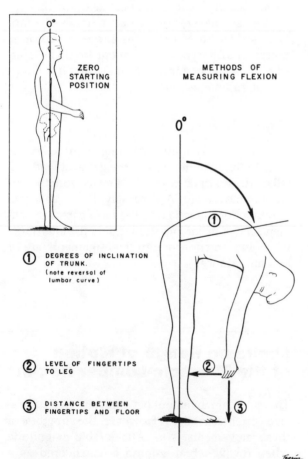

Figure 14.7. The thoracic and lumbar spine (flexion). *Note.* From *Joint Motion Method of Measurement and Recording* (p. 47), 1965, Edinburgh: Churchill Livingstone. Copyright 1965 by The American Academy of Orthopaedic Surgeons. Reprinted by permission.

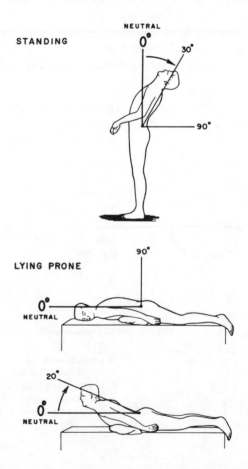

Figure 14.8. The thoracic and lumbar spine (extension). *Note.* From *Joint Motion Method of Measurement and Recording* (p. 53), 1965, Edinburgh: Churchill Livingstone. Copyright 1965 by The American Academy of Orthopaedic Surgeons. Reprinted by permission.

abdominal oblique muscles, and assisted by the erector spinae muscles. Range of motion is limited by contractile insufficiency; tension of the oblique abdominal muscles on the side opposite those being stretched; tension of the annulus fibrosus between the vertebrae, contralateral ligamenta flava, intertransverse ligaments, and anterior longitudinal ligaments; and interlocking of the articular facets on the side of the movement.

The Interrelationship of Stretching the Lower Back, Pelvis, and Hamstrings

Probably one of the most commonly performed, least understood, and potentially dangerous flexibility exercises and/or tests for the hamstring muscles and lower back is hip flexion with the knees extended. Although numerous variations exist, this is often performed in one of four ways:

- a toe-touch from a standing position,
- a toe-touch from a sitting position,
- a toe-touch from a hurdler's stretch position, and
- a toe-touch from a supine position.

When stretching or testing for flexibility, one must be careful to distinguish between tight, normal, and stretched muscles. Equally important, one

must also make sure that only the desired muscle groups are stretched. Often, as will be seen, the true results are masked or obscured (Kendall, Kendall, & Wadsworth, 1971) (see Figure 14.10). Therefore, some additional knowledge of the structures that are involved is necessary.

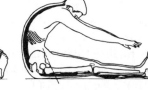
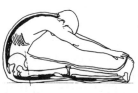

a Normal length of back, hamstring, and gastroc-soleus muscles

b Normal length of back and hamstring muscles, short gastroc-soleus muscles

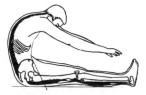
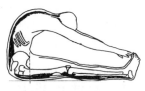

c Stretched upper back and hamstring muscles, slightly short low back muscles, and normal length of gastroc-soleus muscles.

d Stretched upper back muscles, slightly short low back and short hamstring muscles, and normal length of gastroc-soleus muscles.

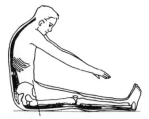
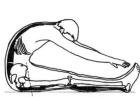

e Normal length of back and hamstring muscles, short gastroc-soleus muscles.

f Normal length of upper back, hamstring, and gastroc-soleus muscles, short low back muscles.

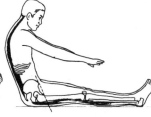
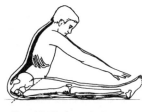

g Normal length of upper back muscles, contracture of low back muscles with paralysis of extremity muscles.

h Normal length of upper back muscles, short low back, hamstring, and gastroc-soleus muscles.

Figure 14.10. Forward-bending test for length of posterior muscles. *Note.* From *Muscles Testing and Function* (2nd ed., pp. 234-235) by H.O. Kendall, F.P. Kendall, and G.E. Wadsworth, 1971, Baltimore: Williams and Wilkins. Copyright 1971 by Williams and Wilkins. Reprinted by permission.

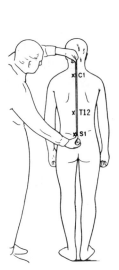
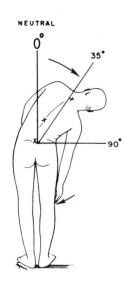

Figure 14.9. The thoracic and lumbar spine (lateral bending). *Note.* From *Joint Motion Method of Measurement and Recording* (p. 51), 1965, Edinburgh: Churchill Livingstone. Copyright 1965 by The American Academy of Orthopaedic Surgeons. Reprinted by permission.

Virtually no forward flexion is present in the thoracic region of the thoracic-lumbar segment (the cervical area will not be considered here, as it does not pertain to the topic in question). This is because the disks in this region are thin, and the direction the facet point. In contrast, most if not all of the forward flexion occurs in the lumbar spine. More specifically, 5 to 10% of flexion is found to occur between L_1 and L_4; 20 to 25% between L_4 and L_5; and 60 to 75% between L_5 and S_1 (see Figure 14.11). Furthermore, most of the spinal flexion occurs by the time the trunk is inclined 45 degrees forward. In actuality, total lumbar flexion is limited to the extent of reversal of the lordosis curve (Cailliet, 1981a). As a matter of fact, Cailliet points out that if a person were to bend forward to touch his or her fingers to the floor without bending at the knees, more flexion would be required than the degree of flexion attributed to the lumbar spine flexion. Hence, were this lumbar curve reversal the only flexion possible, one could not bend even half the distance to the floor. Additional flexion must be possible—but how? The answer is that flexion also occurs at the hip joints.

The flexion possible at the hips is attributed to the mobility of the pelvic girdle. If you recall, the hip is a ball and socket formed by the rounded heads of the femurs fitted into the cuplike acetabular sockets. Consequently, the pelvis is capable of rotation around the fulcrum of the two lateral hip joints. This can be likened to the action of a seesaw or teeter board (Cailliet, 1981; Kapandji, 1982). Therefore, in hip flexion the anterior portion of the pelvis descends and the posterior aspect ascends. With reextension, the pelvis rotates back to its erect stance (see Figure 14.12).

Optimal and safe performance when stretching requires a blending of adequate flexibility, strength, and mechanics. For example, when performing hip flexion with the knees extended, several factors may potentially restrict range of motion. Probably the most common causes are tight low back muscles and tight hamstring muscles. Obviously, with tight low back muscles, lumbar flexion is restricted. However, when the hamstrings are tight, the pelvis is restricted from rotating. This is because the hamstrings are attached to the posterior portion of the knee and the tuberosity of the ischium (Cailliet, 1981a). Other potentially limiting factors include defects in the disks, ligaments, or bony structure; irregular curvature of the spine; impingement of the joints (see Figure 14.13); sciatic nerve irritation (see Figure 14.14); and/or any muscle imbalance (Cailliet, 1981a; Walther, 1981).

When developing flexibility, safety must always come first. For example, when performing a toe-touch with both legs straight from a stand, the body is susceptible to injury and pain. This often occurs when tight muscles in the lower back or hamstrings are overstretched (see Figure 14.15), and is especially true with ballistic stretching. Faulty mechanics can also initiate injury. The mechanics of the lumbar spine are such that any increased weight that is anterior (forward) to the

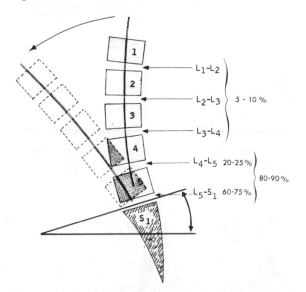

Figure 14.11. Segmental site and degree of lumbar flexion. The degree of flexion noted in the lumbar spine as a percentage of total spinal flexion is indicated. The major portion of flexion (75%) occurs at the lumbosacral joint; 15-20% of flexion occurs at the level L_4-L_5 interspace; and the remaining 5-10% is distributed between L_4 and L_5. The forward-flexed diagram indicates the mere reversal past lordosis of total flexion of the lumbar curve. *Note.* From *Low Back Pain Syndrome* (3rd ed., p. 40) by R. Cailliet, 1981, Philadelphia: F.A. Davis. Copyright 1981 by F.A. Davis Company. Reprinted by permission.

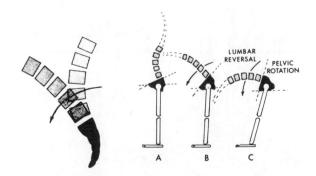

Figure 14.12. Lumbar pelvic rhythm. With pelvis fixed, flexion-extension of the lumbar spine occurs mostly in the lower segments L_{4-5} and L_5-S_1. *Note.* From *Low Back Pain Syndrome* (3rd ed., p. 44) by R. Cailliet, 1981, Philadelphia: F.A. Davis. Copyright 1981 by F.A. Davis Company. Reprinted by permission.

vertebral column greatly increases the forces that are exerted on the lumbar spine. Consequently, the resultant forces at the fulcrum, which is the lower lumbar segment, are very high. This fault is often seen when one performs the movement with the arms horizontal to the floor. To reduce

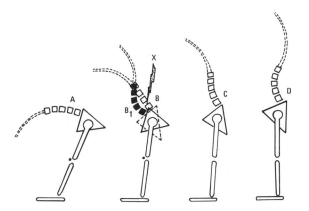

Figure 14.13. Mechanism of acute facet impingement. A, B, C, and D depict the proper physiologic resumption of the erect position from total flexion with reverse lumbar-pelvic rhythm. B shows improper premature lordotic curve which cantilevers the lumbar spine anterior to the center of gravity. This position approximates the facets at X and, coupled with the eccentric leading of the spine, requires greater muscular contraction of the erector spinae group. Facet impingement can occur. *Note.* From *Low Back Pain Syndrome* (3rd ed., p. 64) by R. Cailliet, 1981, Philadelphia: F.A. Davis. Copyright 1981 by F.A. Davis Company. Reprinted by permission.

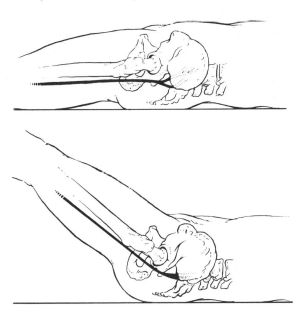

Figure 14.14. Sciatic nerve irritation. The passive straight leg raising test stretches the sciatic nerve as it passes behind the hip joint. If one or several of the nerve roots comprising the sciatic nerve has been stretched or irritated, the result will be a marked increase in pain.

the strain on the back, place the hands on the hips, as shown in Figure 14.16 (Segal, 1983; White & Panjabi, 1978).

As far as twisting and bending the trunk laterally are concerned, research by Schultz et al. (1982) found that these positions did not load the spine more than positions of forward bending. Lateral bending movements can load the spine moderately, but not nearly as much as the flexion movement, for two reasons: (a) the trunk cannot be laterally offset very much, so that the moment imposed cannot become very large, and (b) the lateral abdominal wall muscles act on the spine through a relatively large moment arm, so they need not contract strongly to counterbalance the offset weight moment (Schultz et al., 1982). Nonetheless, the possibility of injury still exists. For example, Segal (1983) points out that in side bending, when one puts the opposite arm overhead, additional and unnecessary stretch is placed on the lower back muscles on the same side as the extended arm (see Exercise #170). The risk of injury can be further compounded if the lateral rotation is combined with excessive rotation and flexion or excessive rotation and extension (Garu, 1986). When this exercise is performed in a ballistic manner, the potential of injury is even greater.

Another potential cause of low back injury and/or pain is faulty reextension from the flexed

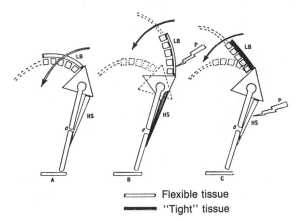

Flexible tissue
"Tight" tissue

Figure 14.15. Mechanism of stretch pain in the "tight hamstring" and the "tight low back" syndromes. A: Normal flexibility with unrestricted lumbar-pelvic rhythm. B: Tight hamstrings (HS) restricting pelvic rotation and thereby causing excessive stretch of low back (LB) resulting in pain (P). C: Tight low back (LB) performing an incomplete lumbar reversal and thus, by placing excessive stretch on the hamstrings (HS), causing pain (P) in both the hamstrings and the low back as well as a disrupted lumbar-pelvic rhythm. *Note.* From *Low Back Pain Syndrome* (3rd ed., p. 65) by R. Cailliet, 1981, Philadelphia: F.A. Davis. Copyright 1981 by F.A. Davis Company. Reprinted by permission.

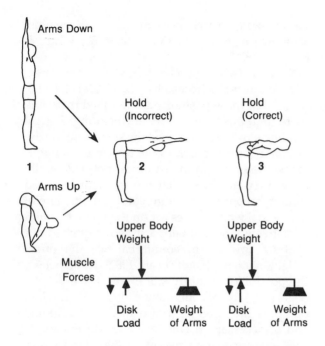

Figure 14.16. The effect of a load anterior to the vertebral body. (1) The greater any load that is anterior to the vertebral bodies, the greater the forces exerted on the lumbar spine. (2) Extending or lowering the arms horizontally increases stress on the lumbar spine. (3) Placing the hands on the hips (fulcrum) decreases the load anterior to the vertebral bodies reducing stress.

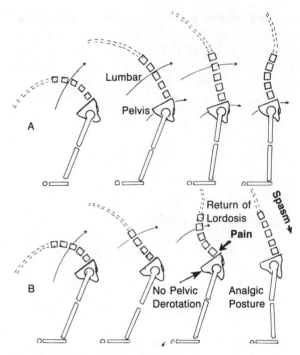

Figure 14.17. Proper versus improper flexion and reextension. A depicts proper simultaneous resumption of the lumbar lordosis with pelvic rotation. B reveals the regaining of pelvic lordosis with no pelvic derotation, thus causing painful lordotic posture with the upper part of the body held ahead of the center of gravity. *Note.* From *Low Back Pain Syndrome* (3rd ed., p. 132) by R. Cailliet, 1981, Philadelphia: F.A. Davis. Copyright 1981 by F.A. Davis Company. Reprinted by permission.

position in which the lordosis is regained before the pelvis is derotated (Cailliet, 1981a). Ideally, in reassuming the erect stance, the lumbar spine should act as an inflexible rod. Therefore, the back should be straight and fully extended. With this type of faulty reextension, the upper portion of the body rises early so the lower back arches and the lordosis curve is in front of the center of gravity (see Figure 14.17). Consequently, this places an excessive stress on the lower back. As further elaborated by Cailliet, normally the lumbar spine is supported by the supraspinous ligaments when in full flexion to extension until the last 45 degrees. Remember, the reextension to the full upright posture is by pelvic derotation. Then, for the last 45 degrees of extension, the erector spinae muscles straighten the spine. Hence, the lower back regains its lordosis. However, due to the short lower arm to which the erector spinae muscles are attached, this portion of reextension is inefficient. Then when the erector spinae muscles fatigue, the task of maintaining and supporting the excessive load falls on the vertebral ligaments. Consequently, once the ligaments give way, the load falls on the joints, and subluxation of the joint results (see Figure 14.18).

A toe-touch from a sitting position or modified hurdler's stretch also requires caution. This is especially apparent when stretching with a partner. Too often, injury occurs when a partner unknowingly imparts that little extra stretch. To prevent such accidents from developing, anticipation and communication must be employed.

The Cervical Vertebrae

The neck's skeletal framework is made up of seven cervical vertebrae. The most well-known are the first and second—the atlas and axis. These vertebrae are unique in structure. The atlas directly supports the head and forms a bony ring. In contrast, the axis features a bony projection which forms a peg-like pivot. Around this peg-like pivot the atlas rotates when the head is turned from side to side. Thus this design determines much of the direction and extent of motion of the head (see Figure 14.19).

Movements of the Neck

The cervical region is capable of flexion, extension, lateral flexion, and circumduction. This region is the most mobile and shows the freest ranges of motion of all the vertebrae because the disks are thickest in relation to the height of the vertebral body. The ratio of disk to body is 2/5, or 40% percent (Kapandji, 1982). Furthermore, since the width of the body is greater than its height or depth, there is a greater capacity for flexion-extension than for lateral bending.

Limits to Range of Motion

The major determinants of the direction and extent of motion reside in the shape of the vertebral bodies and in the contours and orientations of the intervertebral articulations. The ligaments, fascia, and capsules also provide constraints to motion. When their elastic limits are reached, the tension created causes motion to halt. Following is a brief analysis of the limiting factors associated with range of motion in the cervical region.

Flexion.   Cervical flexion is defined as drawing the head forward to the chest (see Figure 14.20A). The primary muscle involved in flexion is the sternocleidomastoideus. Flexion of the neck is limited by contractile insufficiency; tension of the posterior longitudinal ligament, ligamenta flava, and the interspinal and supraspinal ligaments; tension of the posterior muscles and fascia of the neck; the apposition of the lower lips of vertebral bodies anteriorly with the surfaces of the adjacent vertebrae; compression of the intervertebral fibrocartilage in front; and the chin coming to rest on the chest.

Extension.   Cervical extension is the returning of the head from the flexed position (the head forward on the chest) to an upright position. Drawing the head backward beyond the upright position is called cervical hyperextension. This movement is produced by the trapezius, semispinalis capitis, splenius capitis, and splenius cervicis. Range of motion is limited by contractile insufficiency; tension of the anterior longitudinal ligament; tension of the anterior neck muscles and fascia; approximation of the spinous processes; the locking of the posterior edges of the superior atlantal facets in the condyloid fossae of the occipital bone; and contact of the head on the muscle mass of the upper trunk.

Lateral Flexion.   Cervical lateral flexion may be described as tilting the head so that the left ear

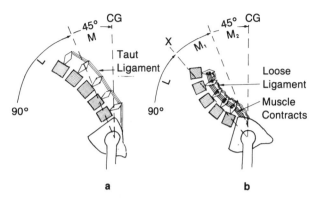

Figure 14.18.   Faulty reextension of the lumbar spine. (a) Correct reextension. Until the last 45 degrees, the lumbar spine is supported (L) by supraspinous ligaments requiring no muscular effort. Muscles normally become active in the last 45 degrees (M) when the carrying angle is close to the center of gravity (CG). (b) Premature lumbar lordosis with pelvis not adequately derotated causes the erector muscles (M₁) to contract before having reached the last 45 degrees. The ligaments loosen, and the muscles take the brunt and contract inefficiently and forcefully, resulting in pain. *Note.* From *Low Back Pain Syndrome* (3rd ed., p. 133) by R. Cailliet, 1981, Philadelphia: F.A. Davis. Copyright 1981 by F.A. Davis Company. Reprinted by permission.

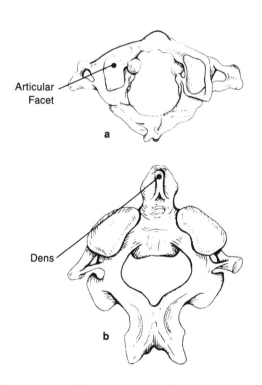

Figure 14.19.   The cervical vertebrae. (a) A superior view of the first cervical vertebrae. (b) A superior view of the axis with the dens. *Note.* From *Living Anatomy* (p. 82) by J.E. Donnelly, 1982, Champaign, IL: Human Kinetics. Copyright 1982 by J.E. Donnelly. Reprinted by permission.

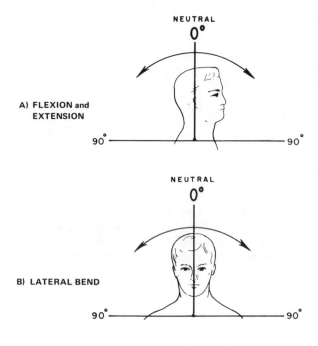

NEUTRAL
0°

A) FLEXION and EXTENSION

90° — 90°

NEUTRAL
0°

B) LATERAL BEND

90° — 90°

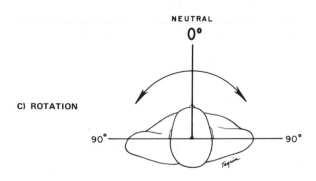

NEUTRAL
0°

C) ROTATION

90° — 90°

Figure 14.20. Motions of the cervical spine. (a) Flexion and extension. (b) Lateral bend. (c) Rotation. *Note.* From *Manual of Orthopaedic Surgery* (p. 115), 1985, Park Ridge, IL: American Orthopaedic Association. Copyright 1972 by The American Orthopaedic Association. Reprinted by permission.

moves nearer the left shoulder or the right ear draws closer to the right shoulder (see Figure 14.20B). Lateral flexion of the neck is produced by the sternocleidomastoideus, splenius capitis, semispinalis capitis, and longus capitis. Range of motion is restricted by contractile insufficiency; tension of the intertransverse ligaments; tension of the neck muscles and fascia on the side opposing flexion; and the articular pillars. Table 14.2 summarizes factors limiting lumbar, thoracic, and cervical movements.

Dangerous Stretching

Probably the most controversial and potentially dangerous stretch for the cervical region is the plough (see Exercises #157, 158, 179). A modified version is the inverted bicycle exercise which is used as a warming-up maneuver, and is performed lying supine and rolling over onto the back portion of the neck and top of the shoulders so that the feet are up in the air. The stretch can be further intensified by extending the feet downward and/or placing the shins flat on the floor with the knees touching the shoulders.

According to Kisner and Colby (1985), there are two major problems with this exercise. First, the region being stretched frequently tends to be flexed from faulty position. Second, the flexed and inverted position compresses the lungs and heart, consequently decreasing their potential effectiveness. Thus Kisner and Colby question "whether the benefits of this exercise outweigh the combined negative effects on the neck and upper back posture, circulation, and respiration" (p. 619).

Review Questions

1. Draw a diagram and label the three types of abnormal vertebral curves.

2. Explain the significance of disk thickness as it relates to flexibility. What is more important, absolute thickness or relative thickness? Explain why.

3. Explain how aging affects vertebral flexibility.

4. Explain the paradox that the annulus fibrosus must receive the ultimate effects of the vertebral compression although it is designed to resist horizontal displacement. Draw a diagram illustrating this concept.

5. Explain how a toe-touching test is apt to be an inaccurate measure of lower back flexibility.

6. Draw a diagram illustrating the lumbar pelvic rhythm.

7. Describe several exercises that should be modified to reduce the potential of injury to the vertebral region.

Table 14.2 Factors Limiting Lumbar, Thoracic, and Cervical Movement

Lumbar region	Flexion Thoracic region	Cervical region
A) The ratio between the height of the intervertebral disks and the height of the bony part of the column (disk thickness).		
B) All posterior ligaments-->		
C) The capsule of the facet joints-->		
D) The direction/orientation of the articular surfaces-->		
E) Tension of the spinal extensor muscles.		Tension of the posterior neck muscles
F) Contact of the last rib with the abdomen.		The chin resting on the chest.

Extension

Lumbar region	Thoracic region	Cervical region
A) The ratio between the height of the intervertebral disks and the height of the bony part of the column (disk thickness).		
B) Tension of the anterior ligament--->		
C) The orientation of the articular surfaces: frontal plane-->		
D) Contact/impingement of the overlapping spinous processes --->		
E)	Attachment of the ribs to the sternum.	
F) Tension of the anterior abdominal muscles.		Tension of the ventral neck muscles

Lateral Flexion

Lumbar region	Thoracic region	Cervical region
A) The ratio between the height of the intervertebral disks and the height of the bony part of the column (disk thickness).		
B) All ligamentous structures lateral to the midline--->		
C) Contact/impingement of the articular processes -->		
D)	Attachment of the ribs to the sternum.	
E)	Tension of the costovertebral ligament.	
F) Tension of the oblique abs opposite the side being stretched		Tension of the neck muscles opposite the side being stretched.

8. Explain the proper body mechanics to use during flexion and reextension. Draw a diagram illustrating the proper and improper technique.

9. You are diagnosing an athlete who can perform a split but cannot bring his or her head onto the thighs while attempting a sitting toe-touching test. Describe how best to facilitate improvement of that skill. Give specific exercises and procedures to follow.

10. Explain the controversy regarding the plough stretch. Would you include it in an exercise program? Explain why or why not.

Answers

1. See Figure 14.2a, b, and c.

2. The amount of movement that can occur in any part of the vertebral column depends in large part upon the ratio between the height of the intervertebral disks and the height of the bony part of the column. However, it can be stated that the ratio of disk thickness to the height of the vertebral body is more important than the absolute thickness of the disk, because the greater the ratio the greater the mobility.

3. Vertebral flexibility diminishes over a period of time.

4. This is because the nucleus pulposus transforms the vertical thrust into a radical or shear force. Then the shear force is restricted by the elastic and tensile strength of the fibers. See Figure 14.5.

5. It is apt to be inaccurate because tightness in the hamstrings can mask flexibility in the lower back.

6. See Figure 14.12.

7. See Exercises #135-158.

8. During flexion, the hands should be placed as close to the fulcrum (i.e., hips) as possible. With reextension, the lumbar spine should act as an inflexible rod. See Figures 14.16 and 14.17.

9. The problem is a lack of flexibility in the lower back. The solution here is to stretch this region by incorporating Exercises #46-51 and 56.

10. The controversy associated with the plough stretch is that it might reinforce a faulty position and the exercise tends to compress the lungs and heart. The plough should be included in a stretching exercise for those who are healthy. However, the degree of stretch should be adapted to the ability of the individual.

Recommended Readings

American Academy of Orthopaedic Surgeons (1975). *Atlas of orthotics. Biomechanical principles and applications.* St. Louis: C.V. Mosby.

Basmajian, J.V. (1975). *Grant's method of anatomy* (9th ed.). Baltimore: Williams and Wilkins.

Daniels, L., & Worthingham, C. (1980). *Muscle testing. Techniques of manual examination* (4th ed.). Philadelphia: W.B. Saunders.

Dunn, B. (1965). Physiotherapy and the ballet. *Physiotherapy*, **51**(4), 125-128.

Rothman, R.H., & Simeone, F.A. (1982). *The spine* (2nd ed.). Philadelphia: W.B. Saunders.

Steindler, A. (1977). *Kinesiology of the human body.* Springfield, IL: Charles C Thomas.

Urbaniak, J.R. (1976). Basic anatomy and biomechanics of the low back in relation to low back pain. *Athletic Training*, **11**(3), 114-118.

Williams, P.L., & Warwick, R. (1980). *Gray's anatomy* (36th British ed.). Philadelphia: W. B. Saunders.

CHAPTER 15

The Upper Extremity

The upper extremity shall be considered here as consisting of the shoulder girdle, shoulder joint, arm, elbow joint, forearm, wrist joint, and hand. It will be analyzed in terms of structure, function, limitation to range of motion, and methodology of stretching.

The Shoulder Girdle and Arm-Complex

The shoulder girdle and shoulder-arm-complex is made up of a pair of clavicle, humerus, and scapula bones, plus the sternum. In combination, they comprise three major joints: the glenohumeral, sternoclavicular, and acromioclavicular. According to Kapandji (1982), there are five joints, with the addition of the subdeltoid and the scapulo-thoracic (see Figure 15.1). Neither of these are anatomical

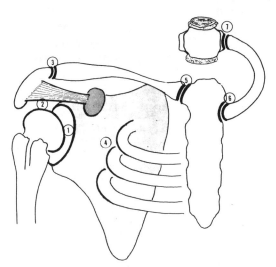

Figure 15.1. Composite drawing of the shoulder girdle. (1) glenohumeral; (2) suprahumeral; (3) acromioclavicular; (4) scapulocostal; (5) sternoclavicular; (6) costosternal; (7) costovertebral. *Note.* From *Shoulder Pain* (p. 2) by R. Cailliet, 1966, Philadelphia: F.A. Davis. Copyright 1966 by F.A. Davis Company. Reprinted by permission.

joints. Although many movements appear to take place in the glenohumeral joint, they often occur simultaneously in others. Without the assistance of these joints, movements of the upper limb would be seriously restricted.

Gross Anatomy

The glenohumeral or scapulohumeral joint is a modified ball and socket joint comprised of the humeral head and the shallow glenoid fossa (i.e., cavity) of the scapula. The joint is one of the most mobile and unstable in the human body. The lack of stability is due primarily to its weak bony architecture. The major stability of the joint is provided by the large, enveloping musculature. Its secondary line of support comes from the capsular-ligamentous complexes. These are the glenoid labrum, fibrous capsule, and glenohumeral, coracohumeral, and transverse humeral ligaments (see Figure 15.2).

Analysis of Movement

The clavicular movements which occur at the sternoclavicular and acromioclavicular joints must always be associated with movements of the scapula, and movements of the scapula are usually accompanied by movements of the humerus and shoulder. These movements include elevation, depression, protraction, and retraction. Similarly, movements of the upper arm at the glenohumeral joint must always be associated with movements of the scapula and the previously cited joints. The movements of the glenohumeral joint are best described in relation to the humeral segment on the trunk. These include flexion, extension, abduction, adduction, medial rotation, lateral rotation, horizontal transverse abduction, and horizontal transverse adduction.

Flexion. Flexion of the glenohumeral joint is defined as movement of the humerus forwards and medially across the front of the chest. Pure flexion ranges from 0 to 90 degrees, and if modified, up to 180 degrees (see Figure 15.3). For purposes of analysis, the movement is divided into three phases. The first phase has been called the setting phase (Inman, Saunders, & Abbott, 1944), and ranges from 0 to 60 degrees. The muscles primarily responsible for this phase are the anterior fibers of the deltoid, the coraco-brachialis, and the clavicular fibers of the pectoralis major. Range of

motion is limited by contractile insufficiency, tension of the coraco-humeral ligament, and tension of the teres minor, teres major, and infraspinatus.

The second phase of flexion is from 60 to 120 degrees. At this point, a constant, delicate, and intrinsic relationship between the humerus and scapula is developed. This is called the scapulo-humeral rhythm. The ratio of motion in the two joints is constant, being 2 humeral and 1 scapular. This implies that for every 15 degrees of motion of the humerus, the scapulothoracic movement is 5 degrees, and the glenohumeral movement is 10 degrees. Thus, when either of these articulations is fixed by injury or disease, the loss of motion is proportionate to the glenohumeral fixation causing twice as much restriction as scapulothoracic fixation (Turek, 1977). The muscles assisting during this phase are the trapezius and infraspinatus. Movement is restricted by contractile insufficiency, tension of the latissimus dorsi, tension of the serratus anterior, and anything that will impede the scapulohumeral rhythm.

During the final phase, the humerus moves from 120 to 180 degrees. When flexion is resisted at the

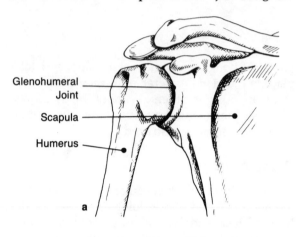

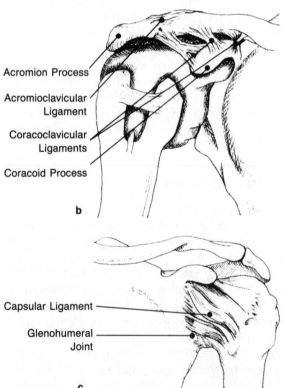

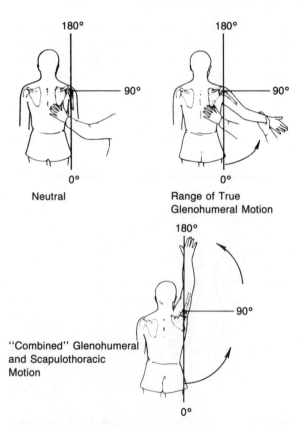

Figure 15.2.   The shoulder girdle ligaments. (a) An anterior view of the acromioclavicular and coracoclavicular ligaments. (b) The capsular ligament, anterior view. *Note.* From *Living Anatomy* (p. 28) by J.E. Donnelly, 1982, Champaign, IL: Human Kinetics. Copyright 1982 by J.E. Donnelly. Reprinted by permission.

Figure 15.3.   Glenohumeral and scapulothoracic motion. *Note.* From *Manual of Orthopaedic Surgery* (p. 139), 1985, Park Ridge, IL: American Orthopaedic Association. Copyright 1972 by The American Orthopaedic Association. Reprinted by permission.

glenohumeral and scapulothoracic joints, movement of the spinal column becomes necessary. This is accomplished by the formation of an exaggeration of the lumbar lordosis (Kapandji, 1982). The muscles responsible for movement and the factors limiting range of motion remain constant. In the final analysis, for a complete 180-degree movement, the humerus moves 120 degrees in relation to the glenoid, and the scapula moves upward and forward on the chest wall 60 degrees. The 60 degrees of scapular motion would be impossible without the 40-degree and 20-degree elevation of the clavicle at the sternoclavicular and acriomio-clavicular joints respectively (see Figures 15.4, 15.5, and 15.6).

Extension and Backward Extension. Extension of the glenohumeral joint involves returning the humerus from the flexed position to its natural hanging position. Backward extension is the upward motion of the humerus in the posterior saggittal plane of the body (i.e., thrusting the arm backward and behind the hip) (see Figure 15.7). Backward extension ranges from 0 to 60 degrees. This movement is produced by the deltoid, latissimus dorsi, and teres major, and is assisted by the teres minor and long head of the triceps. Range of motion is limited by contractile insufficiency, tension of the shoulder flexor muscles, tension of the coraco-humeral ligament, and contact of the greater tubercle of the humerus with the acromion posteriorly.

Abduction. Abduction of the glenohumeral joint is defined as movement that carries the humerus anteriorlaterally away from the trunk (see Figure 15.8). Identical to flexion, the range of abduction at the glenohumeral joint is dependent upon the state of rotation of the humerus. For example, if the humerus is maintained in medial rotation, the humerus will not abduct beyond 60 degrees. However, if the humerus is laterally rotated, abduction can reach 180 degrees. For purposes of analysis, abduction, too, will be divided into three phases.

In the first phase abduction ranges from 0 to 90 degrees. The muscles primarily responsible for this action are the deltoid and supraspinatus. Range of motion is limited by contractile insufficiency, and locking of the shoulder as a result of the greater tuberosity hitting the superior margin of the glenoid. However, when the humerus is laterally rotated, the greater tubercle passes behind the acromion, and abduction is permitted to continue. This action is analogous to a turnout of the hip.

During the second phase, abduction ranges from 90 to 150 degrees. This phase can proceed only with the contribution of the shoulder girdle. The muscles responsible for this movement are the

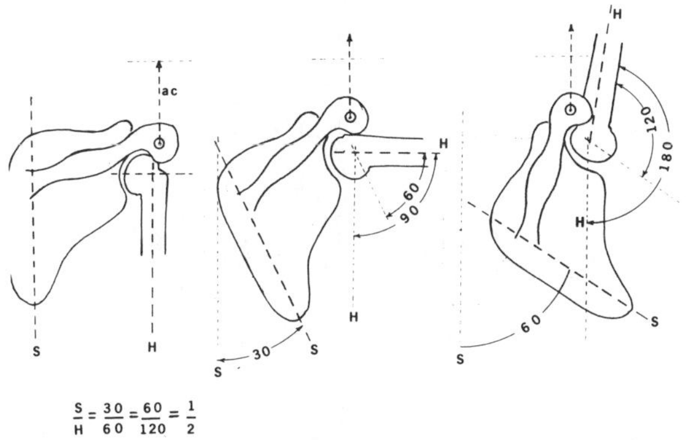

$$\frac{S}{H} = \frac{30}{60} = \frac{60}{120} = \frac{1}{2}$$

Figure 15.4. Scapulohumeral rhythm. The scapula and the humerus at position of rest with the scapula relaxed and the arm dependent, both at position O°. The abduction movement of the arm is accomplished in a smooth, coordinated movement during which for each 15° of arm abduction 10° of motion occurs at the glenohumeral joint and 5° occur due to scapular rotation upon the thorax. The humerus (H) has abducted 90° in relationship to the erect body, but this has been accomplished by 30° rotation of the scapula and 60° of the humerus at the glenohumeral joint, a ratio of 2:1. RIGHT: Full elevation of the arm: 60° at the scapula and 120° at the glenohumeral joint. *Note.* From *Shoulder Pain* (p. 22) by R. Cailliet, 1966, Philadelphia: F.A. Davis. Copyright 1966 by F.A. Davis Company. Reprinted by permission.

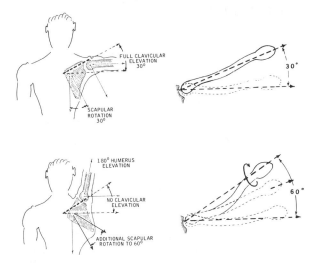

Figure 15.5. Scapular elevation resulting from clavicular rotation. The upper drawing shows the elevation of the clavicle without rotation to 30°. The remaining 30° of scapular rotation, which is imperative in full scapulo-humeral range, occurs by rotation of the "crank-shaped" clavicle about its long axis. *Note.* From *Shoulder Pain* (p. 26) by R. Cailliet, 1966, Philadelphia: F.A. Davis. Copyright 1966 by F.A. Davis Company. Reprinted by permission.

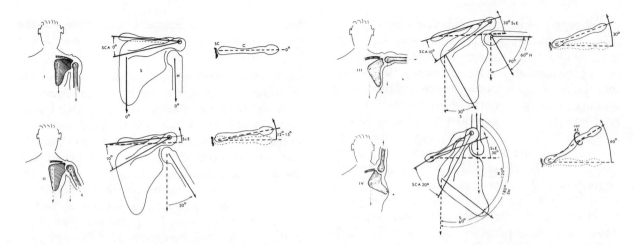

Figure 15.6. Accessory movement of the scapulohumeral rhythm other than the glenohumeral movement. Phase I: The resting arm: 0° scapular rotation, S; 0° spinoclavicular angle, SCA; 0° movement at the sternoclavicular joint, SC; no elevation of the outer end of the clavicle, C; no abduction of the humerus, H. Phase II: Humerus abducted 30°: outer end of the clavicle elevated 12° to 15° with no rotation of the clavicle; elevation occurs at the sternoclavicular joint; some movement occurs at the acromioclavicular joint as seen by increase of 10° of the spinoclavicular angle (angle formed by the clavicle and the scapular spine). Phase III: Humerus, H, abducted to 90° (60° glenohumeral, 30° scapular): clavicle elevated to its final position, 30°; no rotation of clavicle as yet—all movement at the sternoclavicular joint; no change in the SCA. Phase IV: Full overhead elevation (SH 180°, H 120°, S 60°): outer end of clavicle has not elevated further (at the sternoclavicular joint), but the SCA has increased to 20°. Because of the clavicle's rotation and its "cranklike" form, the clavicle elevates an additional 30°. The humerus through this phase has rotated, but this has not influenced the above degrees of movement. *Note.* From *Shoulder Pain* (pp. 30-31) by R. Cailliet, 1966, Philadelphia: F.A. Davis. Copyright 1966 by F.A. Davis Company. Reprinted by permission.

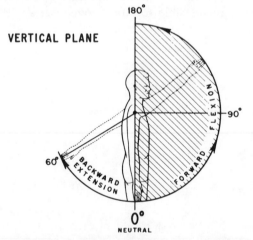

Figure 15.7. Extension and backward extension of the shoulder. *Note.* From *Manual of Orthopaedic Surgery* (p. 136), 1985, Park Ridge, IL: American Orthopaedic Association. Copyright 1972 by The American Orthopaedic Association. Reprinted by permission.

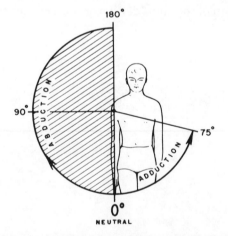

Figure 15.8. Abduction and adduction of the shoulder. *Note.* From *Manual of Orthopaedic Surgery* (p. 136), 1985, Park Ridge, IL: American Orthopaedic Association. Copyright 1972 by The American Orthopaedic Association. Reprinted by permission.

trapezius and serratus anterior. Range of motion is restricted by contractile insufficiency, tension of the adductor muscles (i.e., the latissimus dorsi and pectoralis major), and tension of the middle and inferior bands of the glenohumeral ligament.

The third phase of abduction is from 150 to 180 degrees. To attain a vertical position once more, movement of the vertebral column is required.

This is accomplished by the formation of an exaggeration of the lumbar lordosis (Kapandji, 1982). At the end of abduction, all the abductory muscles are in contraction. All limiting factors are the same as in the second phase.

Adduction. Adduction of the glenohumeral joint is defined as returning the humerus from the abducted position to its naturally hanging position (i.e., the motion of the arm toward the midline of the body) (see Figure 15.8). Adduction is produced primarily by the pectoralis major and latissimus dorsi. Movement is restricted when the humerus makes contact with the body's trunk.

Internal (Inward) or Medial Rotation. Internal or medial rotation of the glenohumeral joint may be measured by three different methods. These include rotation with the arm at the side, rotation with the arm abducted, and rotation with the arm raised posteriorly (see Figure 15.9). The latter is exemplified by tying apron strings behind one's back. Medial rotation is produced by the scapularis, pectoralis major, latissimus dorsi, teres major, and assisted by the deltoid muscle. Range of motion is restricted by contractile insufficiency, tension of the superior portion of the capsular ligament, and tension of the external rotator muscles (i.e., infraspinatus and teres minor).

External (Outward) or Lateral Rotation. External or lateral rotation of the glenohumeral joint is also

measured by the methods previously stated (see Figure 15.9). This movement is limited by contractile insufficiency, tension of the superior portion of the capsular and coraco-humeral ligament, and tension of the internal rotator muscles (i.e., scapularis, pectoralis major, latissimus dorsi, and teres major).

Horizontal Transverse Abduction (Extension). Horizontal transverse abduction may be defined as moving the humerus laterally and backward with the humerus elevated to a horizontal position (see Figure 15.10). Horizontal transverse abduction ranges from 0 to 30 degrees. This movement is produced by the posterior fibers of the deltoid, the infraspinatus, and the teres minor. Range of motion is limited by contractile insufficiency, tension of the anterior fibers of the capsule of the glenohumeral joint, and tension of the pectoralis major and anterior fibers of the deltoid.

Horizontal Transverse Adduction (Flexion). Horizontal transverse adduction may be defined as moving the humerus medially and forward with the humerus elevated to a horizontal position (see Figure 15.10). Horizontal transverse adduction ranges from 0 to 130 degrees. This movement is produced primarily by the pectoralis major and anterior fibers of the deltoid. Range of motion is limited by contractile insufficiency; tension of the glenohumeral's extensor muscles (i.e., latissimus dorsi, teres major, posterior fibers of the deltoid, and teres minor); and contact of the humerus with the trunk.

Elevation of the Scapula. Elevation of the scapula is defined as the scapula moving vertically upward (see Figure 15.11). This movement is brought about by the upper trapezius, levator scapulae,

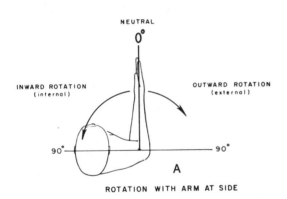

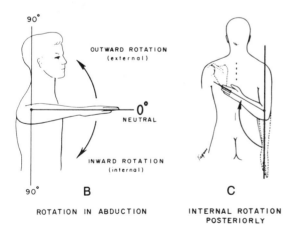

Figure 15.9. Rotary shoulder motion. (a) Rotation with the arm at side. (b) Rotation in abduction. (c) Internal rotation posteriorly. *Note.* From *Manual of Orthopaedic Surgery* (p. 137), 1985, Park Ridge, IL: American Orthopaedic Association. Copyright 1972 by The American Orthopaedic Association. Reprinted by permission.

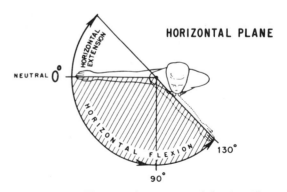

Figure 15.10. Horizontal transverse abduction (flexion) and adduction (extension) of the shoulder. *Note.* From *Manual of Orthopaedic Surgery* (p. 136), 1985, Park Ridge, IL: American Orthopaedic Association. Copyright 1972 by The American Orthopaedic Association. Reprinted by permission.

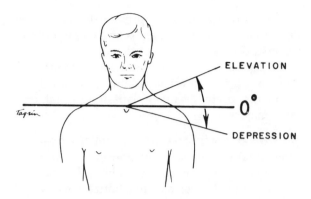

Figure 15.11. Shoulder motions: elevation and depression. *Note.* From *Manual of Orthopaedic Surgery* (p. 134), 1985, Park Ridge, IL: American Orthopaedic Association. Copyright 1972 by The American Orthopaedic Association. Reprinted by permission.

and serratus anterior muscles. The movement is restricted by contractile insufficiency, tension of the antagonistic muscles, tension of the costoclavicular ligament, and tension of the lower part of the capsule.

Depression of the Scapula. Depression of the scapula is defined as the scapula moving downward (see Figure 15.11). When passive, depression is brought about by gravity and the weight of the limb. Depression can be active by pressing downward (or resting on the parallel bars). Simple depression is produced by the pectoralis minor, subclavius, pectoralis major, and latissimus dorsi. Range of motion is limited by contractile insufficiency, tension of the antagonistic muscles, tension of the interclavicular and sternoclavicular ligaments, and the articular disks.

Protraction (Flexion) of the Scapula. Protraction of the scapula is defined as the forward movement of the scapula (see Figure 15.12), which is seen in all forward-pushing or thrusting movements.

Protraction is created by the serratus anterior, pectoralis minor, and levator spinae. Range of motion is restricted by contractile insufficiency, tension of the antagonistic muscles, tension of the anterior sternoclavicular ligament, and tension of the posterior lamina of the costoclavicular ligament.

Retraction (Extension) of the Scapula. Retraction of the scapula is defined as the backward movement of the scapula (see Figure 15.12), and is exemplified by pulling. Retraction is produced by the trapezius and rhomboids, and assisted by the latissimus dorsi. Range of motion is limited by contractile insufficiency, tension of the antagonist muscles, tension of the posterior sternoclavicular ligament, and tension of the anterior lamina of the costoclavicular ligament.

Injuries, Stretching, and Testing

Injuries to the shoulder girdle and shoulder-arm-complex are not uncommon. Preventive actions are identical to those stated earlier with reference to other parts of the body. These include proper warm-up, proper technique, endurance, strength, and flexibility.

Needless to say, flexibility should be developed in all directions and through the full range of movement. However, when stretching or testing this region, one must carefully separate shoulder girdle motion from motion in the vertebral column. For example, to achieve a true stretch and/or test for glenohumeral flexion, one must position the body in hip flexion and lumbar spine flexion. To accomplish this, lie with the lower back flat on the

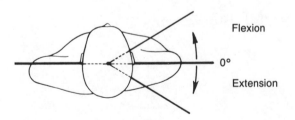

Figure 15.12. Protraction (flexion) and retraction (extension) of the scapula. *Note.* From *Manual of Orthopaedic Surgery* (p. 134), 1985, Park Ridge, IL: American Orthopaedic Association. Copyright 1972 by The American Orthopaedic Association. Reprinted by permission.

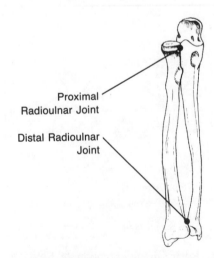

Figure 15.13. An isolated view of the radioulnar joints. *Note.* From *Living Anatomy* (p. 41) by J.E. Donnelly, 1982, Champaign, IL: Human Kinetics. Copyright 1982 by J.E. Donnelly. Reprinted by permission.

floor, both legs flexed, and the heels near the buttocks. Then the humerus should be slowly raised. Once the lower back begins to arch, the maximum range of flexion has been determined. To facilitate additional stretching, a partner needs only to push down on the ribs to keep the back flat on the floor as glenohumeral flexion continues.

The Elbow Joint

The elbow joint is the intermediate joint of the upper extremity between the shoulder and wrist. Three bones form the basic skeletal structure of the elbow: the humerus, radius, and ulna. The elbow is classified as a hinge joint. There are actually three articulations at the elbow joint. However, only two of these will be examined here. They are the humero-ulnar-radial joint, concerned solely with flexion and extension in a sliding fashion; and the other is the radio-ulnar joint concerned solely with pronation and supination (see Figures 15.13 and 15.14).

Analysis of Movements

There are four major movements that can take place at the elbow joint. These are flexion, extension, pronation, and supination. Following is an analysis of these movements.

Flexion. Flexion of the elbow is defined as decreasing the angle between the humerus and forearm of the joint (see Figure 15.15). The primary flexors of the elbow are the biceps brachii, brachialis, and brachioradialis. The following muscles are considered accessory flexors: the pronator teres, wrist and finger flexors, and radial wrist extensors (Turek, 1977). Besides flexion, the short head of the biceps brachii is a major supinator of the forearm. Flexion of the elbow ranges from 0 to 150 degrees when the flexors are hardened by contraction and up to 160 degrees when the muscles are relaxed (Kapandji, 1982). Range of motion is limited by contractile insufficiency; contact of the muscles of the arm on the forearm; impact of the head of the radius against the radial fossa and the coronoid process against the coronoid fossa; tension of the posterior capsular ligaments; and tension developed passively in the triceps.

Extension. Extension of the elbow is defined as returning from the flexed position (see Figure 15.15). The primary extensors of the elbow are the triceps brachii and anconeus. Range of motion varies from 160 to 0 degrees. Extension beyond 0

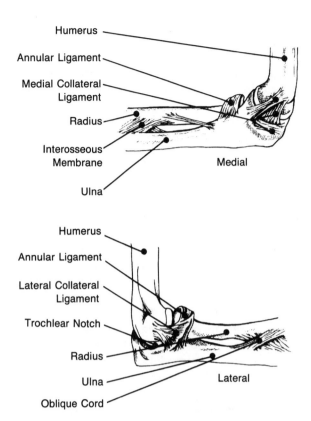

Figure 15.14. Medial and lateral views of the major ligaments of the elbow. *Note.* From *Living Anatomy* (p. 42) by J.E. Donnelly, 1982, Champaign, IL: Human Kinetics. Copyright 1982 by J.E. Donnelly. Reprinted by permission.

degrees is hyperextension. Hyperextension is usually more common in women than men. This condition is a result of a shortened upper curve of the olecranon process of the arm rather than loose ligaments in the joint (Gelabert, 1966). When this condition is present, stretching should not go beyond elbow extension. Range of motion is limited by contractile insufficiency; impact of the olecranon process on the olecranon fossa; tension of the anterior, radial, and ulnar ligaments at the elbow; and tension of the flexor muscles (e.g., biceps brachii).

Pronation. Pronation may be defined as turning the hand from the neutral or palm-up position to the palm-down position (see Figure 15.16). Pronation ranges from 0 to 90 degrees. The movement is seen when top spin is applied in tennis. Pronation is produced by the pronator teres and the pronator quadratus. Range of motion is restricted by contractile insufficiency; tension of the dorsal radioulnar, ulnar collateral, and dorsal radiocarpal ligaments; tension of the lowest fibers of the interosseous membrane; and the radius crossing and impacting against the ulnar.

Supination.   Supination is defined as the outward rotation of the forearm from the neutral or palm-up position (see Figure 15.16). Supination ranges from 0 to 90 degrees. The primary supinators of the forearm are the biceps brachii, supinator, and brachioradialis. Range of motion is limited by contractile insufficiency; tension of the volar radioulnar ligament and ulnar collateral ligament of the wrist; tension of the oblique cord and lowest fibers of the interosseous membrane; and tension of the pronator muscles.

Injuries

Injuries to the musculotendinous and ligament complex of the elbow can be influenced by many factors. Strains, in particular, are commonly associated with activities that demand forceful and repetitive contractions of the forearm muscles. Such injuries are often experienced by tennis, racquetball, and baseball players. Inflammation of the lateral or medial epicondyle is called epicondylitis, or tennis elbow in lay terminology.

Common sense indicates that a preventive approach is the most practical and prudent course to follow. This includes proper warm-up, avoidance of sudden excessive overloading or overuse, optimum technique, and preventive exercises to develop flexibility, strength, and endurance.

The Radiocarpal or Wrist Joint

The radiocarpal, or wrist, is a joint commonly classified as ellipsoid. It is formed by the articulation of the distal end of the radius and three of eight carpal bones in the hand. Ligaments bind the carpals closely and firmly together in two rows of four each. The first or proximal row is comprised of the scaphoid, lunate, triquetum, and pisiform bones. Only the latter does not participate in the formation of the radiocarpal joint. The second, or distal, joint is made up of the trapezium, trapezoid, carpitate, and hammate bones (see Figure 15.17).

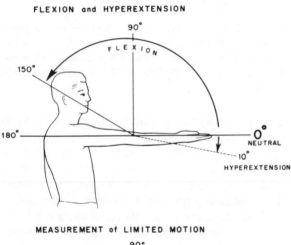

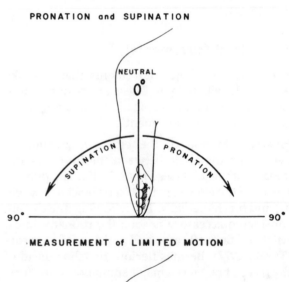

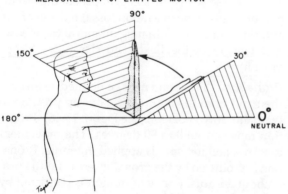

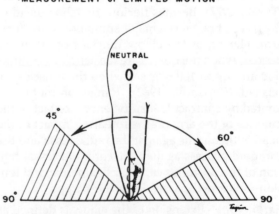

Figure 15.15. Elbow motion: flexion and hyperextension. *Note.* From *Manual of Orthopaedic Surgery* (p. 145), 1985, Park Ridge, IL: American Orthopaedic Association. Copyright 1972 by The American Orthopaedic Association. Reprinted by permission.

Figure 15.16. Pronation and supination. *Note.* From *Manual of Orthopaedic Surgery* (p. 146), 1985, Park Ridge, IL: American Orthopaedic Association. Copyright 1972 by The American Orthopaedic Association. Reprinted by permission.

Stability

The wrist is a very stable joint. Its predominant stabilizing function is carried out by the ligaments of the joint and the numerous muscle tendons that pass over it (see Figure 15.18 and 15.19). However, a portion of this stability is also the result of the bony arrangement. The major ligaments of the wrist are the palmar radiocarpal, palmar ulnocarpal, dorsal radiocarpal, radial collateral, and ulnar collateral.

Anterior

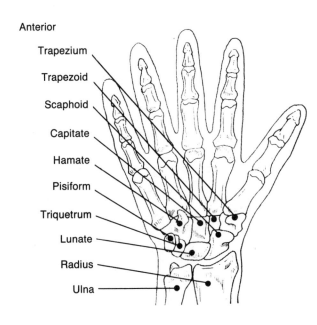

Posterior

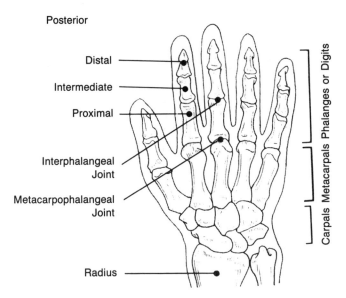

Figure 15.17. Bones of the wrist and hand; anterior and posterior views of the right hand. *Note.* From *Living Anatomy* (p. 48) by J.E. Donnelly, 1982, Champaign, IL: Human Kinetics. Copyright 1982 by J.E. Donnelly. Reprinted by permission.

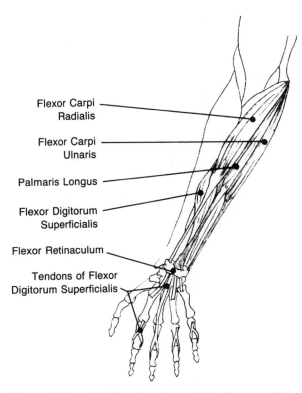

Figure 15.18. An anterior view of the flexors of the wrist. *Note.* From *Living Anatomy* (p. 55) by J.E. Donnelly, 1982, Champaign, IL: Human Kinetics. Copyright 1982 by J.E. Donnelly. Reprinted by permission.

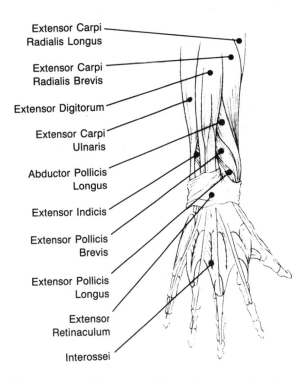

Figure 15.19. Extensors of the wrist, posterior view. *Note.* From *Living Anatomy* (p. 56) by J.E. Donnelly, 1982, Champaign, IL: Human Kinetics. Copyright 1982 by J.E. Donnelly. Reprinted by permission.

Analysis of Movement

The wrist joint allows several active movements. These include flexion, extension, abduction, adduction, and circumduction. However, all but the latter will be examined here.

Flexion.   Flexion of the wrist involves drawing the palm toward the forearm, and ranges from 0 to 90 degrees (see Figure 15.20a). Flexion is greatest when the hand is in the neutral position, neither abducted nor adducted. The chief flexors of the wrist are the flexor carpi radialis, flexor carpi ulnaris, and palmaris longus.

Flexion is limited by contractile insufficiency; tension of the wrist extensor muscles (i.e., extensor carpi radialis longus, extensor carpi radialis brevis, and extensor carpi ulnaris); and tension of the dorsal radiocarpal ligament. Flexion is minimal when the wrist is in pronation (Kapandji, 1982). Movement is also diminished when the fingers are flexed, owing to the increased tension of the extensor muscles.

Extension.   Extension of the wrist occurs when the palm is moved away from the forearm (see Figure 15.20a). This ranges from 0 to 85 degrees. Extension is greatest when the hand is in the neutral position. The main extensors of the wrist are the extensor carpi radialis longus, extensor carpi radialis brevis, and extensor carpi ulnaris. Range of motion is restricted by contractile insufficiency; tension of the wrist flexor muscles (i.e., flexor carpi radialis, flexor carpi ulnaris, and palmaris longus); and tension of the palmar radiocarpal ligament. Extension is minimal during pronation (Kapandji, 1982).

Abduction (Ulnar Deviation).   Abduction of the wrist is defined as flexion of the hand toward the side of the forearm segment where the ulna bone resides (see Figure 15.20b). Abduction takes place almost entirely at the midcarpal joint. It ranges from 0 to 15 degrees. In general, the range of abduction is minimal when the wrist is fully flexed or extended because of the tension developed in the carpal ligaments (Kapandji, 1982). This movement is produced by the flexor carpi radialis, in association with the extensor carpi radialis longus, extensor carpi radialis brevis, abductor carpi radialis longus, and extensor pollicis brevis. Range of motion is limited by contractile insufficiency; tension of the antagonistic muscles; tension of the radial and ulnar collateral radiocarpal ligaments; and impact of the scaphoid on the styloid process of the radius.

Adduction (Radial Deviation).   Adduction of the wrist is defined as flexion of the hand toward the side of the forearm segment where the radius bone resides (see Figure 15.20b). In adduction, most of the movement occurs at the radiocarpal joint and the lunate bone. It ranges from 0 to 45 degrees. The greater range of adduction may be associated with the shortness of the styloid process of the ulna (Williams & Warwick, 1980). Adduction is produced by the flexor carpi ulnaris in association with the extensor carpi ulnaris. Range of motion is restricted by contractile insufficiency, tension of the antagonistic muscles, and impingement of the wrist.

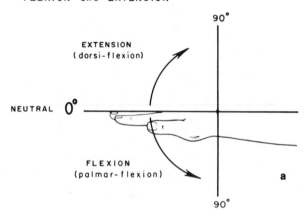

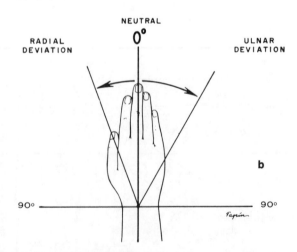

Figure 15.20.   Wrist motions. (a) Flexion and extension. (b) Abduction (ulnar deviation) and adduction (radial deviation). *Note.* From *Manual of Orthopaedic Surgery* (p. 149), 1985, Park Ridge, IL: American Orthopaedic Association. Copyright 1972 by The American Orthopaedic Association. Reprinted by permission.

Review Questions

1. Draw a diagram of the shoulder joint and label the major parts.

2. Compare and contrast the hip to the shoulder joint in terms of flexibility and stability.

3. Explain the concept and significance of the scapulohumeral rhythm.

4. Explain how the concept of the turnout of the hip during abduction can be displayed in the shoulder joint.

5. What action should be taken by a gymnast to facilitate the holding of an iron cross.

6. Explain how the vertebral column can influence flexion of the humerus.

7. What causes natural hyperextension of the elbow? In what group is this most common?

8. Design a program to reduce the chance of tennis elbow for a class of beginning players. Give specific exercises and procedures to follow.

Answers

1. Label: the acromioclavicular, costosternal, costovertebral, glenohumeral, scapulocostal, sternoclavicular, and suprahumeral joints, and the acromion process, clavicle, coracoid process, humerus, and scapula. See Figure 15.1.

2. Although the hip joint possesses considerable flexibility, its chief function is to provide stability. In contrast, the shoulder joint is one of the most mobile and unstable in the human body.

3. If either the humerus or scapula is fixed by injury or disease, the loss of motion is proportionate to the glenohumeral fixation causing twice as much restriction as the scapulothoracic fixation.

4. When the humerus is maintained in medial rotation, the humerus will not abduct beyond 60 degrees. However, if the humerus is laterally rotated, abduction can reach 180 degrees. This is because the greater tubercle will pass behind the acromion.

5. To facilitate the holding of an iron cross one should implement both internal rotation of the humerus and protraction of the scapula.

6. When flexion is resisted at the glenohumeral and scapulothoracic joints, movement of the vertebral column becomes necessary. Hence, anything that may impede movement in the vertebral column will ultimately interfere with the scapulohumeral rhythm and thereby restrict flexion of the humerus.

7. Hyperextension of the elbow is more common in women. This is a result of a shortened upper curve of the olecranon process rather than loose ligaments.

8. Explain to the students at the first meeting the importance of preventing tennis elbow. This can be accomplished by implementing a program that includes proper warm-up, optimum technique, and preventive exercises to develop sufficient flexibility, strength, and endurance. Stretching the medial musculature is accomplished by placing the extended fingertips against the floor with the forearm supinated and the wrist hyperextended. The lateral musculature can be stretched by placing the back of the hand against the floor with the forearm pronated and the wrist hyperextended (Ex. #226). An effective stretch for the supinators is to grasp a stick with one hand in the eagle/elgrip with the elbow flexed (Ex. #227). All stretches should be applied slowly and gradually. Strengthening and endurance should be developed with resistance exercises. This can be achieved through the use of a dumbbell that is flexed, extended, and lateral flexed 10 to 15 times. One or two sets should be performed approximately three times a week.

Recommended Readings

American Academy of Orthopaedic Surgeons. (1975). *Atlas of orthotics. Biomechanical principles and application*. St. Louis: C.V. Mosby.

Basmajian, J.V. (1975). *Grant's method of anatomy* (9th ed.). Baltimore: Williams and Wilkins.

Cummings, G.S. (1984). Comparison of muscle to other soft tissue in limiting elbow extension. *The*

Journal of Orthopaedic and Sports Physical Therapy, **5**(4), 170-174.

Daniels, L., & Worthingham, C. (1980). *Muscle testing* (4th ed.). Philadelphia: W. B. Saunders.

DiStefano, V. (1977). Functional anatomy and biomechanics of the shoulder joints. *Athletic Training,* **12**(3), 141-144.

Hollinshead, W.F., & Jenkins, D.B. (1981). *Functional anatomy of the limbs and back* (5th ed.). Philadelphia: W.B. Saunders.

Kent, B.E. (1971). Functional anatomy of the shoulder complex: A review. *Physical Therapy,* **51**(8), 867-888.

Steindler, A. (1977). *Kinesiology of the human body.* Springfield, IL: Charles C Thomas.

Wilkerson, G.B. (1984). Preventing epicondylitis. *The Physician and Sportsmedicine,* **12**(6), 194-197.

PART III

Stretching Exercises

Prior to undertaking any exercise program, you should obtain a medical examination. You should also obtain examinations at regular intervals throughout the program, or at any time that irregular conditions such as dizziness, pain in the chest, or other such symptoms appear.

Recommendation

It is strongly recommended that chapter 12 be thoroughly reviewed.

Suggestion for Advanced Stretching

The exercises that follow should be executed in a slow, or static, manner. However, those who are more advanced may find it more effective and efficient to incorporate the contract-relax strategy or the hold-relax PNF strategy. These techniques employ stretching a limb or muscle to the point where further motion in the desired direction is prevented by the tension in the antagonist muscle, that is, the muscle being stretched. At this point, either a maximal isotonic or isometric contraction of the antagonist, lasting six seconds, is followed by a period of relaxation. Then, the limb or muscle is again stretched to the point where limitation occurs. This additional stretch can be either passive or active. The entire process is then repeated again. (For additional details, see chapter 11.)

Cross References to Stretching Exercises

The following keys will guide you in selecting stretching exercises for specific parts of the body.

Posterior aspect of toes & plantar arch	1-3
Anterior aspect of toes	4-5
Ankles & lower leg	
Anterior aspect	6-11
Lateral aspect	12-18
Achilles tendon & calf	19-40; 233
Posterior aspect of knee	35-40
Hamstrings	41-62; 75-77; 79-80; 87; 105-110; 155-158
Groin	63-90; 161; 234-235
Quadriceps & hip flexors	91-110; 135-150; 217
Buttocks & hip	111-134
Abdominals	135-150; 215
Lower back	41; 43-44; 46-58; 87; 135-158; 215
Lateral torso	75-76; 121-122; 124-126; 159-172; 211-212; 236-237
Upper back	172-175; 217-218
Posterior aspect of neck	154; 157-158; 176-181
Lateral aspect of neck	182
Anterior aspect of neck	183-185
Chest	186-191; 212; 238-239
Anterior aspect of shoulder	187-190; 192-199; 202-205; 207; 211-218; 220; 238-240
Posterior aspect of shoulder	200-201; 206; 208-210; 219
Biceps	221-222; 242
Triceps	223-226; 241
Wrist extensors	227-228
Wrist flexors	229-232

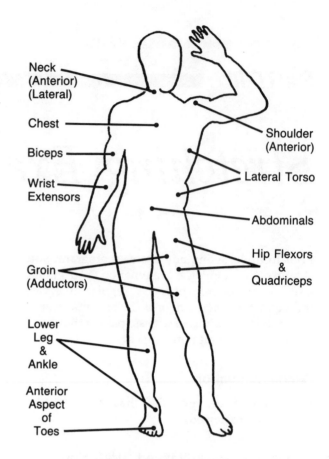

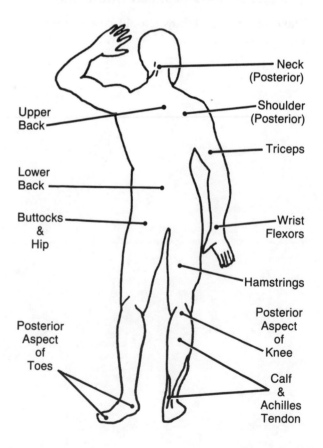

Major Muscles of the Body

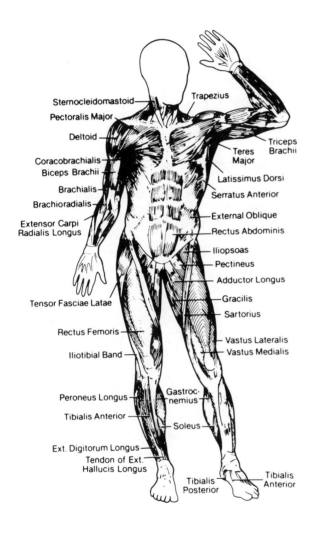

Sternocleidomastoid
Pectoralis Major
Deltoid
Coracobrachialis
Biceps Brachii
Brachialis
Brachioradialis
Extensor Carpi
Radialis Longus
Tensor Fasciae Latae
Rectus Femoris
Iliotibial Band
Peroneus Longus
Tibialis Anterior
Ext. Digitorum Longus
Tendon of Ext.
Hallucis Longus

Trapezius
Triceps
Brachii
Teres
Major
Latissimus Dorsi
Serratus Anterior
External Oblique
Rectus Abdominis
Iliopsoas
Pectineus
Adductor Longus
Gracilis
Sartorius
Vastus Lateralis
Vastus Medialis
Gastroc-
nemius
Soleus
Tibialis
Posterior
Tibialis
Anterior

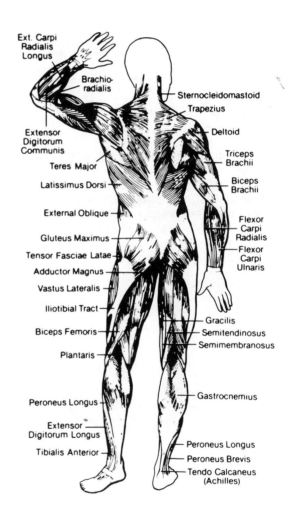

Ext. Carpi
Radialis
Longus
Brachio-
radialis
Extensor
Digitorum
Communis
Teres Major
Latissimus Dorsi
External Oblique
Gluteus Maximus
Tensor Fasciae Latae
Adductor Magnus
Vastus Lateralis
Iliotibial Tract
Biceps Femoris
Plantaris
Peroneus Longus
Extensor
Digitorum Longus
Tibialis Anterior

Sternocleidomastoid
Trapezius
Deltoid
Triceps
Brachii
Biceps
Brachii
Flexor
Carpi
Radialis
Flexor
Carpi
Ulnaris
Gracilis
Semitendinosus
Semimembranosus
Gastrocnemius
Peroneus Longus
Peroneus Brevis
Tendo Calcaneus
(Achilles)

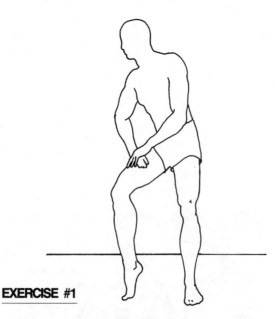

EXERCISE #1

1. Stand upright with one leg slightly in front of the other.
2. Exhale, shift your weight onto the ball of your forward foot, and press downward.
3. Hold the stretch and relax.

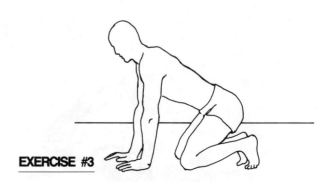

EXERCISE #3

1. Kneel on all fours with your toes underneath you.
2. Exhale and lower your buttocks backward and downward.
3. Hold the stretch and relax.

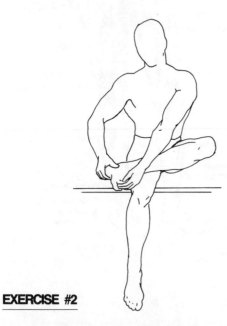

EXERCISE #2

1. Sit upright in a chair or on the floor with one leg crossed over the opposite knee.
2. Grasp hold of your ankle with one hand.
3. Grasp hold of the underside of your toes and ball of the foot.
4. Exhale, and pull your toes backward (extension of the toes).
5. Hold the stretch and relax.

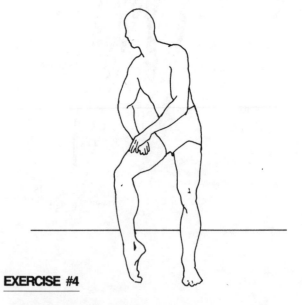

EXERCISE #4

1. Stand upright with one leg slightly in front of the other.
2. Turn your forward foot under so the top portion of your toes contact the floor.
3. Exhale, shift your weight forward, and press your toes down.
4. Hold the stretch and relax.

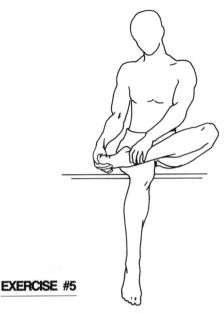

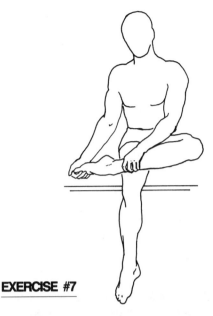

EXERCISE #5

1. Sit upright in a chair or on the floor with one leg crossed over the opposite knee.
2. Grasp hold of your ankle and heel of your foot with one hand.
3. Grasp hold of the top portion of your foot and toes with your other hand.
4. Exhale, and slowly pull the back of your toes to the ball of your foot (flexion).
5. Hold the stretch and relax.

EXERCISE #7

1. Sit upright in a chair or on the floor with one leg crossed over the opposite knee.
2. Grasp hold on/above your ankle or heel of your foot with one hand.
3. Grasp hold of the top portion of your foot with your other hand.
4. Exhale, and slowly pull the bottom of your foot to your body (plantar-flexion).
5. Hold the stretch and relax.

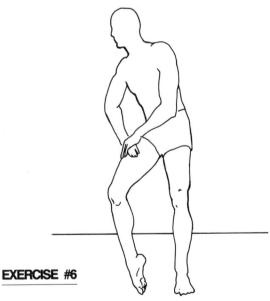

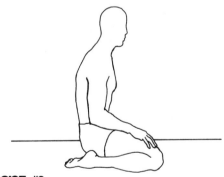

EXERCISE #6

1. Stand upright with one leg slightly in front of the other.
2. Turn your forward foot under so the top portion rests on the floor.
3. Exhale, shift your weight forward, and extend (increase the angle of) the ankle joint.
4. Hold the stretch and relax.

EXERCISE #8

1. Kneel upright with your legs extended.
2. Exhale and slowly lower your buttocks onto your heels (if able).
3. Hold the stretch and relax. *CAUTION:* This should be avoided by those with ''bad knees.'' *NOTE:* Place a blanket or cushion underneath your legs if the position is uncomfortable.

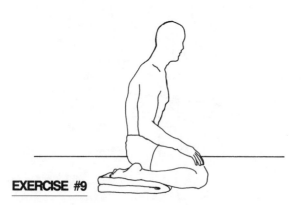

EXERCISE #9

1. Kneel upright on the floor; your toes facing backwards; and your feet elevated by a folded mat or cushion.
2. Exhale and slowly lower your buttocks onto your heels (if able).
3. Hold the stretch and relax. *CAUTION:* This should be avoided by those with "bad knees."

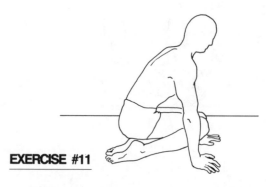

EXERCISE #11

1. Kneel on all fours with your toes facing backwards.
2. Slowly, sit on your heels.
3. Inhale, shift your weight backwards so that your knees lift slightly off the floor.
4. Hold the stretch and relax. *CAUTION:* This should be avoided by those with "bad knees." *NOTE:* Use your hands for support to adjust the proper weight onto the ankle joints.

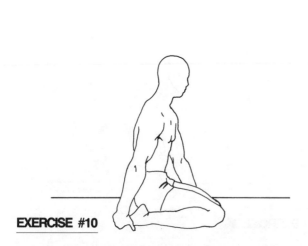

EXERCISE #10

1. Assume the stretch position in exercise #8.
2. Reach around, grasp the top portion of your toes, and pull them toward your head.
3. Hold the stretch and relax. *CAUTION:* This should be avoided by those with "bad knees." *NOTE:* This exercise is used to prevent "shin-splints."

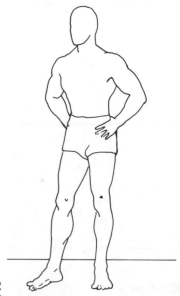

EXERCISE #12

1. Stand upright with either one or both hands on your hips.
2. Turn one foot under so the top outside portion rests on the floor.
3. Exhale, slowly invert your ankle, and press your foot downwards.
4. Hold the stretch and relax.

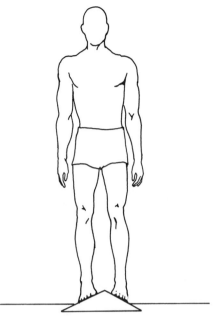

EXERCISE #13

1. Stand upright on an incline board cut at a 45°
   angle.
2. Hold the stretch and relax.

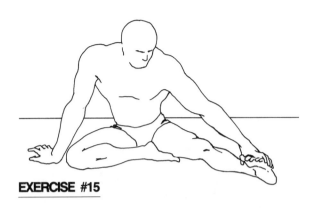

EXERCISE #15

1. Sit upright on the floor with both legs straight.
2. Keep one leg straight and position your opposite
   leg so its heel touches the groin of your extended
   leg.
3. Exhale, bend forward at the waist, and grasp
   your foot.
4. Exhale, and slowly invert your ankle.
5. Relax and hold the stretch. *NOTE:* Use a folded
   blanket if you cannot reach your foot.

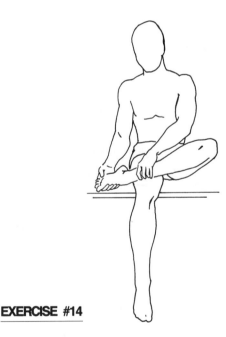

EXERCISE #14

1. Sit upright in a chair or on the floor with one leg
   crossed over the opposite knee.
2. Grasp hold of your ankle and heel of your foot
   with one hand.
3. Grasp hold of the top outside portion of your foot
   with the other hand.
4. Exhale, and slowly invert your ankle.
5. Hold the stretch and relax.

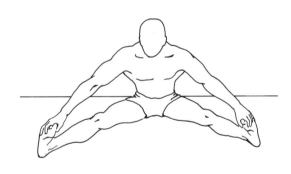

EXERCISE #16

1. Sit upright on the floor with both legs straight
   and straddled.
2. Exhale, bend forward at the waist, and grasp
   both feet.
3. Exhale, and slowly invert both ankles.
4. Hold the stretch and relax. *NOTE:* Use a folded
   blanket if you cannot reach your feet.

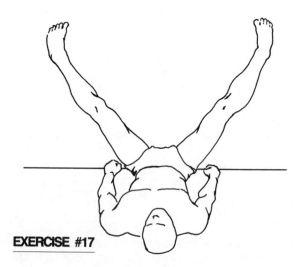

EXERCISE #17

1. Lie flat on your back, both legs raised, and your buttocks against a wall.
2. Straddle both legs.
3. Exhale, and slowly invert both ankles.
4. Hold the stretch and relax.

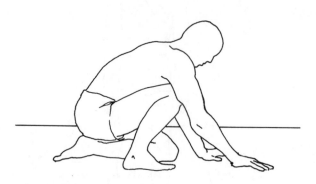

EXERCISE #19

1. Assume a squat position with both hands on the floor for support and balance.
2. Inhale and shift one foot slightly forward and place it flat on the floor.
3. Exhale, and lean your knee beyond the foot.
4. Hold the stretch and relax.

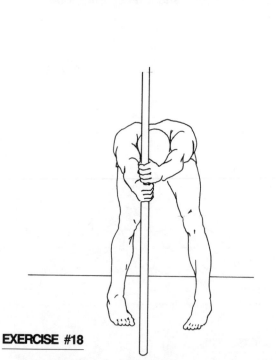

EXERCISE #18

1. Stand upright with both hands grasping a pillar for support.
2. Straddle your feet hip width, feet toed-in, and approximately 1–2 feet from the pillar.
3. Exhale, flex at the waist, and shift your hips backwards to form a 45° angle with your legs.
4. Hold the stretch and relax. *NOTE:* Ideally, your back should be flat and horizontal to the floor.

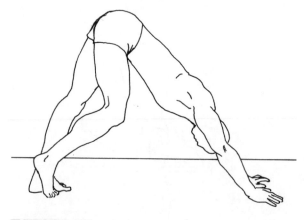

EXERCISE #20

1. Assume a front prone support (push-up) position.
2. Move your hands closer to your feet to raise your hips and form a triangle.
3. At the highest point of the triangle slowly force your heels to the floor, or in an alternating manner flex one knee while keeping your opposite leg extended.
4. Hold the stretch and relax. *CAUTION:* The latter method is commonly employed in a ballistic or rhythmic manner which could result in soreness. *NOTE:* This exercise may be modified with the elbows and/or head resting on the floor.

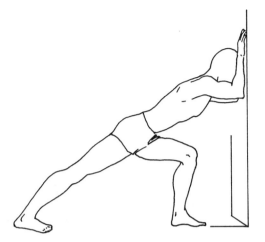

EXERCISE #21

1. Stand upright 4–5 steps from a wall.
2. Bend one leg forward and keep your opposite leg straight.
3. Lean against the wall without losing the straight line of your head, neck, spine, pelvis, right leg, and ankle.
4. Keep your rear foot *down, flat,* and *parallel* to your hips.
5. Exhale, bend your arms, move your chest toward the wall, and shift your weight forward.
6. Hold the stretch and relax.

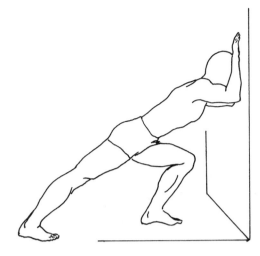

EXERCISE #23

1. Assume the stretch position in exercise #21.
2. Exhale, and flex your forward knee toward the floor.
3. Hold the stretch and relax.

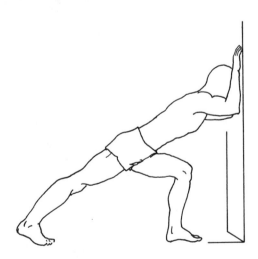

EXERCISE #22

1. Assume the stretch position in exercise #21, except start with the rear foot *raised* and *parallel* to the hips.
2. Exhale, bend your arms, move your chest toward the wall, and shift your weight forward.
3. Exhale, and slowly attempt to force your rear heel to the floor.
4. Hold the stretch and relax.

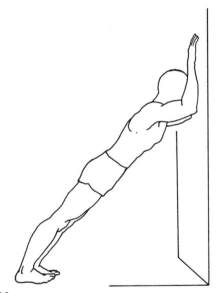

EXERCISE #24

1. Stand upright 4–5 steps from a wall.
2. Lean against the wall without losing the straight line of the head, neck, spine, pelvis, legs, and ankles.
3. Keep both heels *down, flat, together,* and *parallel* to the hips.
4. Exhale, bend your arms, move your chest toward the wall, and shift your weight forward.
5. Hold the stretch and relax.

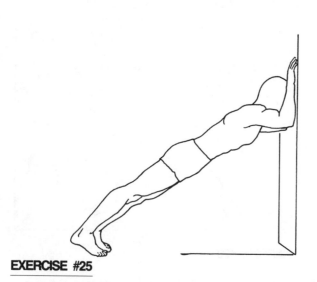

EXERCISE #25

1. Assume the stretch position in exercise #24, except start with the rear feet *raised, together,* and *parallel* to your hips.
2. Exhale, bend your arms, move your chest toward the wall, and shift your weight forward.
3. Exhale, and slowly attempt to force your heels to the floor.
4. Hold the stretch and relax.

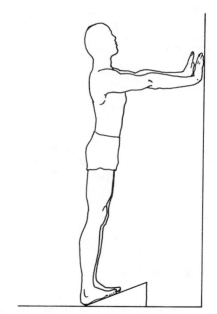

EXERCISE #27

1. Place an incline board facing a wall.
2. Stand upright on the incline board with your hands flat against the wall and lean forward.
3. Hold the stretch and relax.

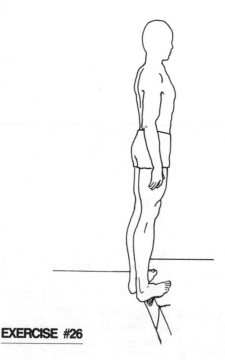

EXERCISE #26

1. Stand upright with the balls of your feet balanced on an edge or step.
2. Exhale, and slowly lower your heels toward the floor.
3. Hold the stretch and relax.

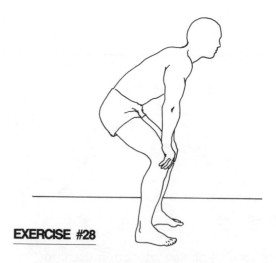

EXERCISE #28

1. Stand upright with both hands on your hips or knees.
2. Keep your heels *down, flat,* and *parallel.*
3. Exhale, and slowly flex your knees, bringing them as close to the floor as possible.
4. Hold the stretch and relax. *NOTE:* If necessary, hold on to a wall for balance.

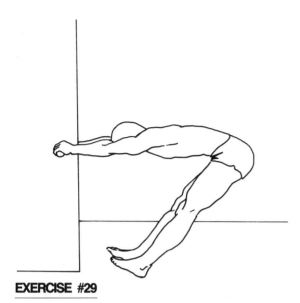

EXERCISE #29

1. Stand upright approximately 2 feet from an opened door.
2. Grasp the door handles with both hands.
3. Lift the front part of your feet and balance on your heels.
4. Exhale, keep both legs straight, and shift your hips backward.
5. Hold the stretch and relax.

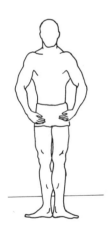
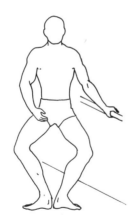

EXERCISE #30

1. Stand upright, feet together, hands on hips.
2. Turn to Position I with your heels together and your toes pointing outward at a 90° angle.
3. Grasp a surface for support and balance.
4. Exhale, and slowly flex your knees.
5. Hold the stretch and relax. *CAUTION:* See the text regarding Demi Pliés. *NOTE:* Concentrate on keeping your weight distributed equally as your heels are maintained flat on the floor.

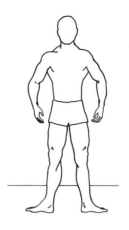
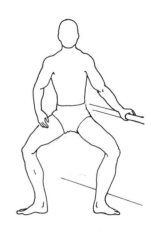

EXERCISE #31

1. Stand upright, feet together, hands by your sides.
2. Turn to Position II with your heels about twelve inches apart, your toes pointing outward at a 90° angle, and your feet in line with each other.
3. Grasp a surface for support and balance.
4. Exhale, and slowly flex your knees.
5. Hold the stretch and relax. *CAUTION:* See the text regarding Demi Pliés. *NOTE:* Concentrate on keeping your weight distributed equally as your heels are maintained flat on the floor.

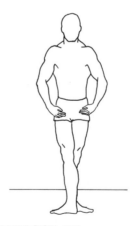
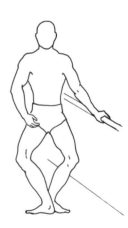

EXERCISE #32

1. Stand upright, feet together, hands on your hips.
2. Turn to Position III so your feet are in line, pressed together, the heel of one foot at the arch or instep of the other foot, and the toes pointing away (in opposite directions of each other).
3. Grasp a surface for support and balance.
4. Exhale, and slowly flex your knees.
5. Hold the stretch and relax. *CAUTION:* See the text regarding Demi Pliés. *NOTE:* Concentrate on keeping your weight distributed equally as your heels are maintained flat on the floor.

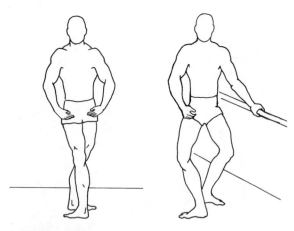

EXERCISE #33

1. Stand upright, feet together, hands on your hips.
2. Turn to Position IV with one foot approximately twelve inches in front of the other, the heel of your forward foot in line with the toes of your back foot, and your feet pointed in the opposite direction.
3. Grasp a surface for support and balance.
4. Exhale, and slowly flex your knees.
5. Hold the stretch and relax. *CAUTION:* See the text regarding Demi Pliés. *NOTE:* Concentrate on keeping your weight distributed equally as your heels are maintained flat on the floor.

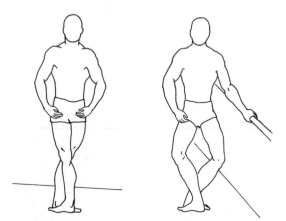

EXERCISE #34

1. Stand upright, feet together, hands on your hips.
2. Turn to Position V with the heel of your front foot flat against the toe of your other foot; at the same time, the toe of your rear foot is against the heel of your front foot; and, your feet are pointed in opposite directions.
3. Grasp a surface for support and balance.
4. Exhale, and slowly flex your knees.
5. Hold the stretch and relax. *CAUTION:* See the text regarding Demi Pliés. *NOTE:* Concentrate on keeping your weight distributed equally as your heels are maintained flat on the floor.

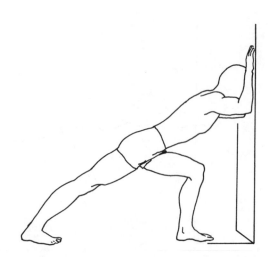

EXERCISE #35

1. Assume the stretch position in exercise #21.
2. Exhale, bend your arms, move your chest toward the wall, and shift your weight forward.
3. Exhale, and slowly contract the quadriceps of your rear leg.
4. Hold the stretch and relax. *NOTE:* Avoid jamming or locking the joint. *CAUTION:* Those with hyperextended knees should avoid.

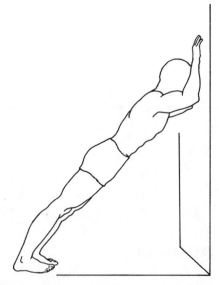

EXERCISE #36

1. Assume the stretch position in exercise #24.
2. Exhale, bend your arms, move your chest toward the wall, and shift your weight forward.
3. Exhale, and slowly contract the quadriceps.
4. Hold the stretch and relax. *NOTE:* Avoid jamming or locking the joint. *CAUTION:* Those with hyperextended knees should avoid.

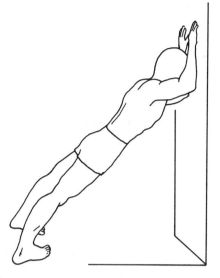

EXERCISE #37

1. Assume the stretch position in exercise #24 with the feet toed in.
2. Exhale, bend your arms, move your chest toward the wall, and shift your weight forward.
3. Exhale, and slowly contract the quadriceps.
4. Hold the stretch and relax. *NOTE:* Avoid jamming or locking the joint. *CAUTION:* Those with hyperextended knees should avoid.

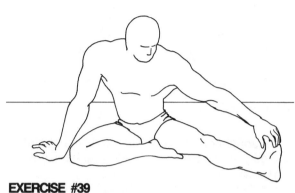

EXERCISE #39

1. Sit upright with both legs straight.
2. Keep one leg straight and position the opposite leg so its heel touches the groin of your extended leg.
3. Exhale, lean forward, and grasp your foot.
4. Exhale, keep your legs straight, and pull on your foot.
5. Hold the stretch and relax. *NOTE:* Use a folded blanket if you cannot reach your feet.

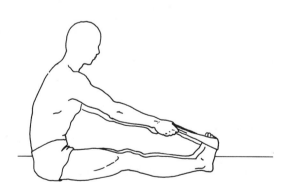

EXERCISE #38

1. Sit upright with both legs straight.
2. Exhale, lean forward, and grasp hold of your feet with your hands, or use a folded towel.
3. Exhale, and pull on your feet.
4. Hold the stretch and relax.

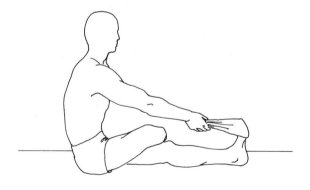

EXERCISE #40

1. Sit upright on the floor with both legs straight.
2. Cross one leg and rest it on the opposing knee.
3. Exhale, lean forward, and grasp hold of your foot or use a folded towel.
4. Exhale, keep your extended leg straight, and pull on your foot.
5. Hold the stretch and relax.

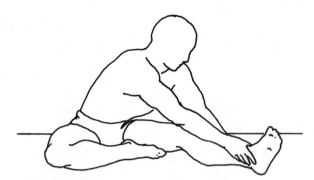

EXERCISE #41

1. Sit upright on the floor with both legs straight.
2. Flex your right knee and slide your heel toward your buttocks.
3. Lower the outer side of your right thigh and calf onto the floor.
4. Place your right heel against the inner side of your left thigh so that a 90° angle is formed between your extended left leg and flexed right leg.
5. Exhale, keeping your left leg straight, bend at the waist, and lower your extended upper torso onto your thigh.
6. Hold the stretch and relax.

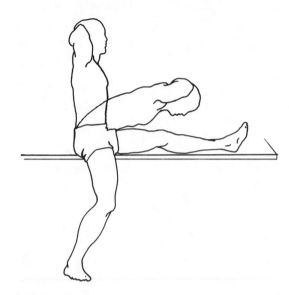

EXERCISE #43

1. Sit upright on a bench with one leg extended, and your opposite foot on the floor.
2. Exhale, extend your upper back and leg resting on the bench, flex at the hips, and lower your trunk onto your thigh.
3. Hold the stretch and relax.

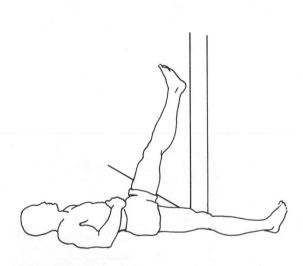

EXERCISE #42

1. Lie flat on your back between a doorway.
2. Position your hips slightly in front of the door frame.
3. Raise one leg and rest it against the door frame while keeping your knee extended and your bottom leg flat on the floor.
4. Hold the stretch and relax. *NOTE:* To increase the stretch, slide the buttocks closer to the doorpost or lift the leg away from the door frame.

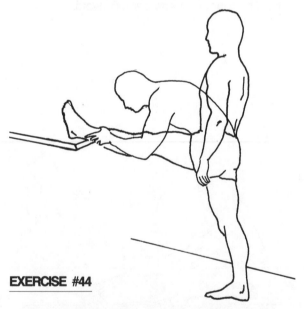

EXERCISE #44

1. Stand upright with one leg raised and resting on an elevated platform.
2. Exhale, keeping both legs straight and your hips squared, extend your upper back, bend forward at the waist, and lower your trunk onto your raised thigh.
3. Hold the stretch and relax.

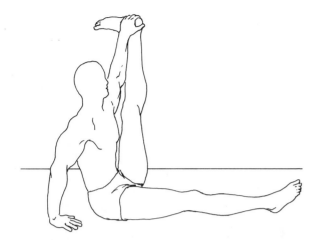

EXERCISE #45

1. Sit upright on the floor, hands behind your hips for support, and your legs extended.
2. Flex one knee and grasp your foot with one hand.
3. Exhale, and slowly extend your leg until it reaches a 90° angle.
4. Hold the stretch and relax.

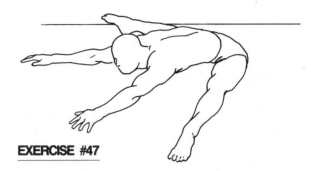

EXERCISE #47

1. Sit upright on the floor with both legs extended.
2. Straddle your legs.
3. Exhale, keeping both legs straight, extend your upper back, bend forward at the waist, and lower your trunk onto the floor.
4. Hold the stretch and relax.

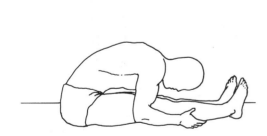

EXERCISE #46

1. Sit upright on the floor with both legs extended.
2. Exhale, keeping both legs straight, extend your upper back, bend forward at the waist, and lower your trunk onto your thighs.
3. Hold the stretch and relax.

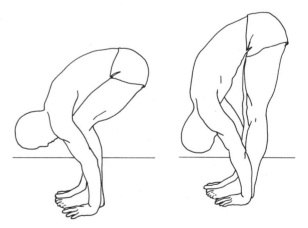

EXERCISE #48

1. Assume a squat position with your hands resting on the floor.
2. Exhale and slowly extend your knees.
3. Hold the stretch and relax. *NOTE:* You will also feel this stretch in the lower back.

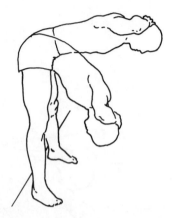

EXERCISE #49

1. Stand upright, legs straddled, and with the back of your heels six inches from a wall.
2. Interlock your hands behind your head.
3. Exhale, keeping both legs straight, extend your upper back, bend forward at the waist, and lower your trunk toward your thighs.
4. Hold the stretch and relax. *NOTE:* Position your buttocks against the wall and feel the pelvis rising as you lower down and vice versa.

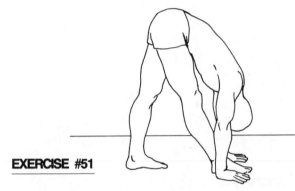

EXERCISE #51

1. Assume the stretch position in exercise #19.
2. Exhale and slowly extend your legs.
3. Hold the stretch and relax.

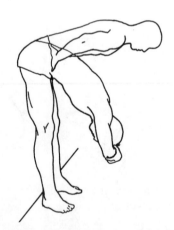

EXERCISE #50

1. Stand upright with the back of your heels six inches from a wall and both hands on your hips.
2. Raise both arms and interlock your hands behind your head.
3. Exhale, keeping both legs straight, extend your upper back, bend forward at the waist, and lower your trunk onto your thighs.
4. Hold the stretch and relax. *NOTE:* Position your buttocks against the wall and feel the pelvis rising as you lower down and vice versa.

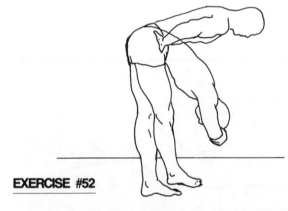

EXERCISE #52

1. Stand upright on the floor with one leg crossed over the other.
2. Exhale, keeping one leg straight, extend your upper back, bend forward at the waist, and lower your trunk onto your thigh.
3. Hold the stretch and relax. *NOTE:* This stretch may be difficult to maintain because of the balancing component.

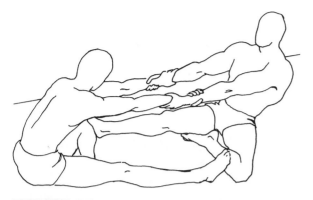

EXERCISE #53

1. Assume the stretch position in exercise #41.
2. Your partner assumes the identical position.
3. Your extended leg will brace against your partner's flexed leg and vice versa.
4. Interlock hands.
5. Exhale, keeping your forward leg straight, extend your upper back, bend forward at the waist, and lower your trunk onto your thigh as your partner leans backward and pulls on your hands.
6. Hold the stretch and relax. *CAUTION:* Communicate and use with great care.

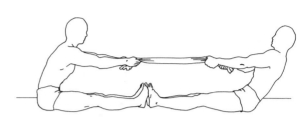

EXERCISE #55

1. Assume the stretch position in exercise #46.
2. Your partner assumes the identical position.
3. Brace your feet against each other, lean forward, and interlock hands. (If unable to do so, use a folded blanket.)
4. Exhale, keeping your legs straight, extend the upper back, bend forward at the waist, and lower your trunk onto your thighs as your partner leans backward and pulls on your hands (or blanket).
5. Hold the stretch and relax. *CAUTION:* Communicate and use with great care.

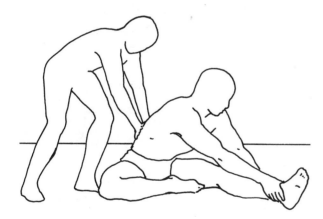

EXERCISE #54

1. Assume the stretch position in exercise #41.
2. Your partner is positioned standing behind you with one hand on the central portion of your upper back, and the other hand on the central portion of your lower back.
3. Exhale, keeping your forward leg straight, extend your upper back, bend forward at the waist, and allow your partner to assist in pushing your upper torso onto your thigh.
4. Hold the stretch and relax. *CAUTION:* Communicate and use with great care.

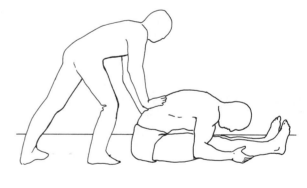

EXERCISE #56

1. Assume the stretch position in exercise #46.
2. Your partner is positioned standing behind you with one hand on the central portion of your upper back, and the other on the central portion of your lower back.
3. Exhale, keeping your legs straight, extend your upper back, bend forward at the waist, and allow your partner to assist in pushing your upper torso onto your thighs.
4. Hold the stretch and relax. *CAUTION:* Communicate and use with great care.

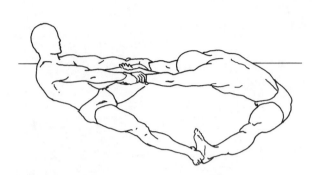

EXERCISE #57

1. Assume the stretch position in exercise #47.
2. Your partner assumes the identical position.
3. Brace your feet against each other, lean forward, and interlock hands.
4. Exhale, keeping your legs straight, extend your upper back, lean forward at the waist, and lower your trunk onto the floor as your partner leans backward and pulls on your hands.
5. Hold the stretch and relax. *CAUTION:* Communicate and use with great care.

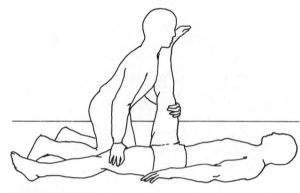

EXERCISE #59

1. Lie flat on your back with your body straight.
2. Inhale, raise one leg, and keep your hips square.
3. Your partner will anchor your lower leg and grasp your raised leg.
4. Exhale, and slowly your partner will raise your leg. (Both legs must remain straight and your hips kept squared.)
5. Hold the stretch and relax. *CAUTION:* Communicate and use with great care.

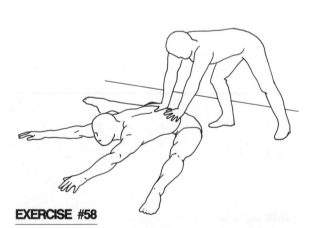

EXERCISE #58

1. Assume the stretch position in exercise #47.
2. Your partner is positioned standing behind with both hands on the central portion of your lower back.
3. Exhale, keeping your legs straight, extend your upper back, lean forward at the waist, and allow your partner to assist in pushing your upper torso onto the floor.
4. Hold the stretch and relax. *CAUTION:* Communicate and use with great care.

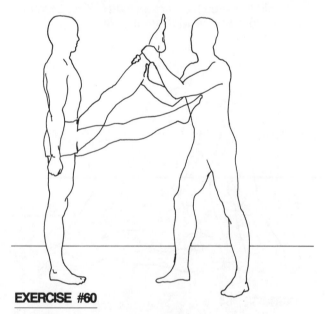

EXERCISE #60

1. Stand upright facing your partner and holding onto a surface for balance and support.
2. Inhale, raise one leg and keep your hips squared.
3. Your partner will grasp your raised leg with one hand above your ankle and the other on your foot.
4. Exhale, and slowly your partner will raise your leg. (Both legs must remain straight and your hips kept squared.)
5. Hold the stretch and relax. *CAUTION:* Communicate and use with great care.

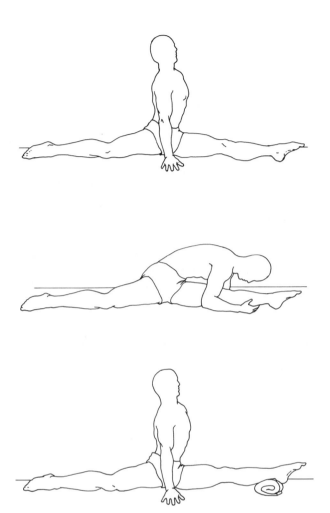

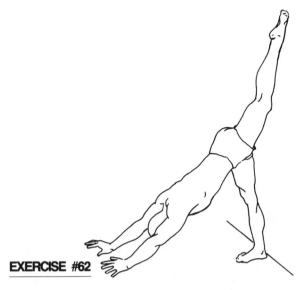

EXERCISE #62

1. Stand upright with your back approximately one foot from a wall.
2. Place your hands on the floor for support and raise one leg against the wall.
3. Exhale, and slowly slide your leg upward against the wall until you attain the split position.
4. Hold the stretch and relax. *NOTE:* Concentrate on using your hands for balance and support, keeping your legs straight, and your hips squared.

EXERCISE #61

1. Kneel on the floor with both legs together and your hands at your side.
2. Lift up your left knee and place your foot a few feet in front for support.
3. Exhale, bend at the waist, lower your upper torso down onto your left thigh, and place your hands a few inches in front of your left foot for support.
4. Exhale, slowly slide your left foot forward and straighten your leg as your rear leg is extended backward.
5. Hold the stretch and relax. *NOTE:* To perform a technically correct split, both legs must be straight, the hips squared, and the buttocks flat on the floor. For aesthetic reasons, some advocate a slight turnout of the rear hip. However, this is usually carried to an extreme. This is primarily due to tight hip flexors and/or improper training. To increase the stretch one can (a) extend the upper torso and lower the chest onto the forward thigh, or (b) perform the split with the forward leg placed on top of some folded blankets.

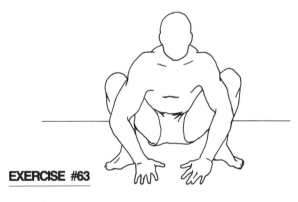

EXERCISE #63

1. Assume a squat position with your feet about twelve inches apart and your toes turned slightly out.
2. Place your elbows on the inside portion of both upper legs.
3. Exhale, and slowly push your legs outward with your elbows.
4. Hold the stretch and relax. *NOTE:* Balancing may be a problem for some. Furthermore, remember the feet must be flat on the floor to reduce strain on the knees.

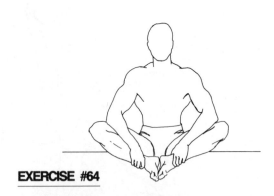

EXERCISE #64

1. Sit upright on the floor.
2. Flex your knees and bring the heels and soles of your feet together as you pull them toward your buttocks.
3. Place your elbows on the inside portion of both upper legs.
4. Exhale, and slowly push your legs to the floor.
5. Hold the stretch and relax. *NOTE:* This stretch is more effective with your back against a wall.

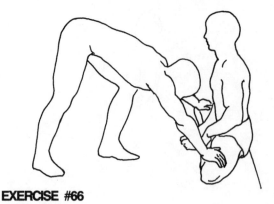

EXERCISE #66

1. Assume the stretch position in exercise #64.
2. Your partner kneels on the floor facing you with his or her hands on the inside portion of both upper legs.
3. Exhale, and allow your partner to assist you in lowering your legs to the floor.
4. Hold the stretch and relax. *CAUTION:* Communicate and use great care.

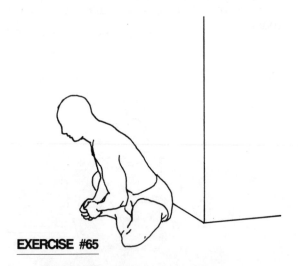

EXERCISE #65

1. Assume the stretch position in exercise #64.
2. Grasp your feet or ankles.
3. Exhale, lean forward from the hips without bending your back and attempt to lower your chest to the floor.
4. Hold the stretch and relax. *NOTE:* To increase the stretch, move the heels closer to your buttocks.

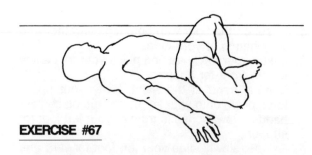

EXERCISE #67

1. Lie flat on your back with your body straight.
2. Flex your knees and bring the heels and soles of your feet together as you pull them toward your buttocks.
3. Exhale, and straddle your knees as wide as possible with the soles of your feet remaining in contact.
4. Hold the stretch and relax.

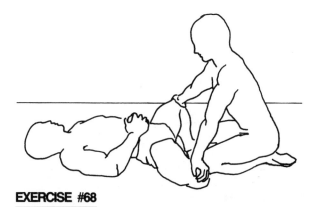

EXERCISE #68

1. Assume the stretch position in exercise #67.
2. Your partner kneels the floor facing you with his or her hands on the upper inside portion of your legs.
3. Exhale, as you allow your partner to gently push your legs to the floor.
4. Hold the stretch and relax. *CAUTION:* Communicate and use great care.

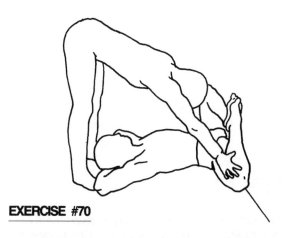

EXERCISE #70

1. Assume the stretch position in exercise #69.
2. Your partner stands facing you with his or her hands on the upper inside portion of your legs.
3. Exhale, as you allow your partner to gently push your legs to the wall.
4. Hold the stretch and relax.

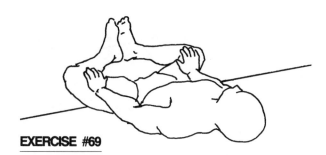

EXERCISE #69

1. Assume the stretch position in exercise #67 with your legs rested against a wall.
2. Place your hands on the upper inside portion of both legs.
3. Exhale, and slowly straddle your legs as wide as possible.
4. Hold the stretch and relax. *CAUTION:* Move further from the wall if you feel pressure building in your lower back.

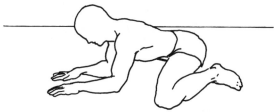

EXERCISE #71

1. Kneel on all fours with your toes facing backward.
2. Bend your arms and rest your elbows on the floor.
3. Exhale, slowly straddle your knees, and attempt to lower your chest to the floor.
4. Hold the stretch and relax. *CAUTION:* This is one of the most intense stretches for the adductors—it's extremely deceptive. *NOTE:* To intensify the stretch, one can (a) adjust the positioning of your feet, or (b) slowly roll your hips.

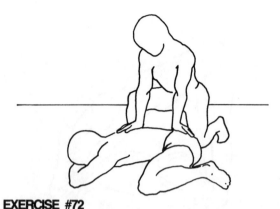

EXERCISE #72

1. Assume the stretch position in exercise #71.
2. Your partner stands either to your side or directly behind you and places his or hands on your hip and upper back.
3. Exhale, as you allow your partner to gently push down to further straddle your legs.
4. Hold the stretch and relax. *CAUTION:* Communicate and use with great care.

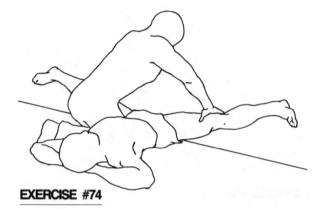

EXERCISE #74

1. Assume the stretch position in exercise #73.
2. Your partner stands facing you and grasps either your ankles or the medial aspect of your thighs.
3. Exhale, as you allow your partner to gently straddle the legs further.
4. Hold the stretch and relax. *NOTE:* The legs must be kept straight.

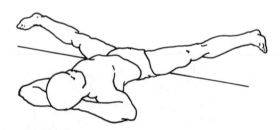

EXERCISE #73

1. Lie flat on your back; legs raised and together, and your buttocks several inches from a wall.
2. Exhale, and slowly straddle your legs as wide as possible.
3. Hold the stretch and relax. *NOTE:* To intensify the stretch, one can wear ankle weights.

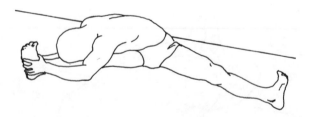

EXERCISE #75

1. Sit upright on the floor with both legs straight.
2. Straddle your legs as wide as possible.
3. Exhale, rotate and extend your trunk onto one leg.
4. Hold the stretch and relax.

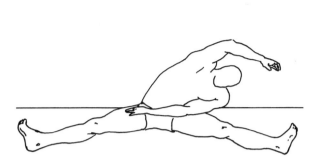

EXERCISE #76

1. Sit upright on the floor with both legs straight.
2. Straddle your legs as wide as possible.
3. Drop one arm and raise your other arm overhead.
4. Exhale, rotate your trunk, and extend your upper torso onto your leg.
5. Hold the stretch and relax.

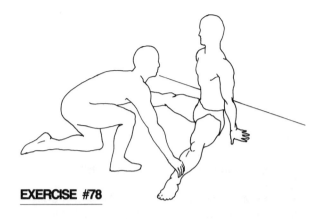

EXERCISE #78

1. Sit upright on the floor with your legs straddled and straight.
2. Your partner kneels facing you and grasps your ankles or the lower part of your legs.
3. Exhale, as you allow your partner to gently straddle your legs further.
4. Hold the stretch and relax.

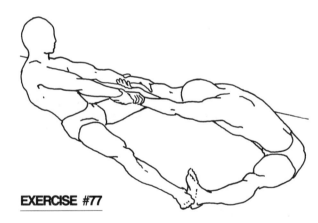

EXERCISE #77

1. Sit upright on the floor with your legs straddled and straight.
2. Your partner assumes the identical position, brace your feet together, and interlock hands.
3. Exhale, keeping your legs straight, bend at the waist, lower your upper torso toward the floor as your partner leans backward and pulls on your hands.
4. Hold the stretch and relax. *CAUTION:* Communicate and use with great care.

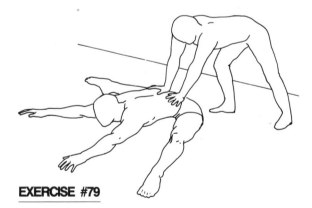

EXERCISE #79

1. Sit upright on the floor with your legs straddled and straight.
2. Your partner stands behind you with his or her hands on the central portion of your back.
3. Exhale, as you allow your partner to gently push your upper torso to the floor.
4. Hold the stretch and relax. *CAUTION:* Communicate and use great care. *Note:* Extend from the hips and do not bend your back.

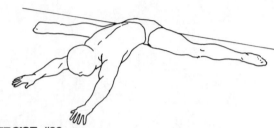

EXERCISE #80

1. Sit upright on the floor with your legs straddled and straight.
2. Exhale, and slowly lower your chest and belly onto the floor while keeping your back flat.
3. Hold the stretch and relax. *NOTE:* Ideally, your legs should form a straight line when executing a straddle or Japanese split. For those with greater flexibility, roll the hips forward and backward.

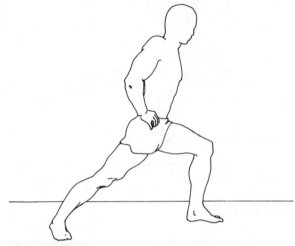

EXERCISE #82

1. Stand upright with the legs straddled about two feet apart.
2. Turn the left foot 90° sideways to the left, keeping the toes and heel in line with the body.
3. Place your hands on your hips.
4. Exhale, slowly lunge forward, and press down on your right hip.
5. Hold the stretch and relax.

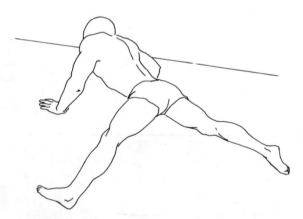

EXERCISE #81

1. Kneel on all fours with your toes facing backward.
2. Extend one leg out sideways.
3. Exhale, bend your arms, lower the hip of the opposite side to the floor, and roll the hip.
4. Hold the stretch and relax. *NOTE:* A similar, yet more intense stretch is to roll your hips in a regular split.

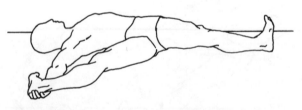

EXERCISE #83

1. Lie flat on your back with your body straight.
2. Flex one leg, grasp the foot, and extend the leg vertically.
3. Exhale, and slowly lower your leg to the floor at your side forming the letter "Y".
4. Hold the stretch and relax.

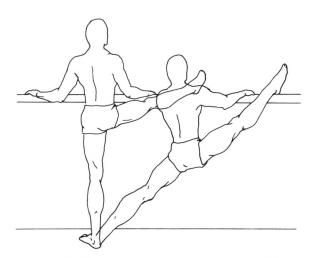

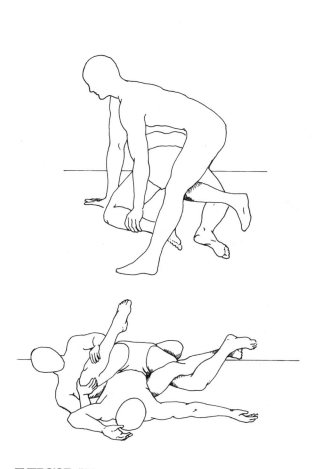

EXERCISE #85

1. Stand upright facing a barre.
2. Raise one leg to the supporting surface and place your heel or instep on top.
3. Exhale, and slowly slide your foot along the surface.
4. Hold the stretch and relax.

EXERCISE #84

1. Kneel on all fours with your toes facing backward.
2. Your partner is positioned on your right side.
3. Your partner slides his or her right leg between your legs through the groin and hooks your right ankle or leg (Grapevine).
4. Your partner reaches across your lower back and grasps your left ankle with his or her hand.
5. Your partner will pull up your left knee from the floor and roll to his or her right with you following. When the roll is completed, your partner will be on his or her back with your back on his or her stomach and your legs straddled. If necessary, your partner can hook his or her left foot over your right foot.
6. Exhale, as you allow your partner to gently pull your legs apart with interlocked hands.
7. Hold the stretch and relax. *CAUTION:* Extreme caution must be used with this *super stretch.* When executing the "banana split" make sure your left knee is completely flexed to avoid excessive stress on the medial part of the knee.

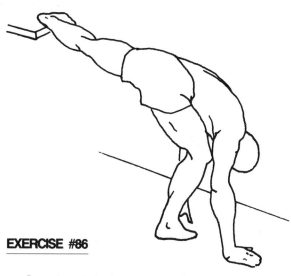

EXERCISE #86

1. Stand upright facing a barre.
2. Keeping both legs straight and your hips squared, raise one leg, and place your heel on the supporting surface.
3. Turnout the foot of the supporting leg.
4. Roll your hips and turn the raised leg medially.
5. Exhale, keeping the raised leg straight, flex the supporting leg, and lower your chest to your knee.
6. Hold the stretch and relax.

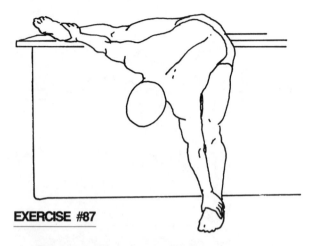

EXERCISE #87

1. Stand upright facing a barre.
2. Keeping both legs straight and your hips squared, raise one leg, and place your heel on the supporting surface.
3. Turnout the foot of the supporting leg.
4. Roll your hips and turn the raised leg medially.
5. Grasp the raised foot with one hand.
6. Exhale, bend forward at the waist, and grasp the foot of the supporting leg.
7. Exhale, keep both legs straight, and lower your upper torso as if performing a straddle split.
8. Hold the stretch and relax. *NOTE:* Concentrate on keeping your back flat.

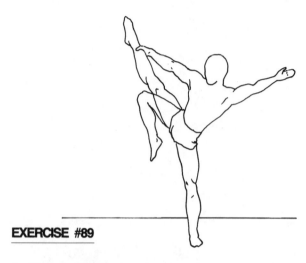

EXERCISE #89

1. Stand upright.
2. Draw the toe of one foot to the opposite ankle, and slide it up the inside of your leg to your knee.
3. Grasp the foot with your hand.
4. Inhale, slowly raise, and straighten your leg sideways.
5. Hold the stretch and relax. *NOTE:* Dancers are capable of performing this skill without the use of their arms for support. For most, muscular insufficiency in the hip flexors will be the limiting factor.

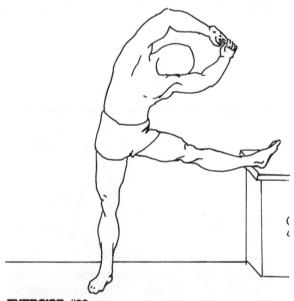

EXERCISE #88

1. Assume the stretch position in exercise #85.
2. Raise your arms overhead and interlock your hands.
3. Exhale, bend sideways, and lower your upper torso toward your raised thigh.
4. Hold the stretch and relax. *NOTE:* Keep your legs straight.

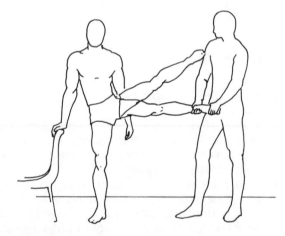

EXERCISE #90

1. Stand upright.
2. Keeping both legs straight, raise one leg sideways.
3. Your partner is positioned to your side, holding your heel with one hand and above your ankle with the other hand.
4. Exhale, as you allow your partner to gently raise your leg.
5. Hold the stretch and relax. *NOTE:* Concentrate on preventing the buttocks from protruding. Also, some may find it easier to hold onto a surface for additional support and balance.

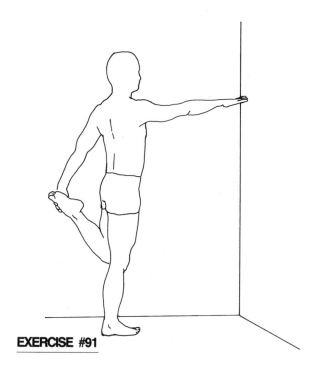

EXERCISE #91

1. Stand upright with one hand against a surface for balance and support.
2. Flex one leg and raise your foot to your buttocks.
3. Slightly flex the supporting leg.
4. Exhale, reach down, grasp your foot with one hand, and pull your heel toward your buttocks.
5. Hold the stretch and relax. *NOTE:* This should be avoided by those with "bad knees."

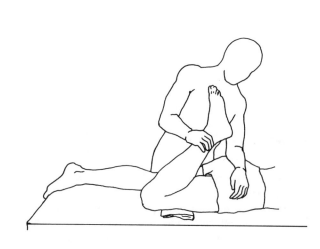

EXERCISE #93

1. Assume the stretch position in exercise #92.
2. Your partner is positioned at your side with one hand anchoring your hips and the other grasping your ankle.
3. Exhale, as you allow your partner to push your heel toward your buttocks.
4. Hold the stretch and relax. *NOTE:* This should be avoided by those with "bad knees." Furthermore, if uncomfortable, place a blanket underneath your thigh.

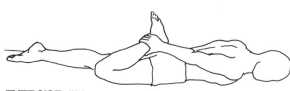

EXERCISE #92

1. Lie face down with your body extended.
2. Flex one leg and bring your heel toward your buttocks.
3. Exhale, swing your arm back to grasp your ankle, and pull your heel toward your buttocks.
4. Hold the stretch and relax. *NOTE:* This should be avoided by those with "bad knees."

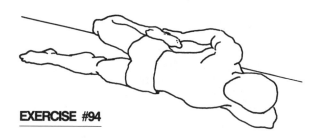

EXERCISE #94

1. Lie on your side with your hips slightly flexed.
2. Flex one leg and bring your heel toward your buttocks.
3. Exhale, swing your arm back to grasp your ankle, and pull your heel toward your buttocks.
4. Hold the stretch and relax. *NOTE:* This should be avoided by those with "bad knees."

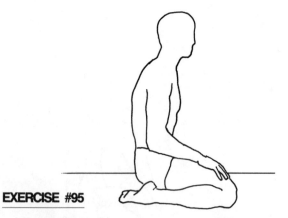

EXERCISE #95

1. Kneel on all fours with your toes facing backward.
2. Exhale, and slowly sit on your heels.
3. Hold the stretch and relax. *CAUTION:* This should be avoided by those with "bad knees." *NOTE:* If uncomfortable, place a blanket underneath your thighs.

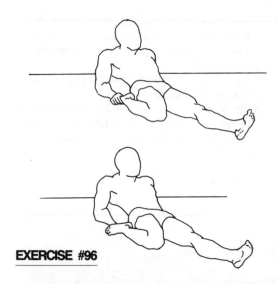

EXERCISE #96

1. Sit upright on the floor with both legs extended.
2. Bend your right leg behind so that the inside of your right knee and thigh is on the floor; and the foot of your rear leg points along the line of the lower leg in a relaxed position.
3. Exhale, slowly lean diagonally back onto your forearm and elbow opposite your rear leg without arching your lower back.
4. Exhale, and continue leaning backward until you are flat on your back.
5. Hold the stretch and relax. *CAUTION:* Do *not* let the foot of the rear leg flare out to the side (B). This will protect the knee. To guard against excessive stress on the lumbar spine, one should keep the forward leg in a slightly flexed position. *NOTE:* To intensify the stretch, one should contract the gluteals and lift the hip off the floor.

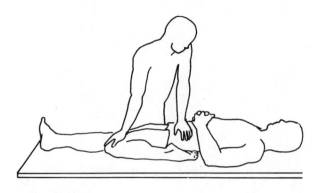

EXERCISE #97

1. Assume the stretch position in exercise #96.
2. Your partner is positioned either kneeling or standing to your side with one hand anchoring your hip.
3. Exhale, as you allow your partner to gently push your leg to the floor.
4. Hold the stretch and relax.

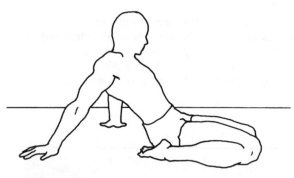

EXERCISE #98

1. Kneel upright, knees together, buttocks on the floor; heels by the side of your thighs; and toes pointing backwards.
2. Exhale and slowly lean backwards.
3. Hold the stretch and relax. *CAUTION:* Do *not* allow the feet to flare out to the side.

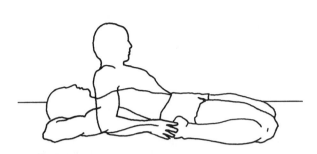

EXERCISE #99

1. Assume the stretch position in exercise #98.
2. Exhale, and continue leaning backward until you are flat on your back.
3. Hold the stretch and relax. *CAUTION:* Do *not* allow the feet to flare out to the side.

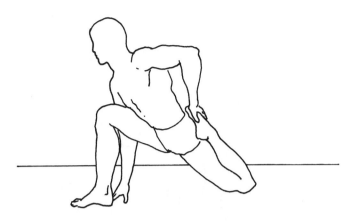

EXERCISE #101

1. Assume the stretch position in exercise #100.
2. Flex your rear leg up to your buttocks.
3. Reach back and grasp your rear foot.
4. Exhale, and slowly pull your heel toward your buttocks.
5. Hold the stretch and relax. *CAUTION:* This should be avoided by those with "bad knees."

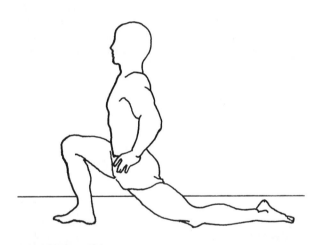

EXERCISE #100

1. Stand upright with the legs straddled two feet apart.
2. Turn your right foot 90° sideways to the right, keeping your toes and heel in line with your body.
3. Flex your right knee and roll your left foot under so the top of the instep rests on the floor.
4. Place your hands on your hips. (Some may prefer placing one hand on the forward knee and one hand on the buttocks.)
5. Exhale, and slowly force your left hip to the floor.
6. Hold the stretch and relax.

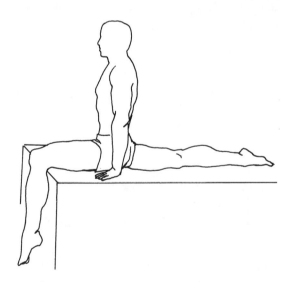

EXERCISE #102

1. Sit upright on an elevated platform (pile of mats or a bed) about three feet above the floor.
2. Position your left leg so it drops over the edge of the platform at the knee and swing your right leg back so as to assume a split position with your leg (thigh, knee, shinbone, and ankle) resting on the platform.
3. Exhale, slowly arch your back, push down on the platform with both hands; and keep your hips squared and turned under.
4. Hold the stretch and relax.

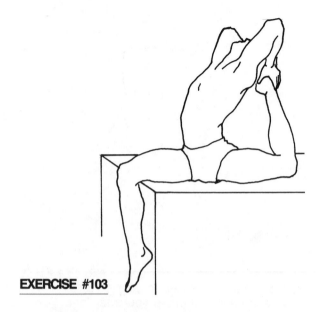

EXERCISE #103

1. Assume the stretch position in exercise #102.
2. Flex your rear leg up to your buttocks.
3. Reach back and grasp your foot.
4. Exhale, and slowly pull your heel toward your buttocks.
5. Hold the stretch and relax. *CAUTION:* This should be avoided by those with ''bad knees.''

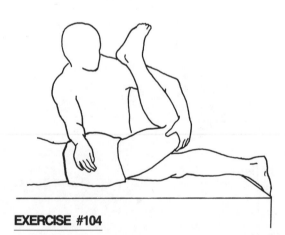

EXERCISE #104

1. Lie face down with your body extended.
2. Your partner is positioned at your side; standing or resting on one knee; with one hand under your knee and the other slightly above the buttocks.
3. Exhale, as you allow your partner to anchor down your belly to the table or floor with one hand, and gently lift your leg higher with the opposite hand.
4. Hold the stretch and relax. *CAUTION:* Contract the gluteals to protect the lower back.

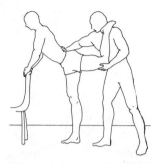

EXERCISE #105

1. Stand upright; slight turnout on the foot to balance on; and holding onto a surface for balance and support.
2. Exhale, bend at your waist, flex one knee, and raise your leg.
3. Your partner is positioned behind you with one hand under your knee and the other hand slightly above your buttocks.
4. Exhale, as you allow your partner to anchor down your body with one hand, and lift your raised leg with the opposite hand.
5. Hold the stretch and relax. *CAUTION:* Hyper-extension of the back when performing an Arabesque can be a potential source of pain and injury. Here, the answer is to spread the extension through all the joints of the spine, instead of forcing it all at the bottom of the spine.

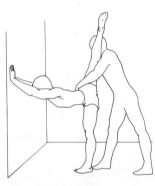

EXERCISE #106

1. Assume the stretched position in exercise #105, but keep your raised leg straight.
2. Your partner is positioned behind you and places his or her shoulder underneath your raised thigh so it can rest on it.
3. Your partner reaches over your raised leg, inter-locks his or her fingers, and places his or her hands on your upper buttocks.
4. Exhale, as you allow your partner to anchor down your body with one hand, and raise your extended thigh up and forward with his or her shoulder.
5. Hold the stretch and relax. *CAUTION:* Hyper-extension of the back when performing an Arabesque can be a potential source of pain and injury. Here, the answer is to spread the extension through all the joints of the spine, instead of forcing it all at the bottom of the spine.

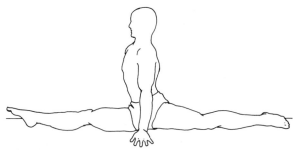

EXERCISE #107

1. Squat on the floor with your hands at your sides for balance and support.
2. Bend your left knee and place your left ankle, shinbone, and knee on the floor.
3. Exhale, slowly slide your right leg forward, and the left leg further back until you are in a split position.
4. Hold the stretch and relax. *NOTE:* As stated earlier, a proper split requires that the legs be kept straight, the hips squared, and the buttocks flat on the floor.

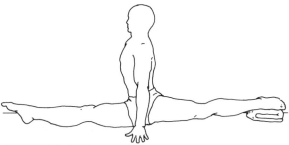

EXERCISE #109

1. Assume the stretch position in exercise #107 with your rear leg elevated on a folded mat.
2. Hold the stretch and relax.

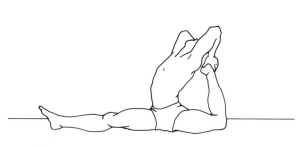

EXERCISE #108

1. Assume the stretch position in exercise #107.
2. Flex your rear leg up to your buttocks.
3. Reach back and grasp your foot.
4. Exhale, and slowly pull your heel toward your buttocks.
5. Hold the stretch and relax. *CAUTION:* This should be avoided by those with "bad knees."

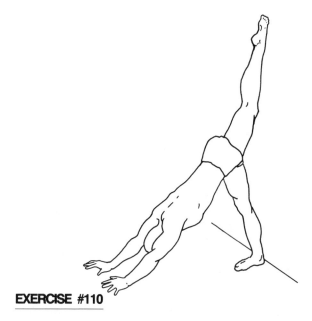

EXERCISE #110

1. Assume the stretch position in exercise #62.
2. Hold the stretch and relax. *NOTE:* This also requires flexibility in the hamstrings.

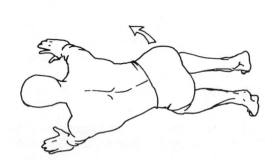

EXERCISE #111

1. Kneel on all fours.
2. Exhale, flex one arm, and slowly rotate your hip out to the same side.
3. Hold the stretch and relax.

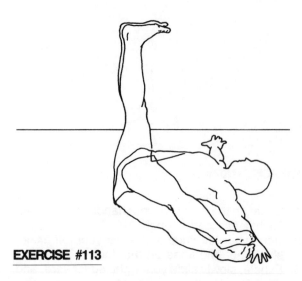

EXERCISE #113

1. Lie flat on your back; your legs raised and straight; and your arms out to the side.
2. Exhale, and slowly lower both legs to the floor on the same side.
3. Hold the stretch and relax. *NOTE:* Keep your elbows, head, and shoulders flat on the floor.

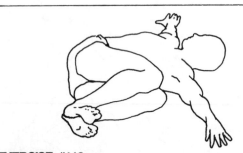

EXERCISE #112

1. Lie flat on your back with your knees flexed and arms out to your sides.
2. Exhale, and slowly lower both legs to the floor on the same side.
3. Hold the stretch and relax. *NOTE:* Keep your elbows, head, and shoulders flat on the floor.

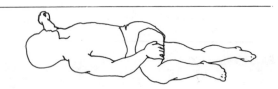

EXERCISE #114

1. Lie flat on your back with your legs extended.
2. Flex one knee and raise it to your chest.
3. Grasp your knee or thigh with one hand.
4. Exhale, and pull your knee across your body to the floor.
5. Hold the stretch and relax. *NOTE:* Keep your elbows, head, and shoulders flat on the floor.

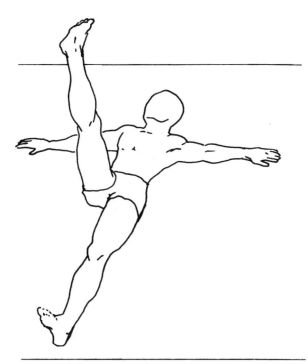

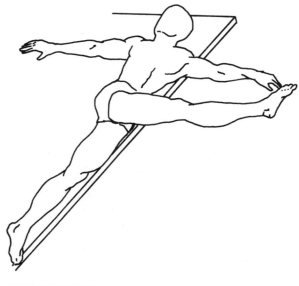

EXERCISE #116

1. Assume the stretch position in exercise #115 while lying on the edge of a table.
2. Exhale, and pull on your hanging leg with the opposite hand.
3. Hold the stretch and relax. *NOTE:* Keep your head and shoulders flat on the table.

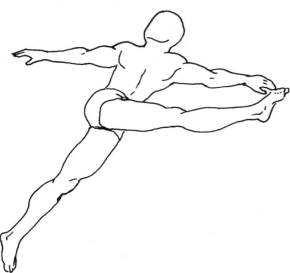

EXERCISE #115

1. Lie flat on your back; one leg raised and straight; and your arms out to your sides.
2. Exhale, and slowly lower your raised leg to the opposite hand.
3. Hold the stretch and relax. *NOTE:* Keep your elbows, head, and shoulders flat on the floor.

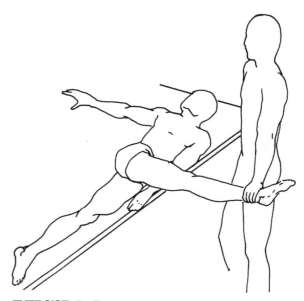

EXERCISE #117

1. Assume the stretch position in exercise #116.
2. Your partner is positioned to your side with one hand grasping your hanging leg.
3. Exhale, as you allow your partner to gently push down your hanging leg. *NOTE:* Keep your head and shoulders flat on the table.

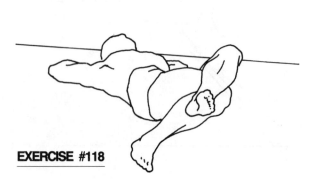

EXERCISE #118

1. Lie flat on your back, knees flexed, and your hands interlocked underneath your head.
2. Lift your left leg over your right leg and hook your leg.
3. Exhale, and use your left leg to force your right leg to the floor.
4. Hold the stretch and relax. *NOTE:* Keep your elbows, head, and shoulders flat on the floor.

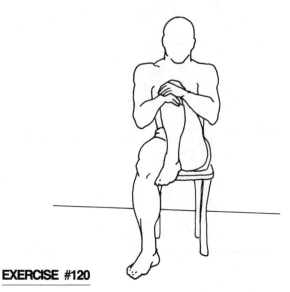

EXERCISE #120

1. Sit upright on a chair with one leg flexed and your heel resting on the edge.
2. Interlock both hands and grasp your raised knee.
3. Exhale, and slowly pull your knee across your body as your heel remains flat on the chair.
4. Hold the stretch and relax.

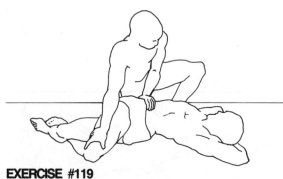

EXERCISE #119

1. Assume the stretch position in exercise #118.
2. Your partner is positioned to your side with one hand on your hip to anchor down your body and the other hand on your flexed knee.
3. Exhale, as you allow your partner to push your leg to the floor.
4. Hold the stretch and relax. *NOTE:* Keep your elbows, head, and shoulders flat on the floor.

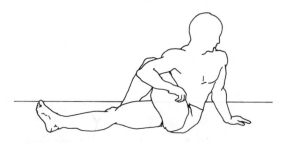

EXERCISE #121

1. Sit upright on the floor, hands behind your hips for support, and your legs extended.
2. Flex your left leg, cross your left foot over your right leg, and slide your heel toward your buttocks.
3. Reach over your left leg with your right arm and place your right elbow on the outside of your left knee.
4. Exhale, look over your left shoulder while twisting your trunk and *pushing back* on your left knee with your right elbow.
5. Hold the stretch and relax.

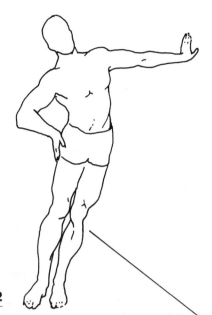

EXERCISE #122

1. Stand upright, feet together, your side facing a wall about an arm's length away.
2. Place one hand on the wall and the heel of your other hand on the back of your hip joint.
3. Exhale, keeping your legs straight, contract your buttocks, rotate your hips slightly forward and in toward the wall.
4. Exhale, and push your hip toward the wall.
5. Hold the stretch and relax.

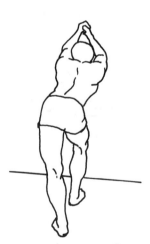

EXERCISE #123

1. Stand upright 4-5 steps from a wall.
2. Bend one leg forward and keep the opposite leg straight.
3. Lean against the wall without losing the straight line of head, neck, spine, pelvis, rear leg, and ankle.
4. Keep your rear heel *down, flat,* and *parallel* to the hips.
5. Exhale, and slowly rotate the hip of the rear leg out sideways.
6. Hold the stretch and relax.

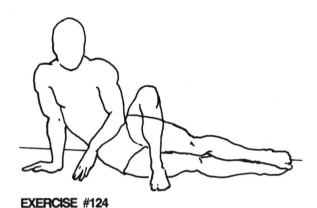

EXERCISE #124

1. Lie on your side with both knees and hips extended and in a straight line with your trunk.
2. Exhale, push-up to a resting position on your hip, placing your arm directly under your shoulder, and bearing weight on your extended arm and hand.
3. Hold the stretch and relax. *NOTE:* It may be necessary to place the opposite foot on the floor to stabilize the pelvis.

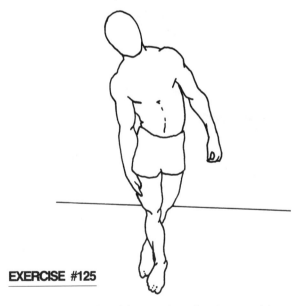

EXERCISE #125

1. Stand upright with your hands at your sides.
2. Extend and adduct your left leg as far as possible.
3. Exhale, and slowly flex your trunk laterally toward your right side with your hands remaining by your hips.
4. Hold the stretch and relax.

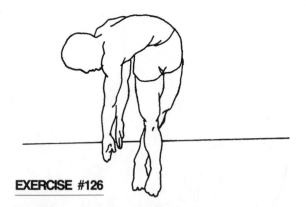

EXERCISE #126

1. Assume the stretch position in exercise #125.
2. Exhale, and slowly flex your trunk laterally toward your right side, and try to touch the heel of your left leg with both hands.
3. Hold the stretch and relax.

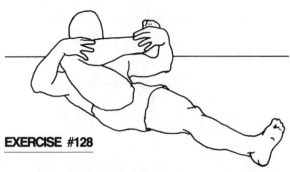

EXERCISE #128

1. Lie on the floor with your body extended.
2. Flex one leg and slide your heel toward your buttocks.
3. Grasp your ankle with one hand and your knee with the opposite hand.
4. Exhale, and slowly pull your foot to the opposite shoulder.
5. Hold the stretch and relax. *NOTE:* Keep your head, shoulders, and back flat on the floor.

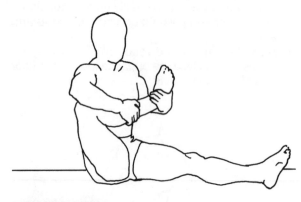

EXERCISE #127

1. Sit upright on the floor with your back flat against a wall.
2. Flex one leg and slide your heel toward your buttocks.
3. Grasp your ankle with one hand and hook your knee with the elbow of the opposite arm.
4. Exhale, and slowly pull your foot to the opposite shoulder.
5. Hold the stretch and relax.

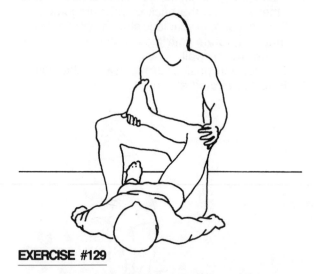

EXERCISE #129

1. Lie flat on your back with your body extended.
2. Raise one leg so your thigh is nearly vertical and your knee is flexed.
3. Exhale, and slowly move your foot in toward your body.
4. Your partner is positioned in front of you and to your side; while resting on one knee, with your opposite foot on the floor; and holding your knee and ankle of the side to be stretched.
5. Exhale, as you allow your partner to slowly move your foot toward your body.
6. Hold the stretch and relax.

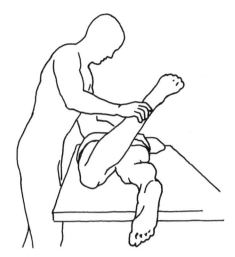

EXERCISE #130

1. Lie face down on a table with your body extended.
2. Flex your leg nearest the table edge.
3. Your partner is positioned to your side with one hand anchoring your body and the other hand grasping your ankle.
4. Exhale, as you allow your partner to push your leg toward the opposite side.
5. Hold the stretch and relax.

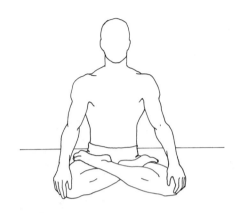

EXERCISE #132

1. Sit upright on the floor with both legs straight.
2. Flex your right knee and place your right foot as high as possible on your left thigh with the sole of your foot turned up.
3. Exhale, flex your left knee, and place it as high as possible on your right thigh with the sole facing up.
4. Hold the stretch and relax. *CAUTION:* Do *not* force this stretch.

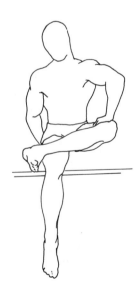

EXERCISE #131

1. Sit upright in a chair or on the floor with one leg crossed over your opposite knee.
2. Place your hand on the medial part of your knee.
3. Exhale and push down on your knee.
4. Hold the stretch and relax. *NOTE:* It may be desired to anchor the leg with the opposite hand.

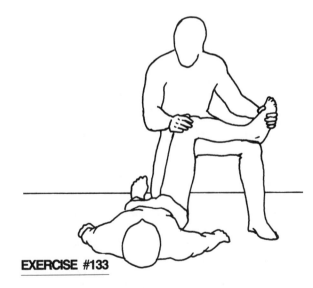

EXERCISE #133

1. Assume the stretch position in exercise #129.
2. Exhale, as you allow your partner to slowly move your foot away from your body.
3. Hold the stretch and relax.

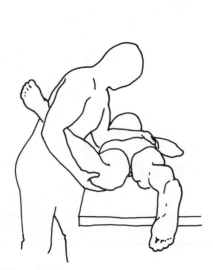

EXERCISE #134

1. Assume the stretch position in exercise #130.
2. Exhale, as you allow your partner to pull your leg away from your body.
3. Hold the stretch and relax.

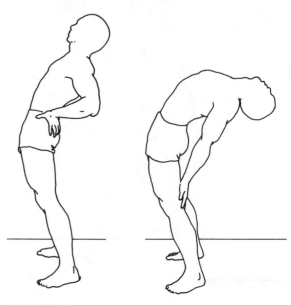

EXERCISE #136

1. Stand upright, legs straddled 2-3 feet, and your hands placed on your hips.
2. Exhale, slowly arch your back, contract your buttocks, and push your hips forward.
3. Exhale, continue arching back, drop your head backward, open your mouth, and gradually slide your hands below your buttocks.
4. Hold the stretch and relax.

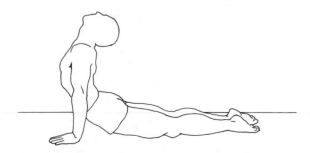

EXERCISE #135

1. Lie face down on the floor with your body extended.
2. Place your palms on the floor by your hips with your fingers pointing forward.
3. Exhale, press down on the floor, raise your head and trunk, contract your buttocks, and arch your back.
4. Hold the stretch and relax. *NOTE:* Concentrate on contracting the gluteals to prevent excessive compression on the lower back.

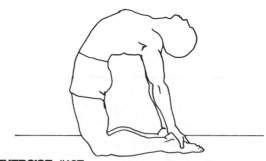

EXERCISE #137

1. Kneel upright on the floor; legs slightly apart and parallel; and your toes pointing backward.
2. Place your palms on your upper hips and buttocks.
3. Exhale, slowly arch your back, contract your buttocks, and push your hips forward.
4. Exhale, continue arching your back, drop your head backward, open your mouth, and gradually slide your hands onto your heels.
5. Hold the stretch and relax.

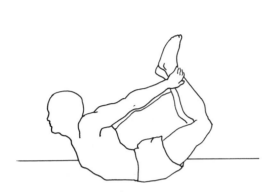

EXERCISE #138

1. Lie face down on the floor with your body extended.
2. Flex your knees and move your heels toward your hips.
3. Exhale, reach back, and grasp both feet.
4. Exhale, contract the buttocks, and lift your chest and knees off the floor.
5. Hold the stretch and relax. *NOTE:* To intensify the stretch, pull the ankles and knees to each other.

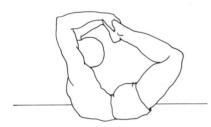

EXERCISE #139

1. Assume the stretch position in exercise #138.
2. Exhale, and pull your feet to your head.
3. Hold the stretch and relax.

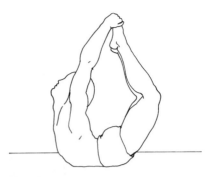

EXERCISE #140

1. Assume the stretch position in exercise #138.
2. Exhale, and pull your legs to a vertical position.
3. Hold the stretch and relax. *NOTE:* This requires extreme suppleness.

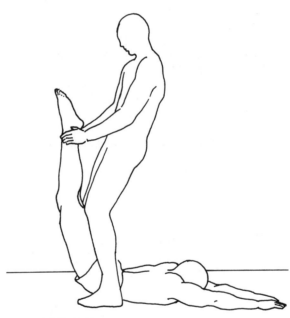

EXERCISE #141

1. Lie face down on the floor; body extended; and your arms parallel and stretched forward.
2. Your partner is positioned straddling your hips and facing your feet.
3. Your partner bends at the hips and knees; reaches under; and grasps both your legs about the lower legs or thighs.
4. Exhale, and contract the gluteals as you allow your partner to slowly lift your thighs off the floor.
5. Hold the stretch and relax. *CAUTION:* Use extreme caution with this super stretch. *NOTE:* Concentrate on contracting the gluteals to prevent compression of the lower back.

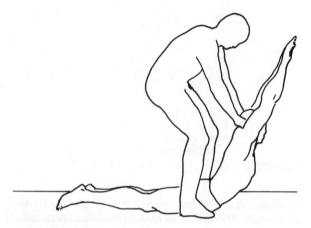

EXERCISE #142

1. Lie face down on the floor; body extended; and your arms parallel and stretched forward.
2. Your partner is positioned straddling your hips and facing your head.
3. Your partner bends at the hips and knees; reaches under and grasps the front part of your chest and shoulders.
4. Exhale, and contract the gluteals as you allow your partner to slowly lift your upper torso off the floor.
5. Hold the stretch and relax. *CAUTION:* Use extreme caution with this super stretch.

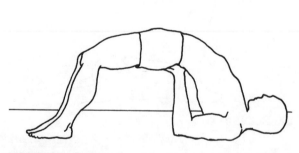

EXERCISE #143

1. Lie flat on your back with your body extended.
2. Flex your knees and slide your heels toward your buttocks, keeping them hip-distance apart.
3. Exhale, grasp your ankles, contract your gluteals, and lift your pelvis off the floor.
4. Hold the stretch and relax. *NOTE:* Concentrate on keeping your feet flat on the floor and contracting your shoulder blades to lift your chest.

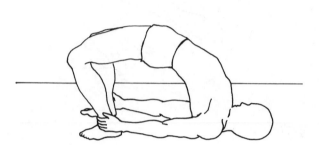

EXERCISE #144

1. Assume the stretch position in exercise #143.
2. Exhale, and grasp your feet.
3. Hold the stretch and relax. *NOTE:* Concentrate on keeping your feet flat on the floor and contracting your shoulder blades to lift your chest.

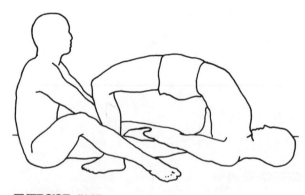

EXERCISE #145

1. Assume the stretch position in exercise #144.
2. Your partner is positioned sitting on the floor; one leg between your straddled legs resting against the middle of your upper back; and grasping both wrists.
3. Exhale, as you allow your partner to pull on your arms and push evenly into both sides of your lower back.
4. Hold the stretch and relax. *NOTE:* Concentrate on keeping your feet and shoulders flat on the floor.

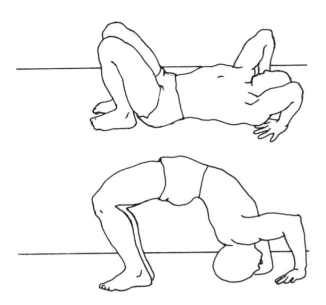

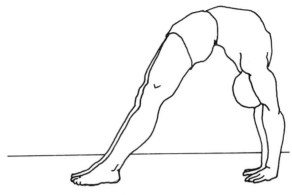

EXERCISE #148

1. Assume the starting position in exercise #146.
2. Exhale, extend your arms and legs, and raise your body into a full bridge.
3. Hold the stretch and relax. *NOTE:* Ideally, your wrists should be parallel to your shoulders.

EXERCISE #146

1. Lie flat on your back; your heels close to your hips; your hands placed on the floor by your neck (under the shoulders); and your fingers pointing toward your feet.
2. Exhale, raise your trunk, and rest your forehead on the floor.
3. Hold the stretch and relax.

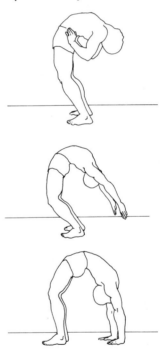

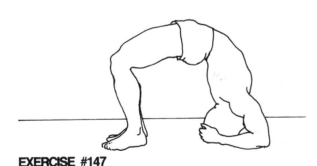

EXERCISE #147

1. Assume the stretch position in exercise #146.
2. Exhale, raise one arm at a time, and place your forearms on the floor.
3. Hold the stretch and relax.

EXERCISE #149

1. Stand upright; feet shoulder width apart; and your palms on your hips.
2. Exhale, push your hips forward, and arch your back.
3. Raise your arms overhead while continuing to arch backward and place your hands on the floor, ending up in a bridge position.
4. Hold the stretch and relax.
5. Flex your arms and lower down onto your shoulders. *CAUTION:* Use a spotter when learning this skill. Remember that your hands must contact the floor with your arms straight and no more than shoulder width. Otherwise, you might land on your head!

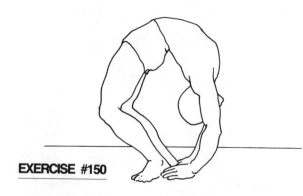

EXERCISE #150

1. Assume the stretch position in exercise #148.
2. Exhale, and slowly close the distance between your hands and your feet until they are touching.
3. Hold the stretch and relax.
4. Separate your hands and feet, flex your arms, and lower down onto your shoulders. *NOTE:* This requires *extreme* flexibility.

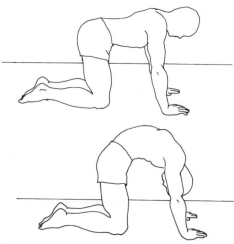

EXERCISE #151

1. Kneel on all fours with your toes facing backward.
2. Inhale, contract your abdominals, and round your back.
3. Exhale, relax your abdominals, and return to the "flat back" position.

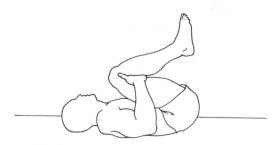

EXERCISE #152

1. Lie flat on your back with your body extended.
2. Flex your knees and slide your feet toward your buttocks.
3. Grasp behind your thighs.
4. Exhale, pull your knees toward your chest/shoulders and elevate your hips from the floor.
5. Hold the stretch and relax. *CAUTION:* Grasping the upper knees may result in their potential hyperextension. Secondly, the legs should be reextended slowly one at a time to prevent possible pain or spasm.

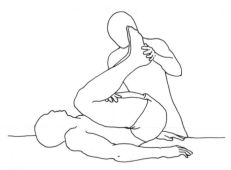

EXERCISE #153

1. Lie flat on your back with your body extended.
2. Flex your knees and slide your feet toward your buttocks.
3. Your partner is positioned to your side with one hand under your hamstrings and the other grasping your heels.
4. Exhale, as you allow your partner to bring your hips to your chest.
5. Hold the stretch and relax.

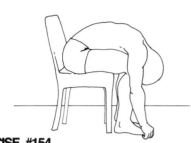

EXERCISE #154

1. Sit upright in a chair.
2. Exhale, extend your upper torso, bend at the waist, and slowly lower your stomach onto your thighs.
3. Hold the stretch and relax.

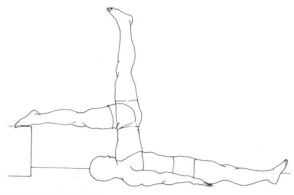

EXERCISE #156

1. Lie flat on your back with your arms by your hips, palms down.
2. Inhale, push down on the floor with your palms, and raise your legs to a vertical position.
3. Exhale, keep your legs straight, and lower your feet onto a chair.
4. Hold the stretch and relax. *CAUTION:* See text on page 138 regarding the plough.

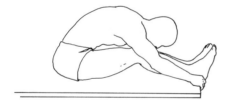

EXERCISE #155

1. Sit upright on a bed or bench with your knees flexed.
2. Exhale, extend your upper torso, bend at the waist, and slowly lower your stomach onto your thighs.
3. Exhale, and slowly extend your legs.
4. Hold the stretch and relax. *NOTE:* After a certain "critical point" the stretch will appear to shift to the hamstrings.

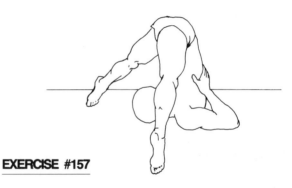

EXERCISE #157

1. Assume the shoulder stand position in exercise #156.
2. Exhale, keep your legs straight and straddled, and lower your feet to the floor.
3. Hold the stretch and relax. *CAUTION:* See text on page 138 regarding the plough.

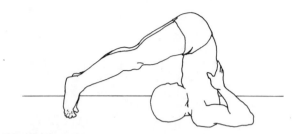

EXERCISE #158

1. Assume the shoulder stand position in exercise #156.
2. Exhale, keep your legs straight and together, and lower your feet to the floor.
3. Hold the stretch and relax. *CAUTION:* See text on page 138 regarding the plough.

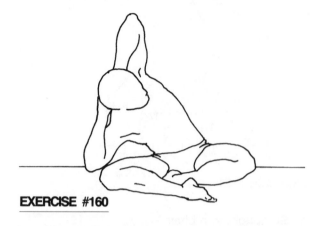

EXERCISE #160

1. Sit upright on the floor with your legs crossed.
2. Interlock your hands behind your head with your elbows lifted.
3. Exhale, bring your right elbow to your right knee, and keep your left shoulder and elbow back.
4. Hold the stretch and relax.

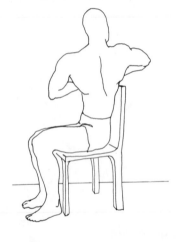

EXERCISE #159

1. Sit upright in a chair.
2. Exhale, turn to your right, and place your hands on the back of a chair.
3. Exhale, keep your feet flat on the floor, push your right hip forward, and press your right elbow into your body.
4. Hold the stretch and relax. *NOTE:* Keep the buttocks flat on the seat.

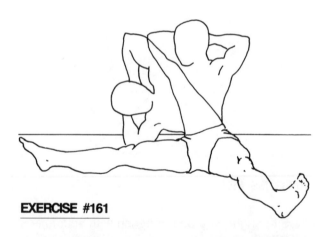

EXERCISE #161

1. Sit upright on the floor with your legs straight and straddled.
2. Interlock your hands behind your head with your elbows lifted.
3. Exhale, bend your torso to the side, attempting to touch your right elbow to the floor outside your right thigh.
4. Hold the stretch and relax.

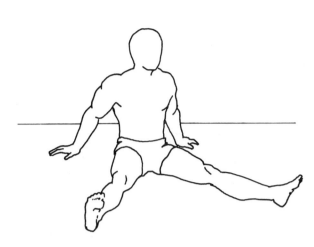

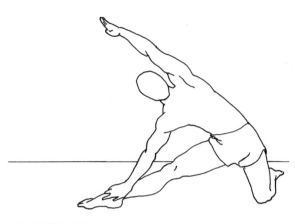

EXERCISE #163

1. Kneel upright on the floor.
2. Extend your right leg out to the side, keeping it in line with your left knee and raise your arms sideways.
3. Exhale, bend from the hips to the right, lower your right hand onto your right foot, and extend your left arm over your left ear.
4. Hold the stretch and relax.

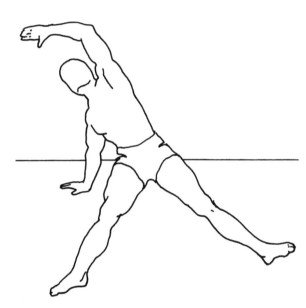

EXERCISE #162

1. Sit upright on the floor with your legs straight and straddled.
2. Lean backward and place your hands behind your hips and on the floor for support.
3. Exhale, support yourself on your heel(s), and swing your left arm up, overhead, and to the right; and, lift your hips off the floor.
4. Hold the stretch and relax. *NOTE:* This is commonly performed in a rhythmic manner.

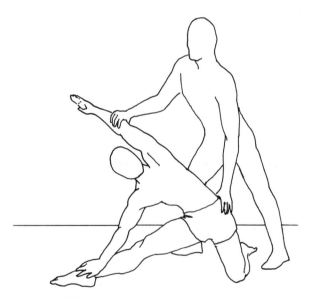

EXERCISE #164

1. Assume the stretch position in exercise #163.
2. Your partner is positioned behind you with one hand anchoring your wrist and the other hand grasping your extended wrist.
3. Exhale, as you allow your partner to stretch your side.
4. Hold the stretch and relax.

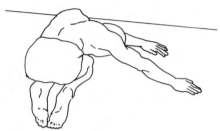

EXERCISE #165

1. Kneel on all fours.
2. Straighten your arms, reach forward as far as possible, and lower your chest to the floor.
3. Exhale, slightly twist your upper torso, and press down with your palms and forearms on the floor.
4. Hold the stretch and relax.

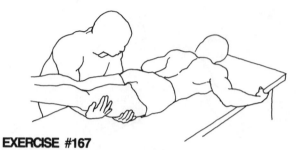

EXERCISE #167

1. Lie face down on a table and hold the sides for stabilization.
2. Your partner is positioned to your side and grasps underneath your thighs.
3. Exhale, as you allow your partner to lift and pull your lower torso laterally away (toward him- or herself).
4. Hold the stretch and relax. *NOTE:* No shoulder movement should occur.

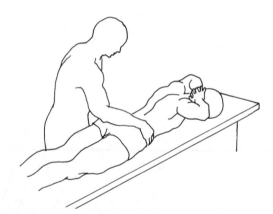

EXERCISE #166

1. Lie face down on a table with your hands interlocked behind your head.
2. Your partner is positioned to your side with his or her hands anchoring your pelvis.
3. Exhale, as you attempt to twist your upper torso sideways.
4. Hold the stretch and relax.

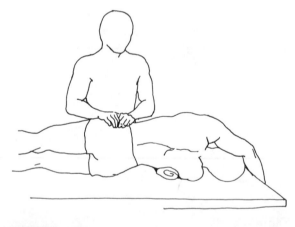

EXERCISE #168

1. Lie sideways on a table with your top arm stretched overhead.
2. Your partner is positioned to your side and achors down your hip.
3. Hold the stretch and relax. *NOTE:* Use a folded towel to reduce discomfort on your side.

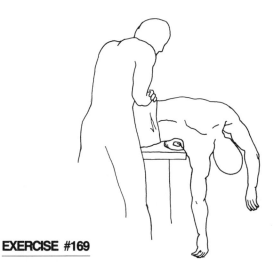

EXERCISE #169

1. Lie over the edge of a table with both arms hanging downward.
2. Your partner is positioned to your side and anchors down your hips.
3. Hold the stretch and relax. *NOTE:* Use a folded towel to reduce discomfort on your side.

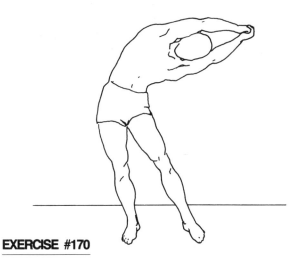

EXERCISE #170

1. Stand upright, feet slightly apart, hands interlocking and overhead.
2. Exhale, drop one ear toward your shoulder, and slowly lower your arms sideways.
3. Hold the stretch and relax. *NOTE:* Contract the buttocks.

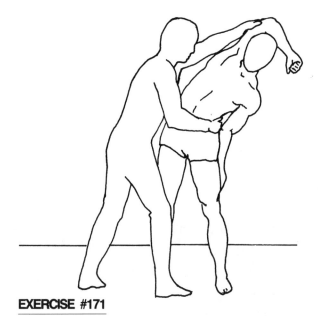

EXERCISE #171

1. Stand upright, feet slightly apart, one arm by your side, and your other arm flexed overhead.
2. Your partner is positioned to your side with one hand on your hip, and your other holding your raised arm on or below your elbow.
3. Exhale, and bend your trunk to one side.
4. Exhale, as you allow your partner to gently push your trunk further to one side.
5. Hold the stretch and relax. *NOTE:* There should be no forward or backward flexing.

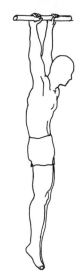

EXERCISE #172

1. Hang from a bar with your arms straight and your body hollow.
2. Exhale, place your chin on your chest and sink in your shoulders.
3. Hold the stretch and relax. *NOTE:* To increase the stretch, one can hang with either one or both hands in an elgrip (the back of the hand faces up and the thumbs grasp under the bar).

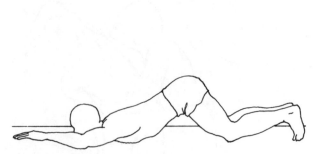

EXERCISE #173

1. Kneel on all fours.
2. Extend your arms forward and lower your chest toward the floor.
3. Exhale, extend your shoulders and press down on the floor with your arms to produce an arch in your back.
4. Hold the stretch and relax.

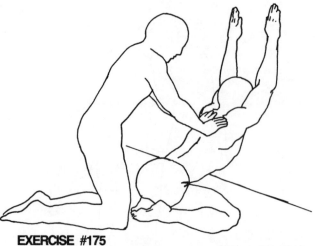

EXERCISE #175

1. Sit upright, knees straddled, facing a wall about an arm's length away.
2. Raise your arms with your elbows straight, lean forward, place arms and hands against the wall shoulder width apart, and your fingers pointing upward.
3. Exhale, extend your shoulders, press down against the wall, open your chest, and produce an arch in your back.
4. Your partner is positioned directly behind with his or her hands placed about the upper portion of your shoulder blades.
5. Exhale, as you allow your partner to gently push downward and away from your head.
6. Hold the stretch and relax.

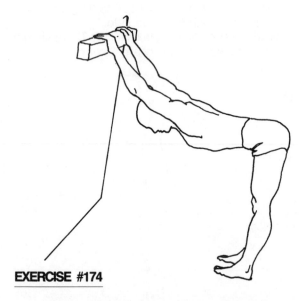

EXERCISE #174

1. Stand upright, feet together, about three feet from a supporting surface approximately waist to shoulder height, and your arms overhead.
2. Exhale, keeping your arms and legs straight, flex at the waist, flatten your back, and grasp the supporting surface with both hands.
3. Exhale, extend your shoulders, and press down on the supporting surface to produce an arch in your back.
4. Hold the stretch and relax.

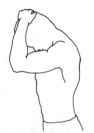

EXERCISE #176

1. Stand or sit upright.
2. Interlock your hands on the back of your head near the crown.
3. Exhale, and pull down on your head, and allow your chin to rest on your chest.
4. Hold the stretch and relax.

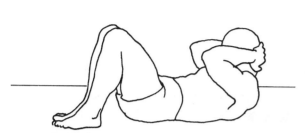

EXERCISE #177

1. Lie flat on the floor with both knees flexed.
2. Interlock your hands on the back of your head near the crown.
3. Exhale, and pull your head off the floor and onto your chest.
4. Hold the stretch and relax.

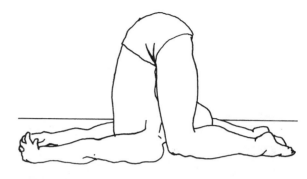

EXERCISE #179

1. Assume the stretch position in exercise #158.
2. Exhale, bring your chin onto your chest, and place your shins flat on the floor with your knees touching your shoulders.
3. Exhale, lower your arms to the floor, and interlock your hands.
4. Hold the stretch and relax. *CAUTION:* See text on page 138 regarding the plough.

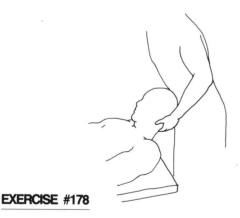

EXERCISE #178

1. Lie flat on the floor or on a table with your head hanging over the edge.
2. Your partner is positioned behind your head with both hands holding your head.
3. Exhale, as you allow your partner to gently lift your head and bring your chin to your chest.
4. Hold the stretch and relax.

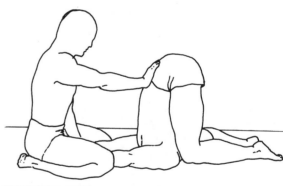

EXERCISE #180

1. Assume the stretch position in exercise #179.
2. Your partner is positioned facing your back, kneeling upright on the floor, his or her legs straddling your arms, and one hand anchoring your arms while the other is placed on your lower back.
3. Exhale, as you allow your partner to gently push your pelvis forward. *CAUTION:* Communicate and use extreme caution. This is a potentially dangerous exercise. See text on page 138 regarding the plough.

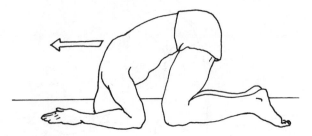

EXERCISE #181

1. Kneel on all fours.
2. Flex your arms and place the crown of your head on the floor.
3. Exhale, roll your head forward, and bring your chin to your chest.
4. Hold the stretch and relax. *NOTE:* This is an essential exercise for all wrestlers.

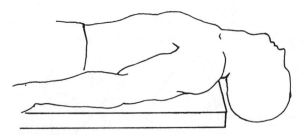

EXERCISE #183

1. Lie flat on a table with your head hanging over the edge.
2. Hold the stretch and relax.

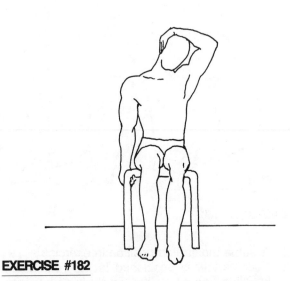

EXERCISE #182

1. Sit or stand upright.
2. Place your left hand on the upper right side of your head.
3. Exhale, and slowly pull the left side of your head onto your left shoulder (lateral flexion).
4. Hold the stretch and relax.

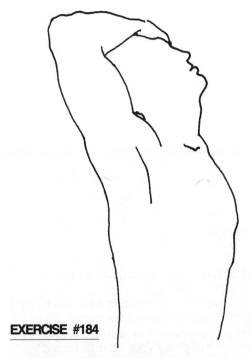

EXERCISE #184

1. Sit or stand upright with your head dropped back.
2. Place your hands on your forehead.
3. Exhale and pull your head backward.
4. Hold the stretch and relax.

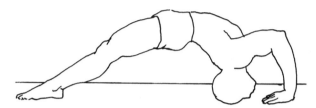

EXERCISE #185

1. Assume the stretch in exercise #146.
2. Exhale, and roll your head backward.
3. Hold the stretch and relax.

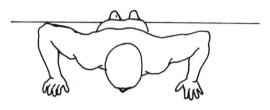

EXERCISE #187

1. Assume a front prone support (push-up) position with your arms as wide as possible.
2. Exhale and slowly lower your chest almost to the floor.
3. Hold the stretch and relax.

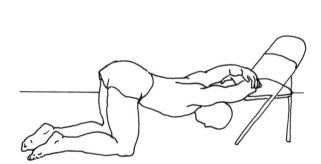

EXERCISE #186

1. Kneel on the floor facing a barre or chair knee height.
2. Flex your arms and rest your interlocked forearms on top of the barre with your head dropping beneath the supporting surface.
3. Exhale, and let your chest and head sink.
4. Hold the stretch and relax.

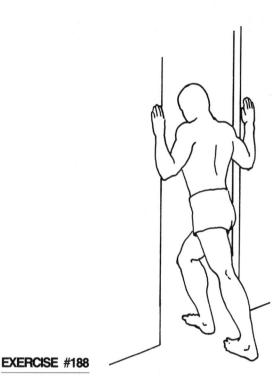

EXERCISE #188

1. Stand upright facing a corner or open doorway.
2. Raise your arms in a reverse "T" (elbows below your shoulders) to stretch the clavicular section of the pectoralis muscles bilaterally.
3. Exhale, and lean your entire body forward.
4. Hold the stretch and relax.

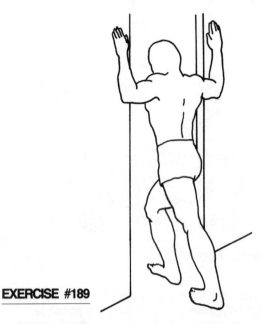

EXERCISE #189

1. Stand upright facing a corner or open doorway.
2. Raise your arms to form the letter "T" (elbows level with your shoulders) to stretch the sternal section of the pectoralis muscles bilaterally.
3. Exhale, and lean your entire body forward.
4. Hold the stretch and relax.

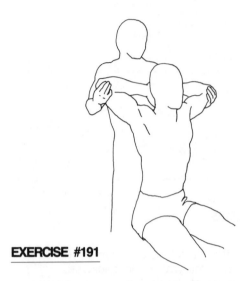

EXERCISE #191

1. Sit upright, both armed flexed, and your hands interlocked behind your head.
2. Your partner is positioned behind you and grasps both elbows.
3. Exhale, as you allow your partner to gently pull your elbows backward toward each other.
4. Hold the stretch and relax.

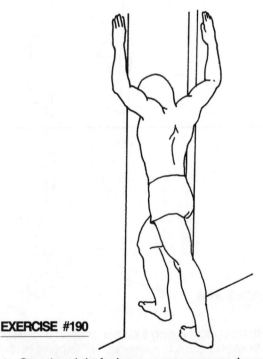

EXERCISE #190

1. Stand upright facing a corner or open doorway.
2. Raise your arms to form the letter "V" (elbows raised above your shoulders) to stretch the costal section of the pectoralis muscles bilaterally.
3. Exhale, and lean your entire body forward.
4. Hold the stretch and relax.

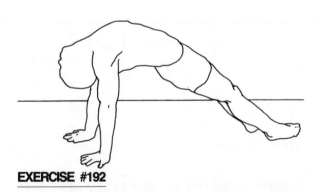

EXERCISE #192

1. Sit upright on the floor, your hands about one foot behind your hips, your fingers pointing away from your body, and your legs extended forward.
2. Inhale, lift your buttocks and lower trunk off the floor, and open your chest as wide as possible.
3. Hold the stretch and relax.

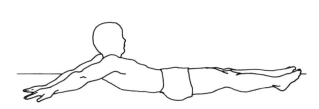

EXERCISE #193

1. Sit upright on the floor, your hands about one foot behind your hips, your fingers pointing away from your body, palms down, and your legs extended forward.
2. Exhale, slide your buttocks forward, and lean backward as far as possible.
3. Hold the stretch and relax.

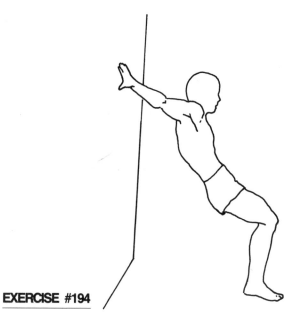

EXERCISE #194

1. Stand upright, your hands behind your hips about shoulder height resting on a wall, and your fingers pointing upward.
2. Exhale, and flex your legs to lower your shoulders.
3. Hold the stretch and relax. *NOTE:* This can also be performed using just one arm.

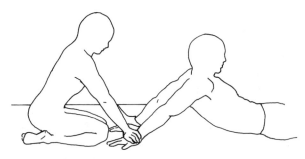

EXERCISE #195

1. Assume the stretch position in exercise #193.
2. Your partner is positioned directly behind you and holding both wrists.
3. Exhale, as you allow the partner to pull your arms backward, upward, and criss-cross.
4. Hold the stretch and relax.

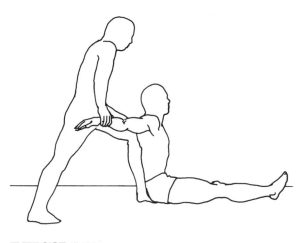

EXERCISE #196

1. Sit upright or kneel on the floor with your arms raised horizontally behind your back.
2. The partner is positioned directly behind you and holding both wrists.
3. Exhale, as you allow your partner to pull your arms backward, upward, and criss-cross.
4. Hold the stretch and relax.

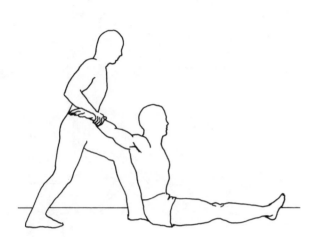

EXERCISE #197

1. Assume the stretch position in exercise #196 but with your arms raised above horizontal.
2. Exhale, as you allow your partner to pull your arms backward, upward, and criss-cross.
3. Hold the stretch and relax.

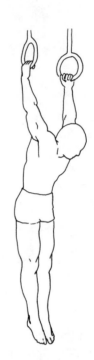

EXERCISE #199

1. Hang from a pair of still rings.
2. Inhale, and raise your body to an inverted hang.
3. Exhale, and slowly lower your legs to the floor (Skin the Cat).
4. Hold the stretch and relax. *NOTE:* Try to sink as low as possible in the shoulders.

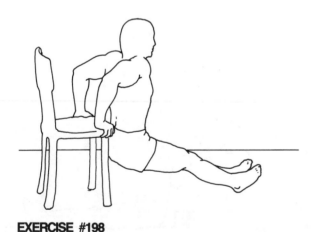

EXERCISE #198

1. Brace yourself on a stable and sturdy chair with your body extended, hips forward, and arms straight.
2. Exhale, flex your arms, and lower your buttocks toward the floor.
3. Hold the stretch and relax. *NOTE:* Use parallel bars if they are available.

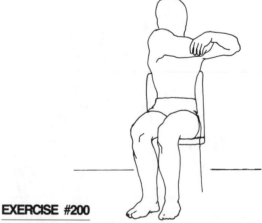

EXERCISE #200

1. Sit or stand upright with one arm raised to shoulder height.
2. Flex your arm across to the opposite shoulder.
3. Grasp your raised elbow with the opposite hand.
4. Exhale, and pull your elbow backward.
5. Hold the stretch and relax.

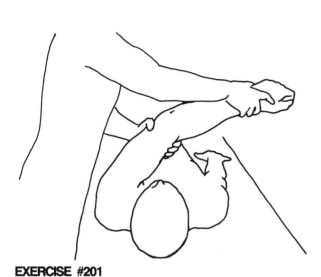

EXERCISE #201

1. Lie on a table with one arm vertically raised.
2. Your partner is positioned to your side with one hand grasping your elbow and the other your wrist.
3. Exhale, as you allow your partner to gently push your extended arm across your chest.
4. Hold the stretch and relax.

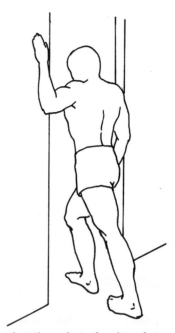

EXERCISE #203

1. Stand upright facing the edge of a door frame.
2. Raise your arm, flex your elbow, and place your hand on the frame.
3. Exhale, and turn away from your fixed arm as it remains against your side.
4. Hold the stretch and relax.

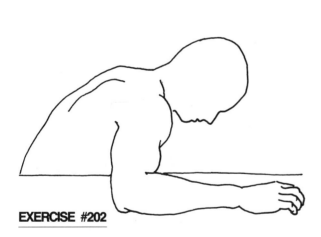

EXERCISE #202

1. Sit upright with your side next to a table.
2. Rest your forearm along the table edge with your elbow flexed.
3. Exhale, bend forward from the waist, and lower your head and shoulder to table level.
4. Hold the stretch and relax.

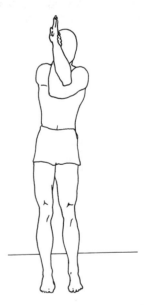

EXERCISE #204

1. Sit or stand upright.
2. Flex your right arm and raise your elbow to chest height.
3. Flex and raise your left arm so its elbow can support your right elbow.
4. Intertwine your forearms so that your left hand grasps your right wrist.
5. Exhale, and pull your wrist outward and downward.
6. Hold the stretch and relax.

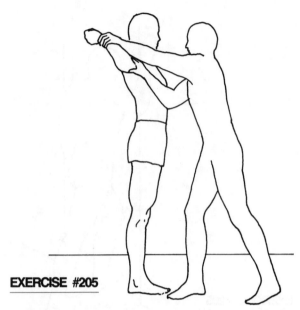

EXERCISE #205

1. Stand upright with your right arm raised to shoulder height and flexed to a right angle.
2. Your partner is positioned in front of you and to your side; grasping your right wrist with his or her left hand; and supporting your right elbow with his or her right hand.
3. Exhale, as you allow your partner to gently push your wrist backward and downward.
4. Hold the stretch and relax.

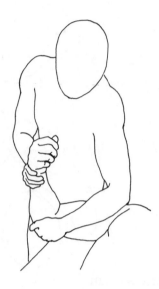

EXERCISE #207

1. Lie flat on your back on a table.
2. Flex your arm and have your elbow rest over the edge.
3. Your partner is positioned to your side with one hand anchoring your elbow and the opposite hand grasping your wrist.
4. Exhale, as you allow your partner to push your hand forward and downward toward your feet.
5. Hold the stretch and relax.

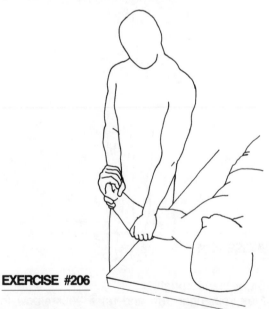

EXERCISE #206

1. Lie flat on your back on a table.
2. Flex your arm with your elbow resting over the edge.
3. Your partner is positioned to your side with one hand anchoring your elbow and the opposite hand grasping your wrist.
4. Exhale, as you allow your partner to gently push downward on your wrist.
5. Hold the stretch and relax.

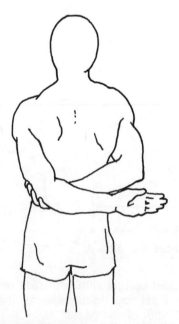

EXERCISE #208

1. Sit or stand upright with one arm flexed behind your back.
2. Grasp the elbow from behind with the opposite hand.
3. Exhale, and pull your elbow across the mid-line of your back.
4. Hold the stretch and relax. *NOTE:* Grasp the wrist if unable to reach the elbow.

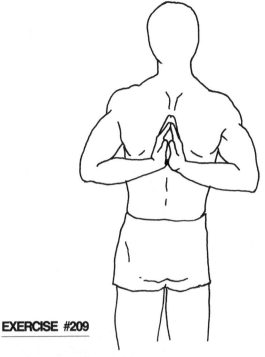

EXERCISE #209

1. Sit or stand upright.
2. Place your palms together behind your back with your fingers pointing downward.
3. Exhale, rotate your wrists so that your fingers are pointing toward your head, and then draw your elbows back.
4. Hold the stretch and relax.

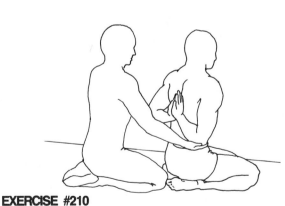

EXERCISE #210

1. Assume the stretch position in exercise #209.
2. Your partner is positioned directly behind you and grasping both elbows.
3. Exhale, as you allow your partner to gently pull your elbows backward.
4. Hold the stretch and relax.

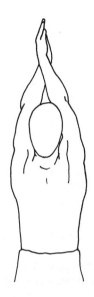

EXERCISE #211

1. Lie flat on your back or sit upright.
2. Cross one wrist over the other and interlock your hands.
3. Inhale, straighten your arms, lower your chin to your chest, and extend your arms behind your head.
4. Hold the stretch and relax. *NOTE:* Your elbows should be behind your ears.

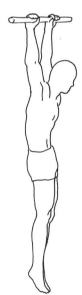

EXERCISE #212

1. Hang from a chin-up bar with your hands in an overgrip, chin on your chest, and your back hollowed.
2. Hold the stretch and relax.

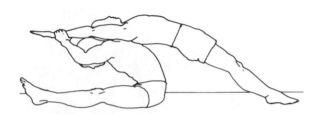

EXERCISE #213

1. Sit upright on the floor, your legs straight, and your arms parallel and overhead.
2. Your partner is positioned on the floor, back to back in the identical position, and grasping your wrists.
3. Exhale, as you allow your partner to lean forward, pull your wrists, and lift your trunk off the floor.
4. Hold the stretch and relax. *NOTE:* Contract your body.

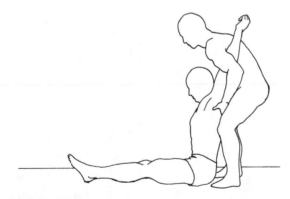

EXERCISE #214

1. Sit upright on the floor, your legs straight, and your arms parallel and overhead.
2. Your partner is positioned directly behind you with his or her knees braced against your spine.
3. Your partner reaches around your arms, hooks his or her elbows in your armpits, and places his or her hands on your upper shoulder blades.
4. Exhale, as you allow your partner to gently push your shoulder blades forward and pull your arms backward.
5. Hold the stretch and relax.

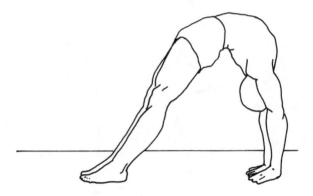

EXERCISE #215

1. Assume the stretch position in exercise #148.
2. Exhale, and force your shoulders past your wrists (vertical).
3. Hold the stretch and relax.

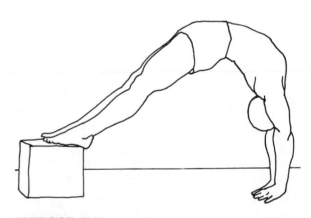

EXERCISE #216

1. Assume the starting position in exercise #148 with your feet resting on a bench.
2. Exhale, and raise your trunk off the floor into a full bridge.
3. Exhale, and force your shoulders past your wrists (vertical).
4. Hold the stretch and relax. *CAUTION:* Make sure the bench is stable and sturdy.

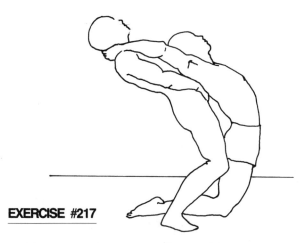

EXERCISE #217

1. Kneel upright on the floor with your arms parallel, overhead, and touching your ears.
2. Your partner straddles your legs from behind and grasps the top side of your shoulder blades or elbows.
3. Grasp your partner around the neck and interlock your hands.
4. Exhale, as your partner lifts up and leans backward.
5. Hold the stretch and relax. *NOTE:* The grasping of the elbows will result in a greater stretch. However, this can be further intensified by having your partner roll his or her pelvis under while pushing in and up with the hips into your hips and lower back.

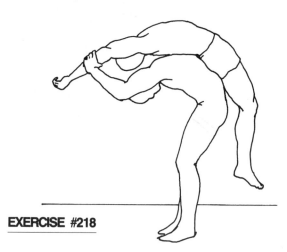

EXERCISE #218

1. Stand upright; feet together; and your arms parallel, overhead, and touching your ears.
2. Your partner is positioned standing back-to-back; his or her knees flexed; and his or her buttocks beneath the one to be lifted.
3. Your partner reaches upward and grasps you on or below the elbows.
4. Exhale, as your partner leans forward, slightly straightens his or her legs, and lifts you off the floor.
5. Hold the stretch and relax. *NOTE:* To increase the stretch, have the hands in an elgrip position.

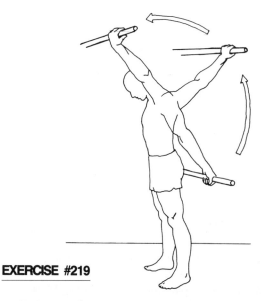

EXERCISE #219

1. Stand upright; feet straddled; and grasping either a pole or towel behind your hips with a reverse grip (your fingers facing upward and the thumb around the pole or towel).
2. Exhale, slowly raise your arms overhead keeping both straight until your arms rotate forward in the shoulder joint and ending in an elgrip.
3. Inhale, then reverse the direction. *NOTE:* The wider the hand placement the easier the dislocation.

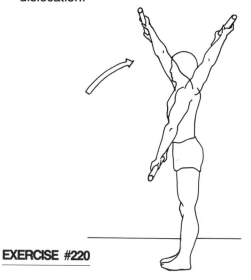

EXERCISE #220

1. Stand upright; feet straddled; and grasping either a pole or towel in front of your hips with an overgrip (regular grip).
2. Inhale, slowly raise your arms overhead keeping both straight until your arms rotate in the shoulder joint, and ending up behind your hips.
3. Inhale, then reverse the direction. *NOTE:* The wider one grasps the pole the easier will be the inlocating action. Remember, the arms must be kept straight and symmetrical—no twisting to the side.

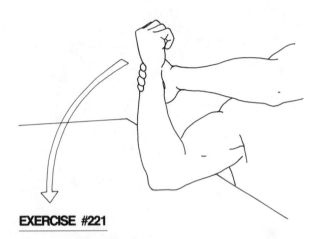

EXERCISE #221

1. Sit upright, one arm flexed 90°, and your elbow resting on a table.
2. Grasp your wrist with the opposite hand.
3. Exhale, and execute a maximal eccentric contraction of the biceps (contract the biceps as they are elongated).

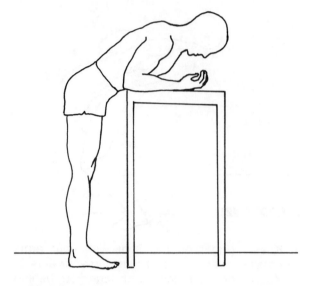

EXERCISE #223

1. Stand upright with your forearms resting on a table.
2. Exhale, bend forward, and bring your shoulders to your wrist.
3. Hold the stretch and relax.

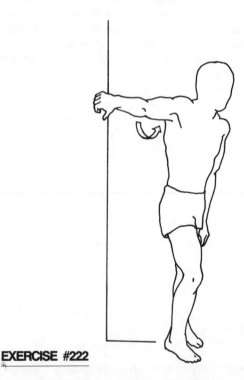

EXERCISE #222

1. Stand upright with your back to a door frame.
2. Rest one hand against the door frame with your arm externally rotated at the shoulder, forearm extended, and your hand pronated with your thumb pointing down.
3. Exhale, and attempt to roll your biceps so they face upward.
4. Hold the stretch and relax.

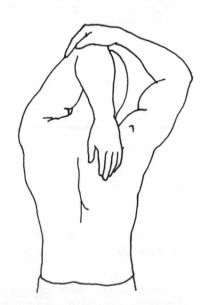

EXERCISE #224

1. Sit or stand upright with one arm flexed, raised overhead next to your ear, and your hand resting on your shoulder blade.
2. Grasp your elbow with the opposite hand.
3. Exhale, and pull your elbow behind your head.
4. Hold the stretch and relax.

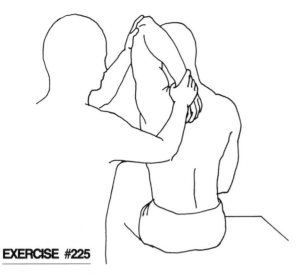

EXERCISE #225

1. Assume the stretch position in exercise #224.
2. Your partner is positioned to your side with one hand grasping your wrist and the other holding your elbow.
3. Exhale, as you allow your partner to raise your elbow and pull your wrist downward.
4. Hold the stretch and relax.

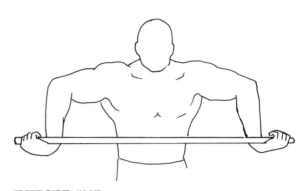

EXERCISE #227

1. Assume the stretch position in exercise #216 (using a pole).
2. Exhale, and flex your elbows.
3. Hold the stretch and relax.

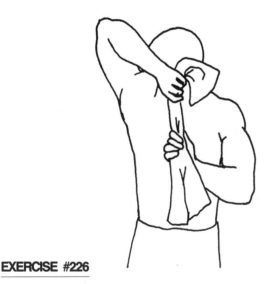

EXERCISE #226

1. Sit or stand upright with one arm placed as far up on your back as possible.
2. Lift your other arm overhead, flex your elbow, and interlock your fingers.
3. Hold the stretch and relax. *NOTE:* Use a folded towel if you cannot interlock the hands.

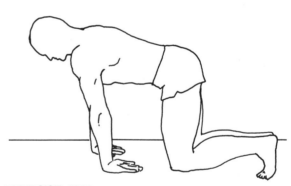

EXERCISE #228

1. Flex your wrist and place the top of your hand against the floor or a wall.
2. Exhale, and lean against the surface.
3. Hold the stretch and relax.

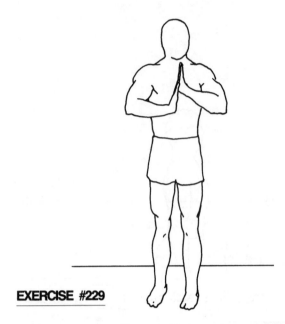

EXERCISE #229

1. Sit or stand upright on the floor with your wrists flexed.
2. Place the heel of one hand against the upper portion of the fingers of your other hand.
3. Exhale, and press the heel of your hand against your fingers.
4. Hold the stretch and relax.

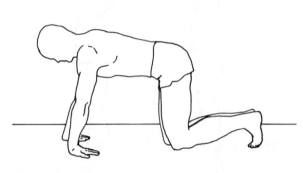

EXERCISE #231

1. Kneel on the floor with your arms extended and your fingers pointed toward your body.
2. Exhale, and lean forward.
3. Hold the stretch and relax.

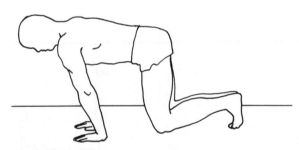

EXERCISE #230

1. Kneel on the floor with your arms extended and your fingers pointed away from your body.
2. Exhale, and lean forward.
3. Hold the stretch and relax.

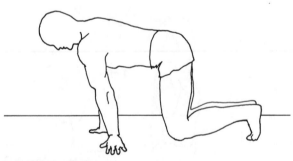

EXERCISE #232

1. Kneel on the floor with your arms extended and the heel of each hand touching the other.
2. Exhale, and lean forward.
3. Hold the stretch and relax.

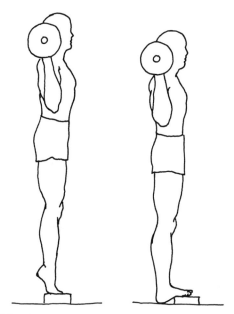

EXERCISE #233

1. Stand upright; toes and balls of your feet on a thick board; and resting a barbell across your shoulders.
2. Exhale, and rise up on your toes as high as possible.
3. Inhale, and lower your heels until they almost touch the floor.
4. Hold the stretch and relax. *NOTE:* This stretch can be varied by turning the toes either in or out.

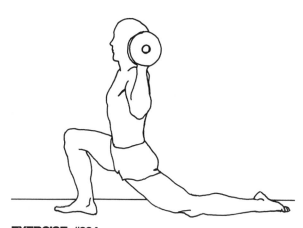

EXERCISE #234

1. Stand upright; your feet parallel and shoulder width; and resting a barbell across your shoulders.
2. Inhale, and lower your body until one knee rests on the floor.
3. Hold the stretch and relax.
4. Exhale, and return to the starting position.

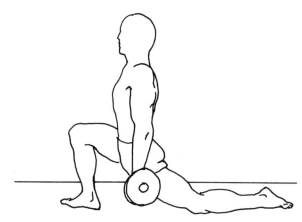

EXERCISE #235

1. Same as exercise #234, but holding a pair of dumbbells.
2. Hold the stretch and relax.
3. Exhale, and return to the starting position.

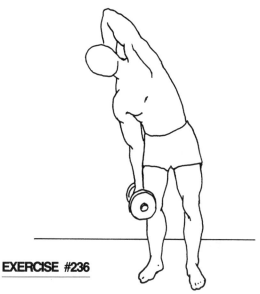

EXERCISE #236

1. Stand upright, your feet parallel and shoulder width apart; one arm flexed behind your head; and your opposite hand holding a dumbbell at your side.
2. Exhale; maintain your body in a lateral plane; and bend sideways as far as possible.
3. Hold the stretch and relax.
4. Exhale, and return to the starting position.

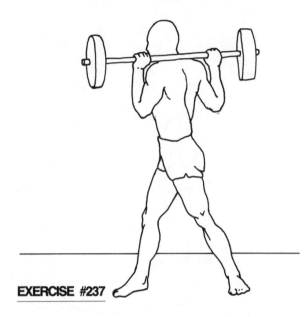

EXERCISE #237

1. Assume the starting position in exercise #234.
2. Exhale, and slowly twist your trunk as far as possible to one side.
3. Hold the stretch and relax.
4. Exhale, and return to the starting position.

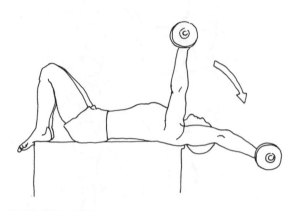

EXERCISE #239

1. Lie flat on your back on a bench; resting a dumbbell on your lower chest; and grasping it with both hands.
2. Exhale and raise the dumbbell off your chest.
3. Inhale; lock your arms straight; and lower the dumbbell over your head as close to the floor as possible.
4. Hold the stretch and relax.
5. Exhale, and return to the starting position.

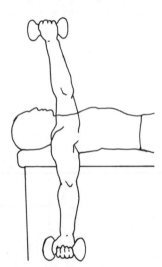

EXERCISE #238

1. Lie on a bench with your legs flexed and your feet resting on its surface.
2. Hold two light dumbbells directly over your chest; your arms straight, and your knuckles facing out.
3. Inhale; keeping your arm flexed; lower the dumbbells sideways and elbows as close to the floor as possible.
4. Hold the stretch and relax.
5. Exhale, and return to the starting position by bringing the dumbbells back up in an arc. *CAUTION:* Do not straighten the arms. *NOTE:* Flys can also be performed on either a decline or incline board.

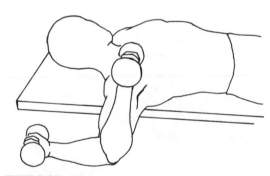

EXERCISE #240

1. Lie flat on a bench or table with your arm resting over the edge and your elbow flexed to 90° while holding a light dumbbell.
2. Inhale and slowly lower the weight downward and parallel to your head.
3. Hold the stretch and relax.
4. Exhale, and return to the starting position.

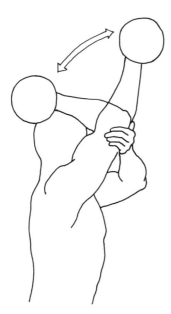

EXERCISE #241

1. Sit upright and hold a dumbbell with both hands overhead.
2. Inhale, and slowly lower the dumbbell behind your head.
3. Hold the stretch and relax.
4. Exhale, and return to the starting position.

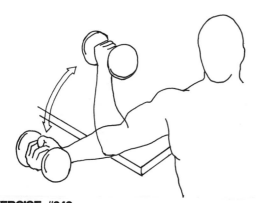

EXERCISE #242

1. Sit or stand by a table with your arm resting on the surface and your elbow flexed to 90° while holding a dumbbell.
2. Inhale, and slowly extend your elbow while contracting your biceps (eccentric action).
3. Hold the stretch and relax.
4. Exhale, and return the weight to the starting position.

References

American Alliance for Health, Physical Education, and Recreation. (1968). *School safety policies with emphasis on physical education, athletics, and recreation.* Washington, DC: Author.

Abraham, W.M. (1977). Factors in delayed muscle soreness. *Medicine and Science in Sports, 9*(1), 11-20.

Abraham, W.M. (1979). Exercise-induced muscular soreness. *The Physician and Sportsmedicine, 7*(10), 57-60.

Abramson, D., Roberts, S.M., & Wilson, P.D. (1934). Relaxation of the pelvic joints in pregnancy. *Surgery Gynecology, 58*(3), 595-613.

Akeson, W.H., Amiel, D., & LaViolette, D. (1967). The connective tissue response to immobility: A study of the chondroitin 4- and 6-sulfate and dermatan sulfate changes in periarticular connective tissue of control and immobilized knees of dogs. *Clinical Orthopaedics and Related Research, 51*, 183-197.

Akeson, W.H., Amiel, D., Mechanic, G.L., Woo, S., Harwood, F.L., & Hammer, M.L. (1977). Collagen crosslinking alterations in joint contractures: Changes in reducible crosslinks in periarticular connective tissue collagen after nine weeks of immobilization. *Connective Tissue Research, 5*(1), 15-20.

Akeson, W.H., Amiel, D., & Woo, S. (1980). Immobility effects on synovial joints: The pathomechanics of joint contracture. *Biorheology, 17*(1/2), 95-110.

American Medical Association Subcommittee on Classification of Sports Injuries. (1966). *Standard nomenclature of athletic injuries.* Chicago: The American Medical Association.

American Orthopaedic Association. (1985). *Manual of orthopaedic surgery.* Chicago: Author.

Anderson, B. (1978). The perfect pre-run stretching routine. *Runners World, 13*(5), 56-61.

Anderson, B. (1980). *Stretching.* Bolinas, CA: Shelter Publications.

Arnheim, D.D. (1971). Stretching. In L.A. Larson (Ed.), *Encyclopedia of sport sciences and medicine* (pp. 165-166). New York: Macmillan.

Asmussen, E. (1956). Observation on experimental muscle soreness. *Acta Rheumatology Scandinavica, 2*, 109-116.

Asmussen, E., & Bonde-Petersen, F. (1974). Storage of elastic energy in skeletal muscles in man. *Acta Physiologica Scandinavica, 91*(3), 385-392.

Astrand, P.O., & Rodahl, K. (1978). *The textbook of work physiology* (2nd ed.). New York: McGraw-Hill.

Aten, D.W., & Knight, K.T. (1978). Therapeutic exercise in athletic training—principles and overview. *Athletic Training, 13*(3), 123-126.

Balaftsalis, H. (1982/1983). Knee joint laxity contributing to footballers' injuries. *Physio Therapy in Sport, 5*(3), 26-27.

Ballantyne, B.T., Reser, M.D., Lorenz, G.W., & Smidt, G.L. (1986). The effects of inversion traction on spinal column configuration, heart rate, blood pressure, and perceived discomfort. *Journal of Orthopaedic and Sports Physical Therapy, 7*(5), 254-260.

Barney, V.S., Hirst, C.C., & Jensen, C.R. (1972). *Conditioning exercises: Exercises to improve body form and function* (3rd ed.). St. Louis: C.V. Mosby.

Barrack, R.L., Skinner, H.B., Brunet, M.E., & Cook, S.D. (1983). Joint laxity and proprioception in the knee. *The Physician and Sportsmedicine, 11*(6), 130-135.

Basmajian, J.V. (1975). Motor learning and control. *Archives of Physical Medicine and Rehabilitation, 58*(1), 38-41.

Basmajian, J.V. (1981). Biofeedback in rehabilitation: A review of principles and practices. *Archives of Physical Medicine and Rehabilitation, 62*(10), 469-475.

Bates, R.A. (1971). *Flexibility training: The optimal time period to spend in a position of maximal stretch.* Unpublished master's thesis, University of Alberta, Edmonton.

Bates, R.A. (1976). Flexibility development: Mind over matter. In J.H. Salmela (Ed.), *The advanced study of gymnastics* (pp. 233-241). Springfield, IL: Charles C Thomas.

Beaulieu, J.E. (1981). Developing a stretching program. *The Physician and Sportsmedicine, 9*(11), 59-69.

Becker, A.H. (1979). Traction for knee-flexion contractures. *Physical Therapy, 59*(9), 1114.

Beighton, P., Grahame, R., & Bird, H. (1983). *Hypermobility of joints.* Berlin: Springer-Verlag.

Bell, R.D., & Hoshizaki, T.B. (1981). Relationship of age and sex with range of motion of seventeen joint actions in humans. *Canadian Journal of Applied Sports Science*, **6**(4), 202-206.

Benson, H. (1980). *The relaxation response*. New York: Avon Books.

Bick, E.M. (1961). Aging in the connective tissues of the human musculoskeletal system. *Geriatrics*, **16**(9), 448-453.

Biesterfeldt, H.J. (1974). Flexibility programs. *International Gymnast*, **16**(3), 22-23.

Billig, H.E., & Lowendahl, E. (1949). *Mobilization of the human body*. Stanford: Stanford University Press.

Bird, H. (1979). Joint laxity in sport. *MediSport the Review of Sports Medicine*, **1**(5), 30-31.

Bird, H.A., Calguneri, M., & Wright, V. (1981). Changes in joint laxity occurring during pregnancy. *Annals of the Rheumatic Diseases*, **40**(2), 209-212.

Bird, H.A., Hudson, A., & Wright, V. (1980). Joint laxity and osteoarthritis: A radiological survey of female physical education specialists. *British Journal of Sports Medicine*, **14**(4), 179-188.

Bloom, W., & Fawcett, D.W. (1975). *A textbook of histology* (10th ed.). Philadelphia: W.B. Saunders.

Bohannon, R., Gajdosik, R., & LeVeau, B. (1985). Contribution of pelvic and lower limb motion to increase in the angle of passive straight leg raising. *Physical Therapy*, **65**(4), 474-476.

Booth, F.W., & Gould, W. (1975). Training and disuse on connective tissue. In J. Whitmore & J. Keogh (Eds.), *Exercise and sports sciences reviews* (Vol. 3, pp. 83-112). New York: Academic Press.

Boscoe, C., Tarkka, I., & Komi, P.V. (1982). Effects of elastic energy and myoelectrical potentiation of triceps surae during stretch-shortening cycle exercise. *International Journal of Sports Medicine*, **3**(3), 137-140.

Brewer, V., & Hinson, M. (1978). Relationship of pregnancy to lateral knee stability. *Medicine and Science in Sports*, **10**(1), 39.

Brodelius, A. (1961). Osteoarthrosis of the talar joints in footballers and ballet dancers. *Acta Orthopaedica Scandinavica*, **30**, 309-314.

Broer, M.R., & Gales, N.R. (1958). Importance of various body measurements in performance of toe touch test. *Research Quarterly*, **29**(3), 253-257.

Bryant, S. (1984). Flexibility and stretching. *The Physician and Sportsmedicine*, **12**(2), 171.

Bryant, W.M. (1977). Wound healing. *Clinical Symposia*, **29**(3), 1-36.

Burkett, L.N. (1970). Causative factors in hamstring strain. *Medicine and Science in Sports*, **2**(1), 39-42.

Burkett, L.N. (1971). Cause and prevention of hamstring pulls. *Athletic Journal*, **51**(6), 34.

Burkett, L.N. (1975). Investigation into hamstring strains: The case of the hybrid muscle. *The Journal of Sports Medicine and Physical Fitness*, **3**(5), 228-231.

Burkhardt, S. (1982). The rationale for joint mobilization. In G.W. Bell (Ed.), *Professional preparation in athletic training* (pp. 101-106). Champaign, IL: Human Kinetics.

Cailliet, R. (1977). *Soft tissue pain and disability*. Philadelphia: F.A. Davis.

Cailliet, R. (1981a). *Low back pain syndrome*. Philadelphia: F.A. Davis.

Cailliet, R. (1981b). *Shoulder pain* (2nd ed.). Philadelphia: F.A. Davis.

Carlson, F.D., & Wilkie, D.R. (1974). *Muscle physiology*. Englewood Cliffs, NJ: Prentice-Hall.

Cavagna, G.A., Dusman, B., & Margaria, R. (1968). Positive work done by a previously stretched muscle. *Journal of Applied Physiology*, **24**(1), 21-32.

Cavagna, G.A., Saibene, F.P., & Margaria, R. (1965). Effect of negative work on the amount of positive work performed by an isolated muscle. *Journal of Applied Physiology*, **20**(1), 157-160.

Cherry, D.B. (1980). Review of physical therapy alternatives for reducing muscle contracture. *Physical Therapy*, **60**(7), 877-881.

Chujoy, A., & Manchester, P.W. (Eds.). (1967). *The dance encyclopedia*. New York: Simon & Schuster.

Ciullo, J.V., & Zarins, B. (1983). Biomechanics of the musculotendinous unit. In B. Zarins (Ed.), *Clinics in sports medicine* (Vol. 2, pp. 71-85). Philadelphia: W.B. Saunders.

Committee on the Medical Aspects of Sports of the American Medical Association and the National Federation. (1975). Muscle soreness can be eliminated. *Athletic Training*, **10**(1), 42.

Consumer Reports. (1975). Chiropractors: Healers or quacks? *Consumer Reports*, **40**(9), 542-547.

Corbin, C.B. (1973). *A textbook of motor development*. Dubuque, IA: William C. Brown.

Corbin, C.B., & Noble, L. (1980). Flexibility: A major component of physical fitness. *The Journal of Physical Education and Recreation, 51*(6), 23-24, 57-60.

Cornelius, W.L. (1981). Two effective flexibility methods. *Athletic Training, 16*(1), 23-25.

Cornelius, W.L. (1983). Stretch evoked emg activity by isometric contraction and submaximal concentric contraction. *Athletic Training, 18*(2), 106-109.

Cornelius, W.L., & Hinson, M.M. (1980). The relationship between isometric contractions of hip extensors and subsequent flexibility in males. *Journal of Sports Medicine and Physical Fitness, 20*(1), 75-80.

Councilman, J.E. (1968). *The science of swimming.* Englewood Cliffs, NJ: Prentice-Hall.

Coville, C.A. (1979). Relaxation in physical education curricula. *The Physical Educator, 36*(4), 176-181.

Cowan, P.M., McGavin, S., & North, A.C. (1955). The polypeptide chain configuration of collagen. *Nature, 176*(4492), 1062-1064.

Craig, T.T. (Ed.). (1973). *American Medical Association comments in sports medicine.* Chicago: American Medical Association.

Crisp, J. (1970). Properties of tendon and skin. In Y.C. Yung, N. Perrone, & M. Anliker (Eds.), *Biomechanics: Its foundations and objectives* (pp. 141-180). Englewood Cliffs: NJ.

Crosman, L.J., Chateauvert, S.R., & Weisberg, J. (1984). The effects of massage to the hamstring muscle group on the range of motion. *Journal of Orthopaedic and Sports Physical Therapy, 6*(3), 168-172.

Davis, E.C., Logan, G.A., & McKinney, W.C. (1965). *Biophysical values of muscular activity with implications for research* (2nd ed.). Dubuque, IA: William C. Brown.

Davson, H. (1970). *A textbook of general physiology* (4th ed.). Baltimore: Williams and Wilkins.

de Vries, H.A. (1961a). Prevention of muscular distress after exercise. *Research Quarterly, 32*(2), 177-185.

de Vries, H.A. (1961b). Electromyographic observation of the effect of static stretching upon muscular distress. *Research Quarterly, 32*(4), 468-479.

de Vries, H.A. (1962). Evaluation of static stretching procedures for improvement of flexibility. *Research Quarterly, 33*(2), 222-229.

de Vries, H.A. (1966). Quantitative electromyographic investigation of the spasm theory of muscle pain. *The American Journal of Physical Medicine, 45*(3), 119-134.

de Vries, H.A. (1975). Physical fitness programs: Does physical activity promote relaxation? *Journal of Physical Education and Recreation, 46*(7), 52-53.

de Vries, H.A. (1980). *Physiology of exercise* (3rd ed.). Dubuque, IA: William C. Brown.

de Vries, H.A., & Adams, G.M. (1972). Emg comparison of single doses of exercise and meprobamate as to effects on muscular relaxation. *American Journal of Physical Medicine, 51*(3), 130-141.

de Vries, H.A., Wiswell, R.A., Bulbulion, R., & Moritani, T. (1981). Tranquilizer effect of exercise. *American Journal of Physical Medicine, 60*(2), 57-66.

Dick, F.W. (1980). *Sports training principles.* London: Lepus Books.

Dickenson, R.V. (1968). The specificity of flexibility. *Research Quarterly, 39*(3), 792-794.

Doherty, K. (1971). *Track and field omnibook.* Swarthmore, PA: Tafmop Publishers.

Dollan, J.P., & Holliday, L.J. (1974). *First-aid management athletics, physical education, recreation* (4th ed.). Danville, IL: Interstate Printers and Publishers.

Donatelli, R., & Owens-Burkhardt, H. (1981). Effects of immobilization on the extensibility of periarticular connective tissue. *Journal of Orthopaedic and Sports Physical Therapy, 3*(2), 67-72.

Donnelly, J.E. (1982). *Living anatomy.* Champaign, IL: Human Kinetics.

Dorland's illustrated medical dictionary (26th ed.). (1981). Philadelphia: W.B. Saunders.

Dowsing, G.S. (1978). Partner exercise. *Coaching Women's Athletics, 4*(2), 18-20.

Dummer, G.M., Vaccardo, P., & Clarke, D.H. (1985). Muscular strength and flexibility of two female master swimmers in the eighth decade of life. *The Journal of Orthopaedic and Sports Physical Therapy, 6*(4), 235-237.

Eldren, H.R. (1968). Physical properties of collagen fibers. In D.A. Hull (Ed.), *International review of connective tissue research* (Vol. 4, pp. 248-283). New York: Academic Press.

Eldred, E., Hutton, R.S., & Smith, J.L. (1976). Nature of the persisting changes in afferent discharge from muscle following its contraction. *Progressive Brain Research, 44*, 157-171.

Elliott, D.H. (1965). Structure and function of mammalian tendon. *Biological Review*, **40**(3), 392-421.

Ende, L.S., & Wickstrom, J. (1982). Ballet injuries. *The Physician and Sportsmedicine*, **10**(7), 101-118.

Fanning, T., & Fanning, R. (1978). *Keep running*. New York: Sovereign Press.

Fardy, P.S. (1981). Isometric exercise and the cardiovascular system. *The Physician and Sportsmedicine*, **9**(9), 43-56.

Farfan, H.F. (1973). *Mechanical disorders of the low back*. Philadelphia: Lea and Febiger.

Farfan, H.F. (1978). The biomechanical advantage of lordosis and hip extension for upright activity. *Spine*, **3**(4), 336-342.

Fisk, J.W., & Rose, R.S. (1977). *A practical guide to management of the painful neck and back*. Springfield, IL: Charles C Thomas.

Flintney, F.W., & Hirst, D.G. (1978). Cross-bridge detachment and sarcomere 'give' during stretch of active frog's muscle. *Journal of Physiology (London)*, **276**, 449-465.

Follan, L.M. (1981). *Lilias and your life*. New York: Collier Books.

Francis, K.T. (1983). Delayed muscle soreness: A review. *The Journal of Orthopaedic and Sports Physical Therapy*, **5**(1), 10-13.

Franzblau, C., & Faru, B. (1981). Elastin. In E.D. Hay (Ed.), *Cell biology of extracellular matrix* (pp. 75-78). New York: Plenum Press.

Fridén, J. (1984). Changes in human skeletal muscle induced by long-term eccentric exercise. *Cell Tissue Research*, **236**(2), 365-372.

Fridén, J., Sjöstrom, M., & Ekblom, B. (1981). A morphological study of delayed muscle soreness. *Experimentia*, **37**(5), 506-507.

Fujiwara, M., & Basmajian, J.V. (1975). Electromyographic study of the two-joint muscles. *The American Journal of Physical Medicine*, **54**(5), 234-242.

Gajdosik, R., & Lusin, G. (1983). Hamstring muscle tightness: Reliability of an active-knee-extension test. *Physical Therapy*, **63**(7), 1085-1089.

Gardner, E.B. (1969, May). Proprioceptive reflexes and their participation in motor skills. *Quest*, **12**, 1-25.

Garu, J. (1986). Exercise do's & don'ts: Side bends. *Dance Exercise Today*, **4**(4), 34-35.

Gelabert, R. (1966). *Raul Gelabert's anatomy for the dancer*. New York: Danad Publishing.

Germain, N.W., & Blair, S.N. (1983). Variability of shoulder flexion with age, activity and sex. *The American Corrective Therapy Journal*, **37**(6), 156-160.

Gilliam, T.B., Villanacci, J.F., Freedson, P.S., & Sady, S.P. (1979). Isokinetic torque in boys and girls ages 7 to 13: Effect of age, height, and weight. *Research Quarterly*, **50**(4), 599-609.

Glazer, R.M. (1980). Rehabilitation. In R.B. Happenstall (Ed.), *Fracture treatment and healing* (pp. 1041-1068). Philadelphia: W.B. Saunders.

Goldspink, G. (1968). Sarcomere length during post-natal growth of mammalian muscle fibres. *Journal of Cell Science*, **3**(4), 539-548.

Goldspink, G. (1976). The adaptation of muscle to a new functional length. In D.J. Anderson & B. Matthews (Eds.), *Mastication* (pp. 90-99). Bristol, England: John Wright and Sons.

Goldspink, G., Tabary, C., Tardieu, C., & Tardieu, G. (1974). Effect of denervation on the adaptation of sarcomere number and muscle extensibility to the functional length of the muscle. *Journal of Physiology (London)*, **236**(3), 733-742.

Goldspink, G., & Williams, P.E. (1978). The nature of the increased passive resistance in muscle following immobilization of the mouse soleus muscle. *Journal of Physiology (London)*, **289**. (Proceedings of the Physiological Society December 15-16, 1978).

Golub, L.J., & Christaldi, J. (1957). Reducing dysmenorrhea in young adolescents. *Journal of Health, Physical Education, and Recreation*, **28**(5), 24-25, 59.

Gomolak, C.W. (1975). Know your joints. *WomenSports*, **2**(3), 62-64.

Gosline, J.M. (1976). The physical properties of elastic tissue. In D.A. Hull & D.S. Jackson (Eds.), *International review of connective tissue research* (Vol. 7, pp. 211-257). New York: Academic Press.

Gowitzke, B.A., & Milner, M. (1980). *Understanding the scientific basis of human movement* (2nd ed.). Baltimore: Williams & Wilkins.

Grana, W.A., & Moretz, J.A. (1978). Ligamentous laxity in secondary school athletes. *Journal of the American Medical Association*, **240**(18), 1975-1976.

Granit, R. (1962). Muscle tone and postural regulation. In K. Rodahl & S.M. Horvath (Eds.), *Muscle as tissue* (p. 190). New York: McGraw-Hill.

Grant, M.E., Prockop, P.D., & Darwin, J. (1972). The biosynthesis of collagen. *New England Journal of Medicine,* **286**(4), 194-199.

Grieve, D.W. (1970, December). Stretching active muscles. *Track Technique,* **42**, 1333-1335.

Grob, D. (1983). Common disorders of muscles in the aged. In W. Reichel (Ed.), *Clinical aspects of aging* (2nd ed., pp. 329-333). Baltimore: Williams and Wilkins.

Gross, J. (1961). Collagen. *Scientific America,* **204**(5), 120-133.

Gutmann, E. (1977). Muscle. In C. E. Finch & L. Hayflick (Eds.), *Handbook of the biology of aging* (pp. 445-469). New York: Van Nostrand Reinhold.

Hamilton, W.G. (1978a, February). Ballet and your body: An orthopedist's view. *Dance Magazine,* p. 79.

Hamilton, W.G. (1978b, April). Ballet and your body: An orthopedist's view. *Dance Magazine,* pp. 126-127.

Hamilton, W.G. (1978c, July). Ballet and your body: An orthopedist's view. *Dance Magazine,* pp. 86-87.

Hamilton, W.G. (1978d, August). Ballet and your body: An orthopedist's view. *Dance Magazine,* pp. 84-85.

Hardy, L. (1985). Improving active range of hip flexion. *Research Quarterly for Exercise and Sport,* **56**(2), 111-114.

Harris, F.A. (1978). Facilitation techniques in therapeutic exercise. In J.V. Basmajian (Ed.), *Therapeutic exercise* (3rd ed., pp. 93-137). Baltimore: Williams and Wilkins.

Harris, M.L. (1969a). Flexibility. *Physical Therapy,* **49**(6), 591-601.

Harris, M.L. (1969b). A factor analytic study of flexibility. *Research Quarterly,* **40**(1), 62-70.

Hartley-O'Brien, S.J. (1980). Six mobilization exercises for active range of hip flexion. *Research Quarterly for Exercise and Sport,* **51**(4), 625-635.

Harvey, V.P., & Scott, F.P. (1967). Reliability of a measure of forward flexibility and its relation to physical dimensions of college women. *Research Quarterly,* **38**(1), 28-33.

Hatfield, F.C. (1982). Learning to stretch for strength and safety. *Muscle & Fitness,* **43**(12), 24-25, 193-194.

Hickok, R.J. (1976). Physical therapy. In F.V. Steinberg (Ed.), *Cowdry's the care of the geriatric patient* (5th ed., pp. 420-432). St. Louis: C.V. Mosby.

Hill, A.V. (1961). The heat produced by a muscle after the last shock of tetanus. *Journal of Physiology* (London), **159**, 518-545.

Hinterbuchner, C. (1980). Traction. In J.B. Rogoff (Ed.), *Manipulation, traction, and massage* (2nd ed., pp. 184-210). Baltimore: Williams and Wilkins.

Holland, G.J. (1968). The physiology of flexibility: A review of the literature. *Kinesiology Review I,* 49-62.

Holt, L.E. (no date). *Scientific stretching for sport (3-s).* Nova Scotia: Sport Research Limited.

Holt, L.E., Travis, T.M., & Okita, T. (1970). Comparative study of three stretching techniques. *Perceptual and Motor Skills,* **21**(2), 611-616.

Hoppenfield, S. (1967). *Scoliosis: A manual of concept and treatment.* Philadelphia: J.B. Lippincott.

Hough, T. (1902). Ergographic studies in muscular soreness. *The American Journal of Physiology,* **7**(1), 76-92.

Houk, J., & Hennemann, E. (1967). Responses of golgi tendon organs to active contraction of the soleus muscle of the cat. *The Journal of Neurophysiology,* **30**, 466-481.

Howse, A.J. (1972). Orthopedist's aide ballet. *Clinical Orthopaedics and Related Research,* **89**, 52-63.

Hsieh, C., Walker, J.M., & Gillis, K. (1983). Straight-leg raising test: Comparison of three instruments. *Physical Therapy,* **63**(9), 1429-1433.

Hubley-Kozey, C.L., & Stanish, W.D. (1984). Can stretching prevent athletic injuries? *Journal of Musculoskeletal Medicine,* **1**(9), 25-32.

Huxley, H.E. (1967). Muscle cells. In J. Brachet & A. Mirsky (Eds.), *The cell* (pp. 367-481). New York: Academic Press.

Huxley, H.E., & Hanson, H. (1954). The s-filament. *Nature,* **173**, 973-976.

Iashvili, A.V. (1983). Active and passive flexibility in athletes specializing in different sports. *Soviet Sports Review,* **18**(1), 30-32.

Inman, V.T., Saunders, J.B., & Abbot, L.C. (1944). Observations on the functions of the shoulder joint. *The Journal of Bone and Joint Surgery,* **26**(1), 1-30.

Iyengar, B.K.S. (1979). *Light on yoga*. New York: Schocken Books.

Jackman, R.V. (1963). Device to stretch the achilles tendon. *Journal of the American Physical Therapy Association, 43*, 729.

Jackson, C.P., & Brown, M.D. (1983, October). Is there a role for exercise in the treatment of patients with low back pain? *Clinical Orthopedics and Related Research, 179*, 39-45.

Jackson, I. (1975). *Yoga and the athlete*. Mountain View, CA: World Publishers.

Jacobs, M. (1976). Neurophysiological implications of slow, active stretching. *The American Corrective Therapy Journal, 30*(8), 151-154.

Jacobson, E. (1938). *Progressive relaxation*. Chicago: University of Chicago Press.

Javurek, J. (1982). Experience with hypermobility in athletes. *Theorie A Praxe Telesne Vychovy, 30*(3), 185.

Jencks, B. (1977). *Your body: Biofeedback at its best*. Chicago: Nelson Hall.

Jenkins, R., & Little, R.W. (1974). A constitutive equation for parallel-fibered elastic tissue. *The Journal of Biomechanics, 7*(5), 397-402.

Johns, R.J., & Wright, V. (1962). Relative importance of various tissues in joint stiffness. *Journal of Applied Physiology, 17*(5), 824-828.

Joint motion: Method of measuring and recording. (1984). Edinburgh: Churchill Livingstone.

Jones, A. (1975). Flexibility and metabolic condition. *Athletic Journal, 56*(2), 56-61, 80-81.

Jones, H.H. (1965). The valsalva procedure. *Journal of the American Physical Therapy Association, 45*(6), 570-572.

Kalenak, A., & Morehouse, C. (1975). Knee stability and knee ligament injuries. *Journal of the American Medical Association, 234*(11), 1143-1145.

Kane, M.D., Karl, R.D., & Swain, J.H. (1985). Effects of gravity-facilitated traction on intervertebral dimensions of the lumbar spine. *The Journal of Orthopaedic and Sports Physical Therapy, 6*(5), 281-288.

Kapendji, I.A. (1982). *The physiology of the joints: Vol. I. Upper limb*. Edinburgh: Churchill Livingstone.

Kapandji, I.A. (1971). *The physiology of the joints: Vol. II. Lower limb*. Edinburgh: Churchill Livingstone.

Kapandji, I.A. (1971). *The physiology of the joints: Vol. III. The trunk and the vertebral column*. Edinburgh: Churchill Livingstone.

Karpovich, P.V., & Sinning, W.E. (1971). *Physiology of muscular activity* (7th ed.). Philadelphia: W.B. Saunders.

Kastelic, J., Galeski, A., & Baer, E. (1978). The multicomposite structure of tendon. *Connective Tissue Research, 6*(1), 11-23.

Kelley, D.L. (1971). *Kinesiology fundamentals of motion description*. Englewood Cliffs, NJ: Prentice-Hall.

Kendall, H.O., & Kendall, F.P. (1948). Normal flexibility according to age groups. *Journal of Bone and Joint Surgery, 30A*(3), 690-694.

Kendall, H.O., Kendall, F.P., & Boynton, D.A. (1970). *Posture and pain*. New York: Robert E. Krieger.

Kendall, H.O., Kendall, F.P., & Wadsworth, G. (1971). *Muscles testing and function* (2nd ed.). Baltimore: Williams and Wilkins.

Kisner, C., & Colby, L.A. (1985). *Therapeutic exercise foundations and techniques*. Philadelphia: F.A. Davis.

Klafs, C.E., & Arnheim, D.D. (1977). *Modern principles of athletic training* (4th ed.). St. Louis: C.V. Mosby.

Klatz, R.M., Goldman, R.M., Pinchuk, B.G., Nelson, K.E., & Tarr, R.S. (1983). The effects of gravity inversion procedures on systemic blood pressure, and central retinal arterial pressure. *The Journal of American Osteopathic Association, 82*(11), 111-115.

Klein, K.K. (1961). The deep squat exercise as utilized in weight training for athletics and its effect on the ligaments of the knee. *Journal of the Association for Physical and Mental Rehabilitation, 15*(1), 6-11.

Klein, K.K., & Allman, F.L. (1969). *The knee in sports*. Austin, TX: Pemberton Press.

Klein, K.K., & Roberts, C.A. (1976). Mechanical problems of marathoners and joggers: Cause and solution. *The American Corrective Therapy Journal, 30*(6), 187-191.

Knapp, M.E. (1982). Massage. In F.J. Kottke, G.K. Stillwell, & J.F. Lehmann (Eds.), *Krusen's handbook of physical medicine and rehabilitation* (3rd ed., pp. 386-388). Philadelphia: W.B. Saunders.

Knott, M., & Voss, D.E. (1968). *Proprioceptive neuromuscular facilitation*. New York: Harper & Row.

Komi, P.V., & Boscoe, C. (1978). Utilization of stored elastic energy in men and women. *Medicine and Science in Sports, 10*(4), 261-265.

Kottke, F.J., Pauley, D.L., & Ptak, K.A. (1966). Prolonged stretching for correction of shortening of connective tissue. *Archives of Physical Medicine and Rehabilitation*, **47**(6), 345-352.

Krahenbuhl, G.S., & Martin, S.L. (1977). Adolescence body size and flexibility. *Research Quarterly*, **48**(4), 797-799.

Kulund, D.W., & Töttössy, M. (1983). Warm-up, strength, and power. In D.N. Kulund & M. Töttössy (Eds.), *Orthopedic clinics of North America* (pp. 427-448). Philadelphia: W.B. Saunders.

Laban, M.M. (1962). Collagen tissue: Implications of its response to stress in vitro. *Archives of Physical Medicine and Rehabilitation*, **43**(9), 461-465.

Larson, L.A., & Michelman, H. (1973). *International guide to fitness and health*. New York: Crown Publishers.

Laubach, L.C., & McConville, J.T. (1966a). Relationship between flexibility, anthropometry, and somatotype of college men. *Research Quarterly*, **37**(2), 241-251.

Laubach, L.C., & McConville, J.T. (1966b). Muscle strength, flexibility, and bone size of adult males. *Research Quarterly*, **37**(3), 384-392.

Leard, J.S. (1984). Flexibility and conditioning in the young athlete. In L.J. Micheli (Ed.), *Pediatric and adolescent sports medicine* (pp. 194-210). Boston: Little, Brown, and Company.

Lehmann, J.F., Mascock, A.J., Warren, C.G., & Koblanski, J.N. (1970). Effect of therapeutic temperature on tendon extensibility. *Archives of Physical Medicine and Rehabilitation*, **51**(8), 481-487.

Lehmann, J.P., & DeLateur, B.J. (1982). Diathermy and superficial heat and cold therapy. In F.J. Kottke, G.K. Stillwell, & J.F. Lehmann (Eds.), *Krusen's handbook of physical medicine and rehabilitation* (3rd ed., pp. 295-330). Philadelphia: W.B. Saunders.

Leighton, J.R. (1956). Flexibility characteristics of males ten to eighteen years of age. *Archives of Physical and Mental Rehabilitation*, **37**(8), 494-499.

Leighton, J.R. (1960). On the significance of flexibility for physical education. *Journal of Health, Physical Education, and Recreation*, **31**, 27-28.

Levaret-Joye, H. (1979). Relaxation and motor capacity. *Journal of Sports Medicine*, **19**(2), 151-156.

Lichtor, J. (1972). The loose-jointed young athlete. *The American Journal of Sports Medicine*, **1**(1), 22-23.

Liemohn, W. (1978). Factors related to hamstring strains. *The Journal of Sports Medicine and Physical Fitness*, **18**(1), 71-75.

Light, K.E., Nuzik, S., Personius, W., & Barstrom, A. (1984). A low-loading prolonged stretch vs high-low brief stretch in treating knee contractures. *Physical Therapy*, **64**(3), 330-333.

Logan, G.A., & Egstrom, G.H. (1961). Effects of slow and fast stretching on the sarco-femoral angle. *The Journal Association for Physical and Mental Rehabilitation*, **15**(3), 86-89.

Luttgens, K., & Wells, K.F. (1982). *Kinesiology*. Philadelphia: W.B. Saunders.

Maigne, R. (1980). Manipulation of the spine. In J.B. Rogoff (Ed.), *Manipulation, traction, and massage* (2nd ed., pp. 59-120). Baltimore: Williams and Wilkins.

Maltz, M. (1970). *Psychocybernetics*. New York: Simon and Schuster.

Mann, R.A., Baxter, D.E., & Lutter, L.D. (1981). Running symposium. *Foot and Ankle*, **1**(4), 190-224.

Marvey, D. (1887). Recherces experimentales sur la morphologie de muscles [Experimental research on the morphology of muscles]. *Comptes Rendus Hebdomadaires du Seances de l'Academie des Sciences* (Paris), **105**, 446-451.

Mason, T., & Rigby, B.J. (1963). Thermal transition in collagen. *Biochemica et Biophysica Acta*, **79**(PN1254), 448-450.

Massey, B.A., & Chaudet, N.L. (1956). Effects of systematic, heavy resistance exercise on range of joint movement in young adults. *Research Quarterly*, **27**(1), 41-51.

Mathews, D.K., Shaw, V., & Bohnen, M. (1957). Hip flexibility of college women as related to body segments. *Research Quarterly*, **28**(4), 352-356.

Mathews, D.K., Shaw, V., & Woods, J.W. (1959). Hip flexibility of elementary school boys as related to body segments. *Research Quarterly*, **31**(3), 297-302.

Mathews, D.K., Stacy, R.W., & Hoover, G.N. (1964). *Physiology of muscular activity and exercise*. New York: Ronald Press.

Matveyev, L. (1981). *Fundamentals of sports training*. Moscow: Progress Publishers.

Mayhew, T.P., Norton, B.J., & Sahrmann, S.A. (1983). Electromyographic study of the relationship between hamstring and abdominal muscles during a unilateral straight leg raise. *Physical Therapy*, **63**(11), 1769-1773.

McCue, B.F. (1963). Flexibility measurements of college women. *Research Quarterly*, **24**(3), 316-324.

McDonough, A.L. (1981). Effects of immobilization and exercise on articular cartilage—a review of the literature. *The Journal of Orthopaedic and Sports Physical Therapy*, **3**(1), 2-5.

Mellerowicz, H., & Hansen, G. (1971). Conditioning. In L.A. Larson (Ed.), *Encyclopedia of sport sciences and medicine* (pp. 1586-1587). New York: Macmillan.

Micheli, L.J. (1983). Overuse injuries in children's sport: The growth factor. In D.N. Kulund & M. Töttössy (Eds.), *Orthopedic clinics of North America* (Vol. 14, pp. 337-360). Philadelphia: W.B. Saunders.

Miller, E.H., Schneider, H.J., Bronson, J.L., & McClain, D. (1975). The classical ballet dancer: A new consideration in athletic injuries. *Clinical Orthopaedics and Related Research*, **111**, 181-191.

Moore, J.C. (1984). The golgi tendon organ: A review and update. *The American Journal of Occupational Therapy*, **38**(4), 227-236.

Moore, M.A., & Hutton, R.S. (1980). Electromyographic investigation of muscle stretching techniques. *Medicine and Science in Sports and Exercise*, **12**(5), 322-329.

Morehouse, L.E., & Miller, A.T. (1971). *Physiology of exercise*. St Louis: C.V. Mosby.

Moretz, A.J., Walters, R., & Smith, L. (1982). Flexibility as a predictor of knee injuries in college football players. *The Physician and Sportsmedicine*, **10**(7), 93-97.

Morgan, W.P., & Horstram, D.H. (1976). Anxiety reduction following acute physical activity. *Medicine and Science in Sports*, **8**(1), 62.

Mountcastle, V.B. (1974). *Medical physiology*. St. Louis: C.V. Mosby.

Myers, M. (1983, June). Stretching. *Dance Magazine*, pp. 66-70.

Nelson, J.K., Johnson, B.L., & Smith, G.C. (1983). Physical characteristics, hip flexibility and arm strength of female gymnasts classified by intensity of training across age. *Journal of Sports Medicine and Physical Fitness*, **23**(1), 95-100.

Newham, D.J., Mills, K.R., Quigley, B.M., & Edwards, R.H.T. (1983). Pain and fatigue after concentric and eccentric muscle contractions. *Clinical Science*, **64**(1), 55-62.

Newham, D.J., McPhail, G., Mills, K.R., & Edwards, R.H.T. (1983). Ultrastructural changes after concentric and eccentric contractions of human muscle. *Journal of the Neurological Sciences*, **61**(1), 109-122.

Nicholas, J.A. (1970). Injuries to knee ligaments: Relationship to looseness and tightness in football players. *Journal of the American Medical Association*, **212**(13), 2236-2239.

Nielsen, A.J. (1981). Case study: Myofascial pain of the posterior shoulder relieved by spray and stretch. *The Journal of Orthopaedic and Sports Physical Therapy*, **3**(1), 21-26.

Nikolic, V., & Zimmermann, B. (1968). Functional changes of the tarsal bones of ballet dancers. *Radovi Medicinskog Fakulteta u Zagrebu*, **16**, 131-146.

Olcott, S. (1980). Partner flexibility exercises. *Coaching Women's Athletics*, **6**(2), 10-14.

O'Neil, R. (1976). Prevention of hamstring and groin strain. *Athletic Training*, **11**(1), 27-31.

Panagiotacopulos, N.D., Knauss, W.G., & Bloch, R. (1979). On the mechanical properties of human intervertebral disc material. *Biorheology*, **16**(4/5), 317-330.

Paris, S.V. (1983). Spinal manipulation. *Clinical Orthopaedics and Related Research*, **179**, 55-61.

Parker, M.G., Ruhling, R.O., Holt, D., Bauman, E., & Drayna, M. (1983). Descriptive analysis of quadriceps and hamstrings muscle torque in high school football players. *Journal of Orthopaedic and Sports Physical Therapy*, **5**(1), 2-6.

Pechtl, V. (1982). Fundamentals and methods for the development of flexibility. In D. Harre (Ed.), *Principles of sports training* (pp. 146-152). Berlin: Sportverlag.

Physician's desk reference (40th ed.). (1986). Oradell, NJ: Medical Economics Company.

Ploucher, D.W. (1982). Inversion petechiae. *The New England Journal of Medicine*, **307**(22), 1406-1407.

Point-Counterpoint. (1983). Gravity boots. *International Gymnast*, **25**(11), 72.

Prentice, W.E. (1982). An electromyographic analysis of the effectiveness of heat or cold and stretching for inducing relaxation in injured muscle. *The Journal of Orthopaedic and Sports Physical Therapy*, **3**(3), 133-140.

Prentice, W.E. (1983). A comparison of static stretching and PNF stretching for improving hip joint flexibility. *Athletic Training*, **18**(1), 56-59.

Prockop, D.J., & Guzman, N.A. (1977). Collagen diseases and the biosynthesis of collagen. *Hospital Practice, 12*(12), 61-68.

Püschel, J. (1930). Der wassergehalt voraler un degenerieter zwischenwirbelschiben. *Beitrage Zur Pathologischen Anatomie und Zur Allgemeinen Pathologie, 84*, 123-130.

Ramachandran, G.W. (1967). Structure of collagen at the molecular level. In G.W. Ramachandran (Ed.), *Treatise of collagen* (Vol. I, pp. 103-179). New York: Academic Press.

Rapoport, R. (1984). Flexibility. *Esquire, 101*(5), 97-103.

Rasch, P.J., & Burke, J. (1978). *Kinesiology and applied anatomy*. Philadelphia: Lea and Febiger.

Rathbone, J.L. (1971). Relaxation. In L.A. Larson (Ed.), *Encyclopedia of sport sciences and medicine* (pp. 1312-1313). New York: Macmillan.

Rigby, B. (1964). The effect of mechanical extension under the thermal stability of collagen. *Biochimica et Biophysica Acta, 79*(SC 43008), 634-636.

Rigby, B.J., Hirai, N., Spikes, J.D., & Eyring, J. (1959). The mechanical properties of rat tail tendon. *Journal of General Physiology, 43*(2), 265-283.

Rockstein, M., & Sussman, M. (1979). *Biology of aging*. Belmont, CA: Wadsworth Publishing.

Ruch, T.C., & Patton, H.D. (1965). *Physiology and biophysics*. Philadelphia: W.B. Saunders.

Rusk, H.A. (1977). *Rehabilitation medicine* (4th ed.). St. Louis: C.V. Mosby.

Ryan, A.J. (1972). *Medical care of the athlete*. New York: McGraw-Hill.

Ryan, A.J. (1976). Ballet dancers pose sports medicine challenge. *The Physician and Sportsmedicine, 4*(11), 44.

Sabiston, D.C. (1972). *Textbook of surgery* (10th ed.). Philadelphia: W.B. Saunders.

Sady, S.P., Wortman, M., & Blanke, D. (1982). Flexibility training: Ballistic, static or proprioceptive neuromuscular facilitation. *The Archives of Physical Medicine and Rehabilitation, 63*(6), 261-263.

Sage, G.H. (1971). *Introduction to motor behavior: A neurophysiological approach*. Reading, MA: Addison-Wesley.

Sands, B. (1984). *Coaching women's gymnastics*. Champaign, IL: Human Kinetics.

Sapega, A.A., Quedenfeld, T.C., Moyer, R.A., & Butler, R.A. (1981). Biophysical factors in range-of-motion exercise. *The Physician and Sportsmedicine, 9*(12), 57-65.

Schneider, H.J., King, A.Y., Bronson, J.L., & Miller, E.H. (1974). Stress injuries and developmental change of lower extremities in ballet dancers. *Radiology, 113*, 627-632.

Schottelius, B.A., & Senay, L.C. (1956). Effect of stimulation-length sequence on shape of length-tension diagram. *American Journal of Physiology, 186*, 127-130.

Schubert, M., & Hamerman, D. (1968). *A primer on connective tissue biochemistry*. Philadelphia: Lea and Febiger.

Schultz, A.B., Andersson, G.B., Haderspeck, K., Örtengren, R., Nordin, M., & Björk, R. (1982). Analysis and measurement of lumbar trunk loads in tasks involving bends and twists. *The Journal of Biomechanics, 15*(9), 669-675.

Schultz, P. (1979). Flexibility: Day of the static stretch. *The Physician and Sportsmedicine, 7*(11), 109-117.

Schwane, J.A., Johnson, S.R., Vandenakker, C.B., & Armstrong, R.B. (1981). Blood markers of delayed-onset muscular soreness with downhill treadmill running. *Medicine and Science in Sports and Exercise, 13*(2), 80.

Segal, D.D. (1983). An anatomic and biomechanical approach to low back health: A preventative approach. *The Journal of Sports Medicine and Physical Fitness, 23*(4), 411-421.

Sermeev, B.V. (1966). Development of mobility in the hip joint in sportsmen. *Yessis Review, 2*(1), 16-17.

Shephard, R.J. (1982). *Physiology and biochemistry of exercise*. New York: Praeger.

Shriber, W.J. (1975). *A manual of electrotherapy*. Philadelphia: Lea and Febiger.

Sigerseth, P.C. (1971). In L.A. Larson (Ed.), *Encyclopedia of sport sciences and medicine* (pp. 280-281). New York: Macmillan.

Sime, W.E. (1977). A comparison of exercise and meditation in reducing physiological response to stress. *Medicine and Science in Sports, 9*(1), 55.

Sloane, E. (1980). *Biology of women*. New York: John Wiley and Sons.

Smith, J.L., Hutton, R.S., & Eldred, E. (1974). Post contraction changes in sensitivity of muscle afferents to static and dynamic stretch. *Brain Research, 78*, 193-202.

Snell, R.S. (1986). *Clinical anatomy for medical students* (3rd ed.). Boston: Little, Brown and Company.

Stamford, B. (1984). Flexibility and stretching. *The Physician and Sportsmedicine, 12*(2), 171.

Steindler, A. (1932). The mechanics of muscular contractures in wrist and fingers. *Journal of Bone and Joint Surgery, 14*(1), 1-16.

Steindler, A. (1977). *Kinesiology of the human body.* Springfield, IL: Charles C Thomas Publishers.

Stevens, M.B., & Wigley, F.M. (1984). Osteoarthritis—practical management in older patients. *Geriatrics, 39*(3), 101-120.

Subotnick, S.I. (1977). *The running foot doctor.* Mountain View, CA: World Publications.

Sullivan, P.D., Markos, P.E., & Minor, M.D. (1982). *An integrated approach to therapeutic exercise theory and clinical application.* Reston, VA: Reston Publishing.

Surburg, P.R. (1981). Neuromuscular facilitation techniques in sportsmedicine. *The Physician and Sportsmedicine, 18*(1), 114-127.

Surburg, P.R. (1983). Flexibility exercise reexamined. *Athletic Training, 18*(1), 37-40.

Sutro, C.J. (1947). Hypermobility of bones due to "overlengthened" capsular and ligamentous tissues. *Surgery, 21*(1), 67-76.

Sutton, G. (1984). Hamstrung by hamstring strains: A review of the literature. *The Journal of Orthopaedic and Sports Physical Therapy, 5*(4), 184-195.

Suzuki, S., & Hutton, R.S. (1976). Postcontractile motorneuron discharge produced by muscle afferent activation. *Medicine and Science in Sports, 8*(4), 258-264.

Tanigawa, M.C. (1972). Comparison of the hold-relax procedure and passive mobilization on increasing muscle length. *Physical Therapy, 52*(7), 725-735.

Taunton, J.E. (1982). Pre-game warm-up and flexibility. *The New Zealand Journal of Sports Medicine, 10*(1), 14-18.

Teitz, C.C. (1982). Sports medicine concerns in dance and gymnastics. In M.C. Korn (Ed.), *Pediatric clinics of North America* (pp. 1399-1421). Philadelphia: W.B. Saunders.

Thompson, C.W. (1981). *Manual of structural kinesiology* (9th ed.). St. Louis: C.V. Mosby.

Toufexis, A. (1974). The price of an art. *Physician's World, 2*(4), 44-50.

Travell, J.G., & Simons, D.G. (1983). *Myofascial pain and dysfunction: The trigger point manual.* Baltimore: Williams and Wilkins.

Troels, B. (1973). Achilles tendon rupture. *Acta Orthopaedica Scandinavica, 152*(Suppl.), 1-126.

Tullson, P., & Armstrong, R.B. (1968). Exercise-induced muscle inflammation. *Federation Proceeding, 37*(3), 663.

Tullson, P., & Armstrong, R.B. (1981). Muscle hexose monophosphate shunt activity following exercise. *Experientia, 37*(12), 1311-1312.

Tumanyan, G.S., & Dzhanyan, S.M. (1984). Strength exercises as a means of improving active flexibility of wrestlers. *Soviet Sports Review, 19*(3), 146-150.

Turek, S.L. (1977). *Orthopaedics principles and their application* (3rd ed.). Philadelphia: J.B. Lippincott.

Tyrance, H.J. (1958). Relationships of extreme body types to ranges of flexibility. *Research Quarterly, 29*(3), 349-359.

Uram, P. (1980). *The complete stretching book.* Mountain View, CA: Anderson World.

Urban, L.M. (1981). The straight-leg-raising test: A review. *The Journal of Orthopaedic and Sports Physical Therapy, 2*(3), 117-134.

Verzar, F. (1963). Aging of collagen. *Scientific America, 208*(4), 104-117.

Verzar, F. (1964). Aging of collagen fiber. In D.A. Hall (Ed.), *International review of connective tissue research* (Vol. 2, pp. 244-300). New York: Academic Press.

Viidik, A., Danielson, C.C., & Oxlund, H. (1982). On fundamental and phenomenological models, structure and mechanical properties of collagen, elastin and glycosaminolycan complexes. *Biorheology, 19*(3), 437-451.

Walker, J.M. (1981). Development, maturation and aging of human joints: A review. *Physiotherapy Canada, 33*(3), 153-160.

Walker, S.M. (1961). Delay of twitch relaxation induced by stress and stress-relaxation. *The Journal of Applied Physiology, 16*(5), 801-806.

Wallis, E.L., & Logan, G.A. (1964). *Figure improvement and body conditioning through exercise.* Englewood Cliffs, NJ: Prentice-Hall.

Walther, D.S. (1981). *Applied kinesiology: Basic procedures and muscle testing.* Pueblo, CO: Systems D.C.

Warren, C.G., Lehmann, J.F., & Koblanski, J.N. (1971). Elongation of rat tail tendon: Effect of load and temperature. *Archives of Physical Medicine and Rehabilitation, 52*(3), 465-474.

Warren, C.G., Lehmann, J.F., & Koblanski, J.N. (1976). Heat and stretch procedures: An evaluation using rat tail tendon. *Archives of Physical Medicine and Rehabilitation, 57*(3), 122-126.

Watrous, B., Armstrong, R.B., & Schwane, J.A. (1981). The role of lactic acid in delayed onset muscular soreness. *Medicine and Science in Sports and Exercise, 13*(2), 80.

Wear, C.R. (1963). Relationship of flexibility measurements to length of body segments. *Research Quarterly, 34*(3), 234-238.

Weiss, L., & Greer, R.O. (1977). *Histology* (4th ed.). New York: McGraw-Hill.

White, A.A., & Panjabi, M.M. (1978). *Clinical biomechanics of the spine.* Philadelphia: J.B. Lippincott.

Wickstrom, R.L. (1963). Weight training and flexibility. *Journal of Health, Physical Education and Recreation, 34*(2), 61-62.

Wiktorssohn-Möller, M., Öberg, B., Ekstrand, J., & Gillquist, J. (1983). Effects of warming up, massage, and stretching on range of motion and muscle strength in the lower extremity. *American Journal of Sports Medicine, 11*(4), 249-252.

Williams, J.C.P., & Sperryn, P.N. (1976). *Sports medicine* (2nd ed.). Baltimore: Williams and Wilkins.

Williams, P.E., & Goldspink, G. (1971). Longitudinal growth of striated muscle fibres. *Journal of Cell Science, 9*(3), 751-767.

Williams, P.E., & Goldspink, G. (1973). The effect of immobilization on the longitudinal growth of striated muscle fibres. *Journal of Anatomy, 116*(1), 45-55.

Williams, P.E., & Goldspink, G. (1976). The effect of denervation and dystrophy on the adaptation of sarcomere number to the functional length of the muscle in young and adult mice. *Journal of Anatomy, 122*(2), 455-465.

Williams, P.E., & Goldspink, G. (1978). Changes in sarcomere length and physiological properties in immobilized muscle. *Journal of Anatomy, 127*(3), 459-468.

Williams, P.L., & Warwick, R. (1980). *Gray's anatomy* (36th ed.). Philadelphia: W.B. Saunders.

Wilmore, J., Parr, R.B., Girandola, R.N., Ward, P., Vodak, P.A., Pipes, T.V., Romerom, G.T., & Leslie, P. (1978). Physiological alterations consequent to circuit weight training. *Medicine and Science in Sports, 10*(2), 79-84.

Woo, S., Matthews, J.V., Akeson, W.H., Amiel, D., & Convery, R. (1975). Connective tissue response to immobility: Correlative study of biochemical and biomechanical measurements of normal and immobilized rabbit knees. *Arthritis Rheumatology, 18*(3), 257-264.

Yu, S.H., & Blumenthal, H. (1967). The calcification of elastic tissue. In B.M. Wagner & D.E. Smith (Eds.), *The connective tissue* (pp. 17-49). Baltimore: Williams and Wilkins.

Zajonc, R.B. (1965). Social facilitation. *Science, 149*(3681), 269-274.

Zierler, K.L. (1974). Mechanism of muscular contraction and its energetics. In V.B. Mountcastle (Ed.), *Medical physiology* (Vol. II, 12th ed., pp. 1128-1171). St. Louis: C.V. Mosby.

Author Index

Stevens, M.B., 54
Subotnick, S.I., 108
Sullivan, P.D., 89–91
Surburg, P.R., 8, 89–91
Sussman, M., 19
Sutro, C.J., 8, 54
Sutton, G., 80, 114, 115
Suzuki, S., 90
Swain, J.H., 93

T
Tabary, C., 19, 20
Tabary, J.C., 19, 20
Tanigawa, M.C., 89, 90
Tardieu, C., 19, 20
Tardieu, G., 19, 20
Tarkka, I., 7
Tarr, R.S., 93
Taunton, J.E., 115
Teitz, C.C., 123
Thompson, C.W., 108
Tottossy, M., 67
Toufexis, A., 58
Travell, J.G., 73
Travis, T.M., 89
Troels, B., 67
Tullson, P., 80
Tumanyan, G.S., 88
Turek, S.L., 54, 142, 147
Tyrance, H.J., 66

U
Uram, P., 99
Urban, L.M., 120

V
Vaccaro, P., 64
Vandenakker, C.B., 82
Verzar, F., 27, 28
Viidik, A., 26
Villanacci, J.F., 114
Vodak, P.A., 67
Voss, D.E., 88–91

W
Wadsworth, G., 65, 66, 120, 121, 133
Walker, J.M., 120, 130
Walker, S.M., 86
Wallis, E.L., 101
Walters, R., 8, 9
Walther, D.S., 17, 18, 134
Ward, P., 67
Warren, C.G., 38, 86
Warwick, R., 54, 150
Watrous, B., 82
Wear, C.R., 64, 66
Weisberg, J., 74
Weiss, L., 27
Wells, K.F., 107
White, A.A., 135
Wickstrom, R.L., 67, 108, 109, 123
Wigley, F.M., 54
Wiktorsson-Moller, M., 74
Wilkie, D.R., 29, 36
Williams, F.M., 80
Williams, P.E., 19, 20
Williams, P.L., 54, 150
Wilmore, J., 67
Wilson, P.D., 64
Wilson, P.K., 114
Wiswell, R.A., 4
Woo, S., 28, 30
Woods, J.W., 64
Wortman, M., 85, 89
Wright, V., 9, 29, 64

Y
Yu, S.H., 28

Z
Zajonc, R.B., 57
Zarins, B., 6, 7, 81
Zierler, K.L., 35
Zimmermann, B., 108

Subject Index

Vertebral trunk
    extension, 131–135
    flexion, 131–136
    lateral flexion, 131–133, 135
Viscosity, 66, 67, 101
Viscous
    component, 35, 46, 47
    deformation, 38, 39, 66

W
Warm-down, 3, 58, 66–68, 80, 83, 85, 101, 111
Warm-up, 3, 6, 58, 66–69, 74, 83, 101, 110, 111, 116, 146, 148

Weight training, 8, 67, 68, 97
Whirlpool, 72, 111
Wrist, 52, 148–150
    abduction, 150
    adduction, 150
    extension, 149, 150
    flexion, 150

Y
Yield point, 34
Yoga, 4, 5, 85, 86, 98, 112, 115, 124

Z
Z-line, 13–15, 36, 80